Second Edition

HUMAN DISEASES

A Systemic Approach

Second Edition

HUMAN DISEASES

A Systemic Approach

Mary Lou Mulvihill, Ph.D.
Professor of Biology
William Rainey Harper College
Palatine, Illinois

Appleton & Lange
Norwalk, Connecticut/Los Altos, California

0-8385-3895-9

Notice: The author(s) and publisher of this volume have taken care that the information and recommendations contained herein are accurate and compatible with the standards generally accepted at the time of publication.

87 88 89 90 / 10 9 8 7 6 5 4 3 2 1

Prentice-Hall of Australia, Pty. Ltd., Sydney
Prentice-Hall Canada, Inc.
Prentice-Hall Hispanoamericana, S.A., Mexico
Prentice-Hall of India Private Limited, New Delhi
Prentice-Hall International (UK) Limited, London
Prentice-Hall of Japan, Inc., Tokyo
Prentice-Hall of Southeast Asia (Pte.) Ltd., Singapore
Whitehall Books Ltd., Wellington, New Zealand
Editora Prentice-Hall do Brasil Ltda., Rio de Janeiro

Library of Congress Cataloging-in-Publication Data

Mulvihill, Mary L.
    Human diseases.

    Bibliography: p.
    1. Pathology. I. Title. [DNLM: 1. Medicine.
WB 100 M961h]
RB111.M83 1987   616   86-14649
ISBN 0-8385-3895-9

Design: Kathleen E. Peters

PRINTED IN THE UNITED STATES OF AMERICA

To
my husband, Jim,
and all my loved ones
who encouraged me in this work.

Contents

Preface

The second edition of *Human Diseases: A Systemic Approach* was designed primarily for students entering a health career. Interest in human diseases, however, transcends the classroom, and any reader interested in the human body's functioning will find this book a helpful reference. It is divided into two parts. Part I treats the general mechanisms of disease and introduces such basic terminology as etiology, prognosis, signs and symptoms. Concepts such as inflammation, immunity, allergy, and neoplasia are explained; hereditary diseases and those diseases caused by deficiencies or excesses are also described. Part II covers the most commonly occurring diseases of each system, e.g., cardiovascular, excretory, digestive, and respiratory. Emphasis is placed on the malfunctioning of an organ or organ system in contrast to the normal anatomy and physiology of each, which is reviewed at the beginning of each chapter. Chapters can be read out of sequence to accommodate the various health career areas. Emphasis has been placed on the meaning of medical terms to facilitate understanding, and a complete glossary of terms is included. The book is heavily illustrated—line drawings help convey concepts and numerous photographs show disease states. Valuable study questions, all of which are answered in the text, conclude each chapter. The writing style is simple, concise, and, I hope, interesting. The first edition of the book was very well-received by students and instructors, which has prompted the publication of this second edition. The text has been totally revised, many photographic slides have been replaced, and much of the artwork has been redrawn.

I am grateful to the many people who contributed to the completion of this edition, particularly the excellent reviewers (Fred Dalske, at the University of Central Arkansas in Conway; Thomas E. Kober, at Cincinnati Technical College; Mary M. Saunders, M.D., in Little Rock, Arkansas; Linda S. Slater, at Orange Coast College in Costa Mesa, California; Margaret Von

Dreele, at Rush University in Chicago; and Lydia Wiley, at the National Education Center, The Thompson Institute of Philadelphia), who offered valuable suggestions after having used the first edition. I want to thank the photographers and research librarians of William Rainey Harper College for their assistance in this effort. Barry A. Goldsmith, M.D., Clinical Associate Professor of Surgery (Oncology) Abraham Lincoln School of Medicine at the University of Illinois, reviewed the chapter on neoplasia and provided excellent photographs of skin cancers. David R. Duffell, M.D., Chief, Department of Pathology at Northwest Community Hospital in Arlington Heights, Illinois, gave me access to the complete photographic file of the hospital and assisted with the selection of slides. I would also like to acknowledge the contribution made by my original typist, Vera Davis, RN, Program Coordinator for the Medical Assistant and Medical Transcriptionist Programs at Harper College, not only for her typing but for suggestions she offered through her clinical experience. Karen Dopke assisted with the typing of the revision.

I extend my gratitude to Stuart Horton, Medical Editor of Appleton & Lange, who encouraged this revision; to Janet Blaustein Kublin, Production Editor, who enhanced the text through excellent editing; and to Joy Schmitt, Advertising and Promotion Manager, who helped bring this text to your attention.

I have truly enjoyed writing this book. Now my hope is that it achieves the purpose for which it was written: that the reader will better understand the human body, in health and in disease.

Mary Lou Mulvihill, Ph.D.

PART I

Mechanisms of Disease

CHAPTER 1

Introduction to Disease

The human body is a masterpiece of art. The more one understands the functioning of the body, the greater appreciation one has for it. Even in disease, the body is quite remarkable in attempting to right what is wrong and compensate for it. Changes constantly occur within the body, and yet a steady state called **homeostasis** is generally maintained. A significant disturbance in the homeostasis of the body triggers a variety of responses that often produce **disease** symptoms. Athletes, for example, develop abnormally high red blood cell counts due to their increased need for oxygen. This is a natural compensatory mechanism to circulate more hemoglobin, but it is a disease symptom in polycythemia, which will be discussed later.

An organ will often enlarge, **hypertrophy,** when it is required to do extra work. The heart enlarges with prolonged high blood pressure as it must continue to pump blood against great resistance. Heart muscle also hypertrophies when the valves are defective because valves that are either too narrow or too wide require extra pumping action. If one kidney fails the other enlarges to meet the needs of the body and compensate for the defective one. When blood flow to the kidneys is inadequate, the kidneys help raise the blood pressure by means of a hormonal secretion. If, however, an organ or body part is not used, it will atrophy or decrease in size.

Blood plays several roles in maintaining homeostasis. When tissue is traumatized, injured, or becomes infected, blood flow increases to the damaged site. This is vital because the blood carries cells that are specialized to remove harmful substances and cellular debris. Other cells in the blood produce antibodies against invading organisms that cause disease.

Disease is the unhealthy state of a body part, a physiological system, or the body as a whole. Diseases have characteristic signs and symptoms.

Signs are objective evidence of disease observed on physical examination, such as abnormal pulse or respiratory rate, fever, and pallor, whereas **symptoms** are indications of disease perceived by the patient, such as pain, dizziness, and itching. A disease may be a structural **anomaly,** such as a congenital heart defect, or a functional condition, such as hypertension, high blood pressure, or **trauma.** The abnormal tissue or function is referred to as a **lesion.**

An important aspect of any disease is its **etiology,** or cause. Many familiar diseases are caused by infectious agents: The common cold and flu are viral infections, but abscesses and strep throat are caused by bacteria; fungi and parasites are infectious agents that cause athlete's foot and worm diseases, respectively.

Many diseases are due to **heredity;** they are transmitted by a defective gene. Hemophilia, sickle cell anemia, and color blindness are examples of genetic diseases. **Congenital** birth defects, mental or physical, may be due to a developmental error resulting from a maternal infection during pregnancy, the use of a drug such as thalidomide, or the mother's excessive consumption of alcohol. Some congenital birth defects result from an accident at the time of delivery such as an interference with oxygen supply.

Environmental factors are the cause of many diseases. Skin cancer, for example, can result from excessive exposure to the ultraviolet light rays of the sun, especially in fair-skinned people. The development of leukemia is an occupational hazard for radiologists, as is the development of cancer for asbestos workers.

Malnutrition causes many diseases that are not always due to the unavailability of food, but rather the inability of the person to use it. This will be explained later. Signs of nutritional deficiency diseases frequently accompany chronic alcoholism.

Stress is the cause of several diseases that affect the gastrointestinal system such as peptic ulcers and ulcerative colitis. Stress also aggravates respiratory ailments, asthma for example, and other allergic conditions. If the cause of a disease is not known, it is said to be **idiopathic.**

Another important aspect of disease is the way it manifests itself: the signs and symptoms. An attempt will be made throughout this book to relate the signs and symptoms of a disease to the specific malfunctioning of the ailment. For example, why does the anemic person feel weak, fatigued, and short of breath? How does a hyperactive thyroid cause weight loss, nervousness, and excessive sweating? Why are the ankles swollen in certain heart conditions?

Certain signs and symptoms occur concurrently in some diseases and the combination of symptoms is referred to as a **syndrome**. Mongolism, or

Down's syndrome, is an example of a disease with concurrent signs; the most prominent are mental retardation, an enlarged, protruding tongue, and a characteristic appearance of the eyes.

Diagnosis, the determination of the nature of a disease, is based on many factors, including the signs, symptoms, and, often, laboratory findings. A physician also derives information for making a diagnosis from a physical examination, from interviewing the patient or a family member, and from a medical history of the patient and family. The physician, having made a diagnosis, may state the possible **prognosis** of the disease, the predicted course, and outcome of the disease.

The treatment considered most effective is prescribed and may include medication, surgery, radiation therapy, or possibly psychiatric counseling. A patient may be advised to change habits of life style such as overeating, smoking, or alcohol abuse.

The course of a disease varies. It may have a sudden onset and short term, in which case it is an **acute** disease. A disease may begin insidiously and be long-lived, which is the **chronic** state. Diseases that will end in death are called terminal. The symptoms of a chronic disease at times subside, during a period known as **remission.** They may recur in all their severity in a period of **exacerbation.** Certain diseases, leukemia and ulcerative colitis, for example, are characterized by periods of remission and exacerbation. A **relapse** at times occurs when a disease returns weeks or months after its apparent cessation.

Complications frequently occur, meaning that a disease develops in a patient already suffering from another disease. Patients confined to bed with a serious fracture frequently develop pneumonia as a complication of the inactivity. Infection of the testes may be a complication of mumps, particularly after puberty. Anemia generally accompanies leukemia, cancer, and chronic kidney disease. Bacterial infection frequently follows certain predisposing factors such as kidney stones, heart defects, and an enlarged prostate gland. The relationships between the diseases that develop secondarily and the original disease will be discussed in later chapters.

The aftermath of a particular disease is called the **sequela,** a sequel. The permanent damage to the heart after rheumatic fever is an example of a sequela, as is the paralysis of polio. The sterility resulting from severe inflammation of the fallopian tubes is also a sequela.

Diseases can be classified in many ways, but in this book they will be considered according to the general mechanisms of disease and in the physiologic systems in which they are a factor. General health problems include allergies, malnutrition, obesity, and alcoholism.

An understanding of disease, its cause, the way it affects the body, effective treatments, and its possible prognosis should enable the health professional to alleviate suffering, anxiety, and fear in those who are ill.

SUMMARY

The body attempts to maintain homeostasis in the midst of ever-changing conditions. It senses a deficiency in the working of an organ and tries to compensate for it. The response to a significant disturbance in the body's homeostasis can resemble the symptom of disease. Many factors can cause disease: infectious agents, heredity, environmental conditions, malnutrition, and stress. The cause of a disease is sometimes unknown.

Disease manifests itself by signs and symptoms, objective and subjective indications of its presence. Diagnoses are based on these, together with laboratory findings, medical histories, and physical examinations; the most suitable treatment is then prescribed. Understanding the various aspects of disease enables the health professional to serve those who are ill in a comprehensive manner.

CHAPTER 2

Inflammation, Immunity, and Allergy

INFLAMMATION AND REPAIR

Tissues react to local injury, foreign invasion, or irritation by producing an inflammatory response. Although inflammation is painful, it is nature's way of correcting a disorder. Every disease ending in *itis* is an inflammatory disease, such as appendicitis, bronchitis, and colitis.

The cause of the inflammation may be a trauma or injury, such as a sprained ankle or a severe blow. A physical irritant in the tissue—a piece of glass, a wasp sting, or an ingrown toenail—will trigger the response. **Pathogenic organisms** will do the same. Figure 2–1 shows various agents that are capable of stimulating an inflammatory response.

Inflammation should not be confused with infection. Invading pathogenic organisms—bacteria, viruses, fungi, or parasites—are necessary to produce an infection. Inflammation, however, is a protective tissue response to injury or invasion by disease-producing organisms.

Vascular changes occur when tissue is traumatized or irritated. Local blood vessels, arterioles, and capillaries dilate, resulting in increased blood flow to the injured area. This increased amount of blood, **hyperemia,** causes the heat and redness associated with inflammation. As the blood flow to the site of the injury or infection increases, more and more **leukocytes,**

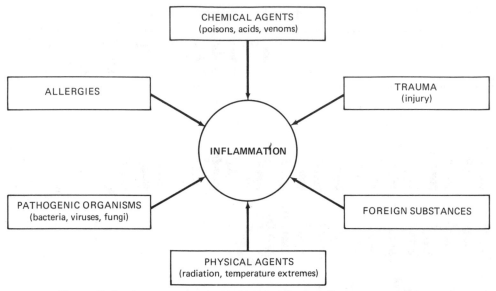

Figure 2-1. Agents capable of stimulating an inflammatory response.

white blood cells, reach the area. Certain of these white cells, the neutrophils or **polymorphs,** line up within the capillary walls. The polymorphs are specialized to fight against the invading agent or injury.

The damaged tissue releases a substance called **histamine** that causes the capillary walls to become more permeable. This increased permeability enables plasma and neutrophils to move out of the blood vessels into the tissue. Neutrophils are **phagocytes** that have the ability to engulf and digest bacteria and cellular debris. The root word, *phag(o)*, means to eat. Figure 2–2 shows the vascular changes that occur with inflammation and the movement of the polymorphs to the infected site.

The plasma and white cells that escape from the capillaries comprise the **inflammatory exudate.** This exudate in the tissues causes the swelling associated with inflammation. The excess of fluid in the tissues (**edema**) puts pressure on sensitive nerve endings, causing pain. The chief signs and symptoms of inflammation are redness, swelling, heat, and pain. It is the increased blood flow to the damaged or irritated area that causes the redness and heat. The inflammatory exudate is responsible for the swelling and pain.

Bacterial infection may be the cause of an inflammation. Organisms such as **staphylococci** and **streptococci** that produce **toxins** (substances damaging to the tissues) will initiate an inflammatory response. To increase the power of the white cells fighting the infection, the bone marrow and lymph nodes release very large quantities of leukocytes. This increased

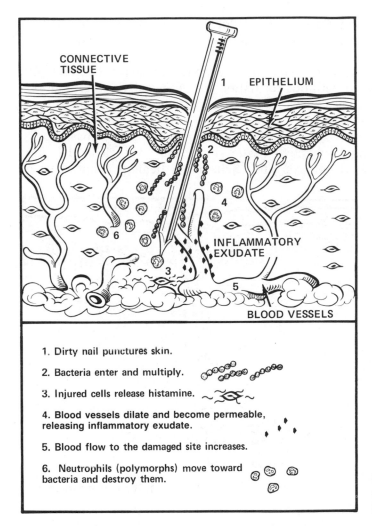

CONNECTIVE
TISSUE

EPITHELIUM

INFLAMMATORY
EXUDATE

BLOOD VESSELS

1. Dirty nail punctures skin.

2. Bacteria enter and multiply.

3. Injured cells release histamine.

4. Blood vessels dilate and become permeable,
releasing inflammatory exudate.

5. Blood flow to the damaged site increases.

6. Neutrophils (polymorphs) move toward
bacteria and destroy them.

Figure 2-2. Vascular
changes that occur with
inflammation.

production of white cells accounts for the elevated white cell count associated with infection. The count may rise to 30,000 or more from the
normal range of 7000 to 9000 per cubic **millimeter** of blood (mm³). The
excessive production of white cells is called **leukocytosis.**

The polymorphs soon die after ingesting bacteria and toxins. Substances are released from the dead cells, now called pus cells, that liquefy
the tissue affected by the toxins. This liquefied tissue—dead polymorphs,
inflammatory exudate, and bacteria—make up the thick, yellow fluid known
as pus. Other phagocytic white cells, the **monocytes** or macrophages, follow
the polymorphs in the process of clearing debris. Inflammatory exudate

contains a plasma protein, **fibrin,** essential for the blood-clotting mechanism. Fibrin acts in the damaged tissue by forming a clot, thus walling off the infection and preventing its spread.

Bacteria that cause pus formation are called **pyogenic** bacteria. An inflammation associated with pus formation is a **suppurative** inflammation. Abscesses, boils, and styes are examples of inflammations with suppuration.

Wound healing and repair can occur only when bacteria have been destroyed. Cut edges of tissue will grow together as connective tissue cells (**fibroblasts**) producing connective tissue fibers that will close the gap. Figure 2–3 shows the fibroblasts and their fibers healing a cut. This is

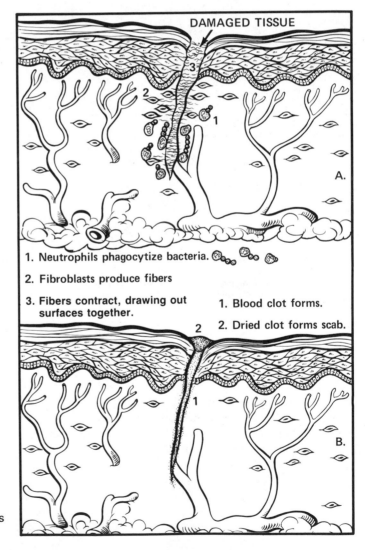

DAMAGED TISSUE

A.

1. Neutrophils phagocytize bacteria.

2. Fibroblasts produce fibers

3. Fibers contract, drawing out
   surfaces together.

1. Blood clot forms.

2. Dried clot forms scab.

B.

Figure 2–3. Fibroblasts
healing a wound.

known as scar tissue. Sometimes the connective tissue fibers will anchor adjacent structures together, such as loops of intestine, causing **adhesions.** The problems associated with adhesions will be explained in later chapters.

A scar following surgery or a severe burn is often raised and hard. This is known as **keloid** healing and is really a benign tumor that is harmless. Surgery to remove such a scar is usually ineffective, as the subsequent incision will have a tendency to heal in the same way.

IMMUNITY: THE ANTIGEN-ANTIBODY REACTION

The immune reaction of the body provides a strong line of defense against invading organisms. The body recognizes bacteria, viruses, molds, and toxins as something foreign to itself and produces substances to counteract them. The foreign element, generally a protein, that triggers this response is called an **antigen.** The substance produced to fight against the antigen is an **antibody.** The two fit together like a lock and key; this union makes the antigen harmless. Once antibodies are formed, a person attacked by the bacteria or virus is **immune** to it. Figure 2–4 illustrates the concept of the antigen–antibody reaction.

It is chiefly plasma cells in **lymphoid tissue,** lymph nodes, thymus gland, and spleen that form antibodies, immunoglobulins. The plasma cells are

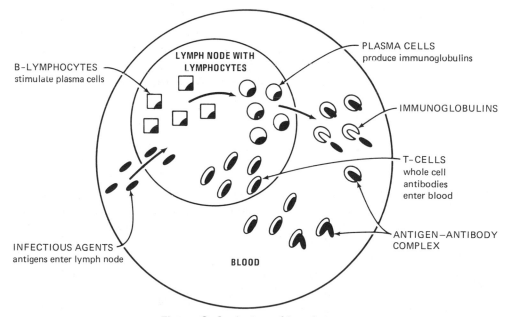

Figure 2-4. Action of lymphocytes.

stimulated to produce immunoglobulins by **B-lymphocytes** in the lymphoid tissue. Other **lymphocytes** called T-cells take on the characteristic of whole cell antibodies and produce a longer-lasting type of immunity. The thymus gland in early life is important in programming the **T-cells** or **T-lymphocytes.**

Everyone is born with a certain amount of immunity. Most immunity, however, is acquired either naturally by exposure to a disease or artificially by immunization.

There are two types of artificial immunity, active and passive. In **active immunity** the person is given a vaccine or a toxoid as the antigen, and he or she forms antibodies to counteract it. A **vaccine** consists of a low dose of dead or deactivated bacteria or viruses. Because the organisms have been specially treated to deactivate them, they cannot cause disease. As protein foreign to the body, these antigens do trigger antibody production against them. A **toxoid** works similarly. It consists of a chemically altered toxin, the poisonous material produced by a pathogenic organism. Having been treated chemically, the toxin will not cause disease. It will, however, stimulate antibody production against it.

This type of immunity, in which cells are exposed to an antigen and begin to form the corresponding antibodies, is long-lived. This kind of protection is given to prevent smallpox, polio, and diphtheria. Time is required to build up immunity, and a booster shot is frequently given for a stronger effect. Once cells have been sensitized to these viruses, bacteria, or toxins, they will continue to produce antibodies against them.

What if a person is exposed to a serious disease such as hepatitis, tetanus, or rabies and has no immunity against it? It takes time to build antibodies and time is limited. In this case, the person is given **passive immunity,** doses of preformed antibodies from immune serum of an animal, usually a horse. This type of immunity is short-lived but acts immediately. Figure 2–5 constrasts active and passive immunity.

HYPERSENSITIVITY—ALLERGIES

Closely related to the concept of immunity is **allergy** or hypersensitivity. Allergies are, in a way, a side effect of the immune response. There are three basic types of allergies. The first serious allergic reaction can occur in anyone. It involves the introduction of large quantities of antigen intravenously when large numbers of antibodies are already present. The best example of this allergic reaction is an incompatible blood transfusion. A person with type A blood has A antigens on the red cells, and antibodies against type B blood in the serum. If the person receives a type B transfusion, the antigens and antibodies will interact. The red blood cells will **agglutinate,** or clump together, and **hemolyze** (rupture). See Figure 2–6A.

ACTIVE IMMUNITY	PASSIVE IMMUNITY
PERSON FORMS ANTIBODIES	PREFORMED ANTIBODIES RECEIVED (usually in immune horse serum)
VACCINE (deactivated bacteria or virus) OR TOXOID (chemically altered toxin)	
LONG-LIVED IMMUNITY (requires time)	SHORT-LIVED IMMUNITY (acts immediately)

Figure 2-5. Differences between active and passive immunity.

The cellular damage triggers the release of histamine from mast cells, causing blood vessels to dilate and thus drastically reducing blood pressure. In addition the capillaries become very permeable and plasma leaks out, reducing blood volume. This further reduces blood pressure. Low blood pressure causes a poor return of venous blood to the heart and cardiac output is drastically reduced. Blood pools rather than circulates, and death can follow. This serious type of allergic reaction is known as **anaphylactic shock.** Figure 2–6B shows this sequence of vascular events.

The second type of allergic reaction can also occur in anyone but is a delayed reaction. Initial exposure to an antigen is required before any antibodies are formed. For example, the first time one contacts poison ivy there will be no reaction. However, the cells may become sensitized to it and will begin making antibodies against the poison ivy antigen. On the next exposure the typical rash and irritation associated with poison ivy will develop.

Another example of the delayed allergic reaction would be an Rh positive (Rh$^+$) blood transfusion to an Rh negative (Rh$^-$) recipient. Rh$^-$ blood means that the Rh antigen or factor is not present. This transfusion would cause no trouble, but in the transfusion the Rh$^-$ recipient is exposed or sensitized to the **Rh factor** and begins to form antibodies against this foreign protein. Subsequent Rh$^+$ transfusions would cause clumping and rupture of red blood cells. Rh incompatibility during pregnancy is also a

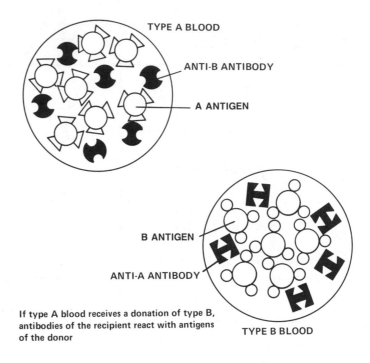

If type A blood receives a donation of type B, antibodies of the recipient react with antigens of the donor

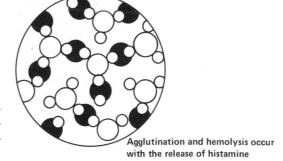

Figure 2-6. A. Anaphylactic shock (incompatible blood transfusion).

Agglutination and hemolysis occur with the release of histamine

delayed allergic reaction. An Rh⁻ mother can become sensitized by the fetus' Rh⁺ blood and make antibodies that destroy the fetal red blood cells. This does not generally occur during the first pregnancy, as the mother has not yet become sensitized. Rh incompatibility is examined closer in Chapter 6.

The third type of allergic reaction occurs only in persons with a certain genetic make up. These people have an abnormal sensitivity to pollens, dust, dog hair, certain foods, and possibly drugs. It is thought that antibodies,

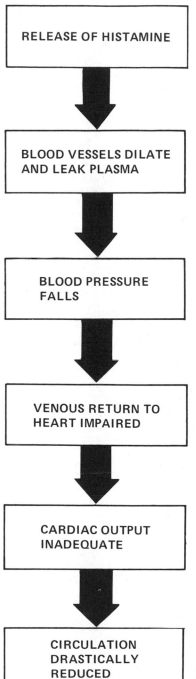

Figure 2-6. B. Sequence of vascular events in anaphylactic shock.

immunoglobulins, against these antigens are improperly made by the genetically allergic person. The abnormal immunoglobulins, IgE rather than IgG, have an affinity for certain cells and attach to them. As the antigen attaches to the antibody, the cells break down and release histamine, which causes dilation of the blood vessels and makes them susceptible to plasma leakage. The leakage of plasma into the tissues causes edema, or swelling, which when localized in the nasal passages results in the familiar congestion and

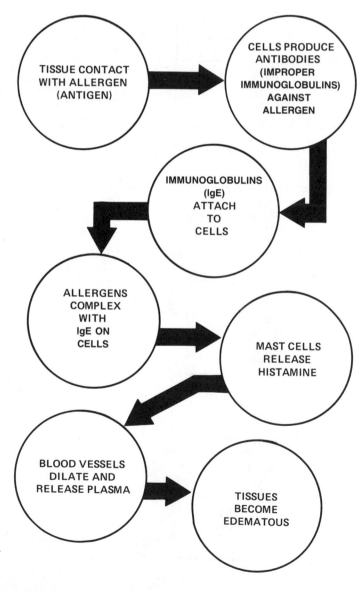

Figure 2-7. Typical allergic reaction.

irritation of hay fever. If the tissue damage and edema are near the skin, the welts and itching of hives may appear. **Antihistamines** are quite effective in the treatment of hives but less so for hay fever. A typical allergic reaction is illustrated in Figure 2–7.

Allergy shots can desensitize the hypersensitive person. Small amounts of the offending antigen are administered and concentrations gradually increased. This gives the allergic person time to build proper antibodies, subsequently reducing the amount of tissue damage.

SUMMARY

Blood plays an essential role in the protective mechanisms of the body. Some white blood cells engulf and digest invading microorganisms and toxins, whereas others produce antibodies against foreign antigens. Vascular changes that occur at the site of damaged tissue or infection increase blood flow to the area.

Inflammation, although painful, is the body's way of counteracting tissue injury. The cardinal signs and symptoms of inflammation—redness, swelling, heat, and pain—result from the increased blood flow and inflammatory exudate. Diseases with names ending in *itis* indicate inflammation of a particular organ or structure.

Antigen–antibody reactions are an important means of body defense. When antibodies against a particular antigen are present, the person, is immune to the disease caused by that antigen. This immunity can be acquired naturally, by exposure to the disease, or artificially by injection.

Allergies are closely related to the immune response. Certain allergic reactions can occur in anyone, but some people are hypersenitive to allergens that are normally harmless. Allergies of the latter type have a genetic basis.

STUDY QUESTIONS

1. What are the four principal signs and symptoms of inflammation? What is the cause of each?
2. Explain the differences between inflammation and infection.
3. Describe the vascular changes that occur in inflammation. What causes these changes?
4. What is the principal function of the various leukocytes in an inflammatory response?

5. What is the significance of leukocytosis?
6. Explain one way that infection is kept from spreading.
7. What does pus consist of?
8. Explain the antigen–antibody reaction.
9. What is the principal site of antibody production?
10. What are the functions of (a) B-lymphocytes and (b) plasma cells?
11. Explain the significant differences between active and passive immunity.
12. What is the relationship between immunity and allergy?
13. Why is anaphylactic shock such a serious allergic reaction?
14. Explain the delayed allergic reaction.
15. A second transfusion of Rh$^+$ blood to an Rh$^-$ recipient causes a transfusion reaction. The reverse is not true. Why?

CHAPTER 3

Neoplasia

The discovery of a lump or a mass can be a frightening experience as one's first thought is often the possibility of cancer. The swelling or tumor may indicate a serious condition or it may be relatively harmless. Formation of such tumors is called *neoplasia*. Swelling caused by new and abnormal growth is called a **neoplasm.** A neoplasm is a mass of new cells that grows in a haphazard fashion with no control and serves no useful function. Neoplasms are divided into two classes: malignant and benign. There is a great difference in the growth rate of various tumors. At times there may be a period of remission when the progress of the growth seems to be temporarily halted. Remission can occur spontaneously or may follow a type of therapy.

MALIGNANT TUMORS

Cancer is a malignant tumor, a growth that can affect any organ. It is often fatal and is the second leading cause of death in the United States. The exact cause of cancer is not known. One of many different factors may trigger the initial cellular change that leads to the tumor formation. Cancer is an invasive type of tumor, and many forms send fingerlike projections into underlying tissue. This manner of penetration resembles the claws of a crab. The Latin word for crab is cancri; the Greek word, karkinos. As the tumor continues to grow, normal cells are destroyed.

The malignancy can grow into a normally open space and then block the lumen of an organ. This pattern of growth can obstruct the esophagus, the intestines, or the respiratory tract.

The surface of the mass often ulcerates, which can lead to a fatal hemorrhage. The key features of malignant tumors are their uncontrolled growth and tendency to *metastasize.*

The rapid growth of the malignant tumor uses up the body's nutrients, its supply of glucose, and amino acids. This factor, coupled with the patient's inability to eat, causes severe weight loss. Frequently there is an accompanying infection and blood loss, and the patient becomes weak and emaciated in appearance. This weakened condition is referred to as **cachexia.**

Causes of Cancer

What are some of the possible causes of this disease? Environmental agents may be a factor. In various geographic areas there is a higher frequency of certain types of cancer than in others. Air or water pollutants may be such agents. There may be a genetic predisposition for a particular cancer, as certain family histories of the disease indicate. Radiation is known to cause skin cancer in certain people who are overexposed to the ultraviolet light of the sun. The people affected may have an inherited sensitivity to solar radiation. A combination of genetic makeup and radiation may cause the cancer.

Workers in the field of radiation must take great precautions to prevent exposure to the harmful rays. This includes x-ray technicians and people using radioactive material in laboratories. Survivors of the atom bomb have shown a high incidence of leukemia as a result of the radiation they received. Certain chemicals used in industry have caused cancer in many workers. A large number of persons working with a particular dye developed cancer of the bladder. Inhalation of asbestos, benzedrine, and arsenic is known to have caused lung cancer. These cancer-causing substances are called **chemical carcinogens.**

Intensive research is being done today to study relationships between food preservatives, elements of cosmetics, and plastics in the development of cancer. Cigarette smoking has been implicated in lung cancer, and cigar and pipe smoking with cancer of the mouth and lip, respectively.

Hormones are related to certain forms of cancer. A benign mole never becomes malignant before puberty, the time when the sex hormone level increases. Cancer of the prostate gland is stimulated by the male hormone testosterone, but its growth is inhibited by estrogen therapy. The ovaries are sometimes removed after breast cancer surgery to prevent estrogen stimulation of other tumors. Many forms of cancer are more common in either men or women, which seems to indicate a hormonal relationship. A virus has been shown to cause at least one kind of cancer in humans.

Viruses invade cells and may alter the genetic material of the cell. This could account for the abnormal cell divisions and rapid growth observed in malignant tumors. Possible causes of cancer are summarized in Figure 3–1.

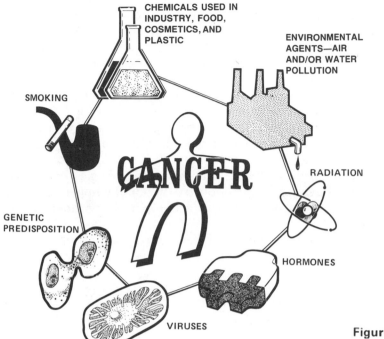

CHEMICALS USED IN
INDUSTRY, FOOD,
COSMETICS, AND
PLASTIC

ENVIRONMENTAL
AGENTS—AIR
AND/OR WATER
POLLUTION

SMOKING

RADIATION

GENETIC
PREDISPOSITION

HORMONES

VIRUSES

Figure 3-1. Possible causes of cancer.

Symptoms of Cancer

Symptoms vary with the site of the malignancy. Pain is usually not an early sign of cancer. It is only when the mass has grown, causing an obstruction or putting pressure on nerve endings, that pain is experienced. Infection frequently accompanies cancer and may cause pain.

There are certain warning signs that a cancerous tumor might be present. Abnormal bleeding or discharge from a natural body opening such as the rectum or vagina may be an indication of a malignancy. Blood in the urine, sputum, or vomitus is cause for investigation. This bleeding may not be due to cancer at all, but it is a precautionary measure to have it checked.

A thickening or lump, particularly in the breast, indicates a tumor or a cyst. A **cyst** is a sac or capsule containing fluid and is usually harmless. The tumor might well be benign, but the possibility of a malignancy exists, and it should be examined by a physician. The American Cancer Society urges women to perform monthly self-examinations of each breast as so much can be gained by early detection of a malignancy.

Another sign of a possible cancer is a persistent cough or hoarseness. A growth in the respiratory tract, or one pressing on it, acts as an irritant in stimulating the cough reflex.

A change in bowel activity, intermittent constipation and diarrhea, may indicate an obstruction in the colon. Difficulties in urination such as urgency, burning sensations, and the inability to start the stream of urine may signal a tumor in the urinary system. In men, it may signal a tumor of the prostate gland.

Normally the body has excellent healing ability. If a sore or an ulceration fails to heal after a period of time there is some reason for it, and the lesion should be examined. A mole may change color, darken, enlarge, or become itchy. This can signal a transition from a benign growth to one that is malignant.

A person experiencing difficulty in swallowing (**dysphagia**) or loss of appetite (**anorexia**) may have some kind of obstruction in the upper gastrointestinal tract. These symptoms, particularly if accompanied by rapid weight loss, are significant.

A severe anemia may indicate internal bleeding from a malignant lesion or malfunctioning of the bone marrow due to a cancerous growth. Exces-

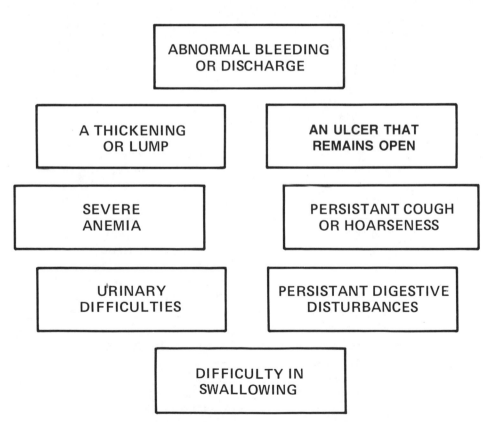

Figure 3-2. Warning signs of cancer.

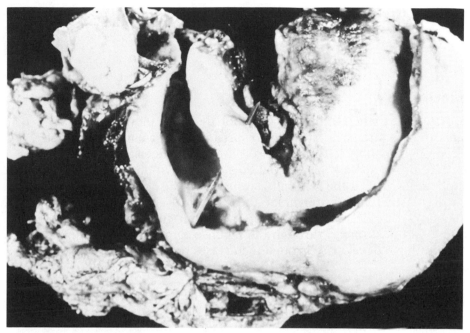

Figure 3-3. Adenocarcinoma of the stomach. White area is the greatly thickened stomach wall. (*Courtesy of Dr. David R. Duffell.*)

sive production of a hormone can signal a tumor, benign or malignant, of an endocrine gland. Figure 3-2 illustrates warning signs that may indicate a malignancy.

Types of Cancer

There are two major types of cancer, carcinoma and sarcoma; the suffix *oma* means a tumor. **Carcinoma** is the more common form, affecting epithelial tissues, skin, and mucous membranes lining body cavities. Tumors of the skin are called **epidermoid carcinomas.** Carcinoma is also the malignancy of glandular tissue such as the breast, liver, and pancreas. Cancerous glandular tumors are known as **adenocarcinomas;** the prefix *adeno* always refers to a gland. Although these tumors develop in either epithelial or glandular tissue, they invade deeper and surrounding tissues. Cancer of the mouth, lung, and stomach are examples of carcinoma. Figure 3-3 shows an adenocarcinoma of the stomach.

Sarcoma is the less common cancer, but it spreads more rapidly and is highly malignant. Connective tissue tumors, such as tumors of bone, muscle, and cartilage, are sarcomas. Rapidly growing tumors show little differentiation, and this lack of form is referred to as **anaplasia,** the prefix *an* meaning without and *plasia,* form. These rapidly growing, undifferentiated tumors are the most responsive to radiation treatment. Figure 3–4 contrasts carcinoma and sarcoma.

Metastasis

Unfortunately, when a malignant tumor develops in an organ such as the breast or prostate gland, it tends to spread to other parts of the body. This spread of the cancer to distant sites is known as **metastasis.**

Carcinoma spreads principally through the lymph vessels, affecting the lymph nodes. This is the reason for removal of the axillary lymph nodes in a radical mastectomy (removal of the breast). Regional lymph nodes are removed in surgical operations for malignant tumors of the colon. Carcinoma can also spread through the bloodstream. Malignant tumors of the liver that have developed through metastases are seen in Figure 3–5.

	CARCINOMA	SARCOMA
AFFECTS	EPITHELIAL AND GLANDULAR TISSUE	CONNECTIVE TISSUE
EXAMPLES	SKIN, BREAST, AND LIVER CANCER	CANCER OF BONE, MUSCLE, AND CARTILAGE
INCIDENCE	MORE COMMON	LESS COMMON
GROWTH RATE	SLOWER	FASTER
METASTASIS	PRINCIPALLY THROUGH LYMPH VESSELS	PRINCIPALLY THROUGH THE BLOOD

Figure 3-4. Distinctions between carcinoma and sarcoma.

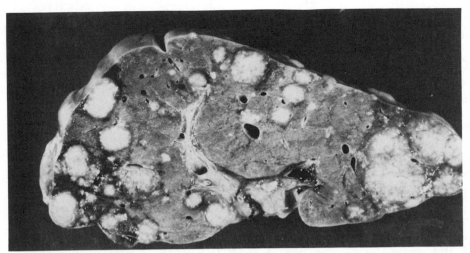

Figure 3-5. Malignant tumors of the liver that have metastasized from other sites. (*Courtesy of Dr. David R. Duffell.*)

The metastasis of sarcoma is generally through the blood vessels. Clusters of cancer cells can break off from the primary sites and travel as emboli to the liver, lungs, brain, or other organs. Frequently, it is a secondary site of cancer that is discovered first.

Diagnosis of Cancer

X-ray techniques, particularly those using contrast dyes, can show the site of a mass or tumor. The tumor can only be diagnosed as malignant through microscopic examination of the cells and tissue. All tumors removed surgically must be sent to a pathology department for this study. When a suspected tumor is **biopsied,** a small sample is removed and examined microscopically for abnormalities. A technique known as the frozen section enables the pathologist to immediately determine whether the sample is malignant. This is extremely helpful during surgery. A sample of the tissue is sent to the laboratory, the surgeon waits for the result, and then determines the extent of the surgery required based on the report.

Another means of obtaining cells for microscopic examination is through scrapings, washings, and secretions from suspected areas. This is called **exfoliative cytology.** It takes advantage of the fact that cancer cells in the early stages tend to be cast off or shed. This technique is helpful in diagnosing early cancer of the bronchus and uterus. It is the principle of the Papanicolaou (Pap) smear, which was named for its originator, Dr. George N. Papanicolaou.

There are different stages of cancer development. The pre-invasive stage means that the tumor has not yet penetrated into underlying tissues. If cancer of the cervix can be determined at this stage through the Pap smear, surgical removal offers good prognosis.

Once the cancer has become invasive its total removal is very difficult. The edges of the malignant tumor are poorly defined and if it is not entirely removed the cancer will recur. If the tumor has metastasized surgery is of little benefit.

Treatment of Cancer

Surgery is very effective in the early stages of certain cancers. Breast cancer is well treated by surgery, as is skin cancer. Fast-growing, undifferentiated tumors respond best to radiation therapy. Radiation has a greater destructive action on fast-growing cells than on normal cells. Hodgkin's disease, a malignancy of the lymph nodes and lymphoid tissue, is a cancer of this type. Hormonal therapy is used to treat cancer of the prostate, either by removal of the androgen sources, which stimulate the tumor growth, or by administration of estrogens, which inhibit it. **Chemotherapy,** the use of **antineoplastic agents** such as nitrogen mustard, is in some cases effective in controlling leukemia.

BENIGN TUMORS

Benign tumors are different from malignant tumors. Benign growths are generally encapsulated with clearly defined edges, which makes their removal from surrounding tissue relatively easy. **Benign** tumors do not metastasize nor do they recur after surgical removal. Only rarely do these tumors ulcerate and bleed. A benign tumor differentiates somewhat in its development and resembles the structure from which it grew.

This does not mean that benign tumors pose no threat. A tumor on the brain or in the spinal cord, even if it is benign, puts pressure on nerves and seriously affects the functioning of the nervous system. Any tumor can obstruct a passageway such as the trachea, shutting off the air supply, or the esophagus, making it impossible to swallow. A benign tumor of a gland can cause oversecretion of its hormone with very serious effects. If a tumor of the anterior pituitary gland develops before puberty, the increased secretion of growth hormone leads to the development of a giant. An adrenal gland tumor produces an oversecretion of androgens (male sex hormones) and causes masculinization of females.

Types of Benign Tumors

Tumors are classified according to the tissue in which they develop. A common benign tumor is the **lipoma**, a soft, fatty tumor that develops in adipose (fat) tissue. As it grows it pushes normal tissue aside. Lipomas are commonly found on the neck, back, and buttocks—anyplace where there is fat.

A **myoma** is a tumor of the muscle; the prefix *myo* refers to muscle. These tumors are rare in voluntary muscle but do develop in smooth muscle. Myomas are the tumors of the uterus referred to as fibroids. Fibroid tumors are also called **leiomyomas,** specifying a tumor of smooth muscle. Leiomyomas are the tumors most commonly found in women. If they are small they may cause no symptoms, but if they become large they can cause menstrual problems or difficulties during a pregnancy, even abortion.

The typical red birthmark, or "port-wine" stain, is another type of benign tumor. It is an **angioma,** a tumor composed of blood vessels. Lymph vessels can also comprise an angioma, but since lymph is colorless a tumor of this type is colorless. An angioma is one type of benign tumor that is not encapsulated.

The common mole is a benign tumor called a **nevus.** Like the angioma it is not encapsulated. This tumor of the skin contains a black pigment called melanin and is sometimes called a melanoma. There is also a cancerous condition known as **malignant melanoma,** so the name nevus is better used when the tumor is benign. The nevus is congenital but may not be apparent until later in life; it usually enlarges at puberty. This benign tumor can change to a malignant melanoma, especially if it is continuously irritated. An increase in size and pigmentation, bleeding, or itchiness may indicate this transformation to the malignant type.

An epithelial tumor that grows as a projecting mass on the skin, or from an inner mucous membrane, is a **papilloma** or polyp. The common wart is an example of a papilloma. This tumor has a fixed base with a stalk growing from it. A growth of this type in the intestinal tract or uterus can be moved back and forth on the stalk and become irritated. It may then become malignant. Figure 3–6 shows a patient with an enlarging mole on the back aggravated by bra irritation.

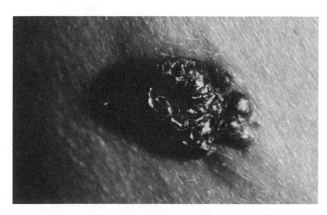

Figure 3-6. Forty-eight-year-old woman with enlarging mole on back, increasing in size over 2 or 3 months. Patient died in 10 months despite radical surgery. (*Courtesy of Dr. Barry A. Goldsmith.*)

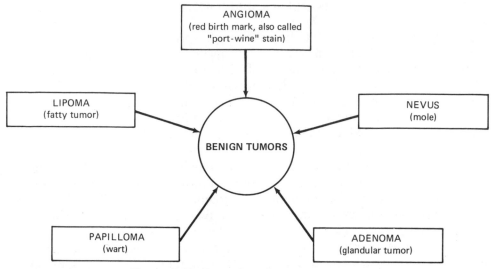

Figure 3-7. Examples of benign tumors.

A benign tumor of glandular tissue is the **adenoma.** It often develops in the breast, thyroid gland, or in mucous glands of the intestinal tract. The adenoma is an example of a benign tumor that resembles the structure from which it develops. Glands and ducts are found within the tumor, and it may be secretory. Various benign tumors are indicated in Figure 3-7.

A unique benign tumor of the ovary is the **teratoma,** or dermoid cyst. Lining the cyst is epidermis; skin with its usual appendages: hair, oil and sweat glands, even teeth. The cyst contains oily material from the sebaceous, oil, glands. The teratoma probably stems from some primitive cell that has the potential of developing in several directions. When these cysts develop on a long pedicle, or stalk, twisting may occur and cause acute abdominal pain. Surgical removal is then necessary.

DIFFERENCES BETWEEN MALIGNANT AND BENIGN TUMORS

Malignant tumors are usually larger and more irregular in shape than benign tumors. Benign tumors are generally encapsulated and malignant ones are not. A malignancy is invasive and penetrating, destroying underlying tissue. This is not characteristic of benign tumors. Malignant tumors grow at a faster rate than benign tumors and metastasize, setting up new colonies of cells at distant sites. Benign tumors resemble the tissue in which they developed, but malignant tumors lack form.

SUMMARY

There are many different kinds of cancer and proposed causes. These causes might be environmental, genetic, viral, or chemical, but some factor stimulates the initial abnormal cell growth. Malignant tumors are best treated when diagnosed in the early stages, so warning signs are important. Abnormal bleeding, a persistent cough, a lump or swelling, or difficulty in swallowing are some of the symptoms that were discussed.

Differences exist between carcinoma and sarcoma, each arising from different tissues of the body and spreading by different channels. The growth rates of carcinoma and sarcoma differ, and the treatments to which each responds best differ.

Malignant tumors are diagnosed by microscopic examination of a tissue biopsy or by cancer cells scraped off or shed from a body surface. Treatment depends on the type of cancer and the location. Some benign tumors can become malignant; others are a danger because of their location; and some are harmless. Malignancies of specific organs will be studied with the disease of the various systems.

STUDY QUESTIONS

1. What are the differences between normal cell growth and growth of a neoplasm?
2. What are some of the dangers of cancer?
3. Name five possible causes of cancer.
4. Name six warning signs of cancer.
5. What is the distinction between carcinoma and sarcoma? Which tends to spread faster?
6. What is the more common route of metastasis in each type?
7. Name some examples of (a) carcinoma and (b) sarcoma.
8. Why is the Pap smear of great value?
9. When is surgery the most effective treatment for cancer?
10. In what type of cancer is radiation therapy most effective?
11. When is a benign tumor dangerous?
12. What is the difference between an adenoma and adenocarcinoma?
13. Describe a dermoid cyst.
14. Name five differences between a benign and malignant tumor.

CHAPTER 4

Hereditary Diseases

Have you ever been startled by observing a particularly strong family resemblance? How is this similarity between brothers and sisters, children and parents, and even between cousins explained? You can say, "It's because of their genes," which is true, but what about two brothers of the same parents who do not resemble each other at all? How does this phenomenon called inheritance work?

All genetic information is contained in the nucleus of each cell, and each time the cell divides, in growth and repair, the information is passed on to the daughter cells. The vehicle of transmission is the DNA molecule, which duplicates itself when a cell is about to divide, providing an exact copy for each daughter cell.

DNA, which stands for deoxyribonucleic acid, is the blueprint for protein synthesis within the cell. Proteins form a structural part of the cell and comprise the enzymes, the biological catalysts, that control cellular activity. Some of the genetic disorders that will be discussed result from the lack of a particular enzyme and are referred to as inborn errors of metabolism.

At the time of cell division, the DNA is assembled into units called chromosomes. Each human cell contains 46 chromosomes divided into 23 pairs. Half of the chromosomes were inherited from each parent. The chromosomes contain thousands of genes, each of which is responsible for the synthesis of one protein. Forty-four of the chromosomes are called **autosomes,** and two are called the X and Y, or the sex, chromosomes, the ones that determine the sex of the person. A combination of XY chromosomes results in a male, and XX chromosomes in a female. This chromosomal composition of the nucleus is called the **karyotype** of the cell. The karyotype can be visualized microscopically and photographed to determine chromosomal abnormalities.

The genes inherited from each parent for a particular trait such as eye color, hair color, and hair type occupy a particular site on a chromosome and are called **alleles.** If the pair of genes are similar, the person is **homozygous** for that trait. If the genes are different, one for dark and one for light hair, for example, the person is **heterozygous.** Some genes always produce an effect and are said to be **dominant.** The result of the dominant gene is the same whether a person is homozygous or heterozygous. The gene for brown eyes, for example, is dominant to that for blue eyes. Other genes are **recessive** and only manifest themselves when the person is homozygous for the trait. This is significant in many hereditary diseases.

Certain factors may cause a deviation from the basic principles of inheritance that have been described. Some genes are codominant, so that both are expressed. An example of codominant genes is found in blood type AB. The gene for the A factor is inherited from one parent and that for the B factor from the other, but both genes are expressed. At times a dominant gene is not fully expressed, a condition known as reduced penetrance.

Spontaneous **mutations** or changes in the DNA structure occur at times, and they become permanent hereditary alterations if the gonads are affected. Mutations can result from viral activity, chemical action, and radiation. The effect of the mutation may be slight and go unnoticed or it may be lethal. Serious mutations are generally incompatible with life and cause the death of a fetus and spontaneous abortion.

The environment interacts with heredity, as seen in certain diseases. A predisposition to develop allergies is inherited, but contact with an offending antigen is required for sensitization to it. As an example, a person is not born allergic to ragweed but develops the hypersensitivty on exposure, and a fair-skinned person can develop cancer when overexposed to the ultraviolet light of the sun. Obesity develops through a combination of heredity and dietary habits.

TRANSMISSION OF HEREDITARY DISEASE

Many of the diseases described throughout this book are called hereditary or familial diseases. In this chapter, the mechanism of transmission will be explained. Some diseases are inherited from a single autosomal dominant gene. One such defective gene causes Huntington's chorea, a disease described in Chapter 15, and another causes familial polyposis, explained in Chapter 10. Other diseases are inherited as autosomal recessives, with one defective gene being inherited from each parent, making the person homozygous for that trait. Cystic fibrosis is such a disease. A third type of inheritance is sex-linked, with the defective gene on the X or Y chromosome. Color blindness and hemophilia are examples of sex-linked inherited diseases.

Autosomal Dominant Disorders

A defective dominant gene is usually transmitted from a parent who is heterozygous for the trait. If the other parent is normal for the particular condition, 50 percent of their children have the chance of being affected and manifesting the genetic defect. The remaining children will be homozogous for the recessive gene and be normal. This is illustrated in Figure 4–1. The disease appears in every generation, with males and females being equally affected. Exceptions to the rule are minimal.

Polydactyly, extra fingers or toes, is an example of an autosomal dominant disorder. A boy or girl inheriting the defective gene from either parent will have the abnormality. **Achondroplasia** is another disorder resulting from one defective dominant gene (Fig. 4–2). The word element *chondro* refers to cartilage, *plasia* to formation, and the prefix *a* means a lack. In this disease, cartilage formation in the fetus is defective. Normally, the fetal skeleton develops as cartilage that is gradually replaced by bone. In achondroplasia the defective cartilage formation results in improper bone development and **achondroplastic dwarfism.** The long bones of the arms and legs are short, the trunk of the body is normal in size, the head is large, and the forehead very prominent. The person develops sexually, has normal intelligence, and is muscular and agile.

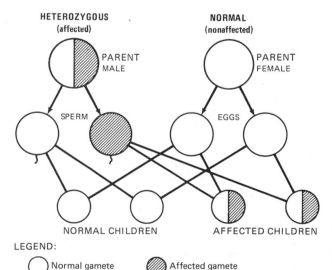

Figure 4-1. Transmission of autosomal dominant disorders (50 percent chance for an affected child).

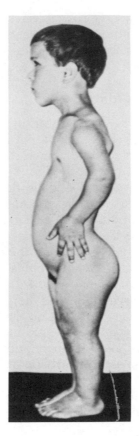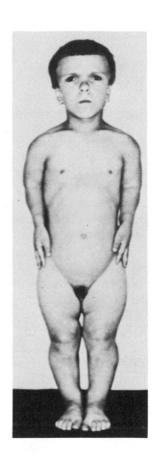

Figure 4-2. A 12-year-old achondroplastic dwarf. Note the disproportion of the limbs to the trunk, the curvature of the spine, and the prominent buttocks. (From Kosowicz. Atlas of Endocrine Diseases, 1978. *Courtesy of The Charles Press*).

DISEASES INHERITED FROM RECESSIVE GENES

These diseases manifest themselves only when a person is homozygous for the defective gene. Two parents who are both carriers of the recessive gene are themselves heterozygous for the trait and do not have the disease. There is a 25% chance that their children will be affected. Two out of four will be carriers and one will be normal. This is shown in Figure 4–3. The recessive gene appears more frequently in a family, and close intermarriage, as between first cousins, increases the risk of the particular disease.

Phenylketonuria, also called PKU, is an example of autosomal recessive gene inheritance. The PKU patient lacks a specific enzyme that converts one amino acid, phenylalanine, to another, tyrosine. This mechanism is illustrated in Figure 4–4. As a result, high levels of phenylalanine and its derivatives build up in the blood and are toxic to the brain, interfering with normal brain development. If the condition is not diagnosed and treated early, severe mental retardation results. Physical development proceeds normally,

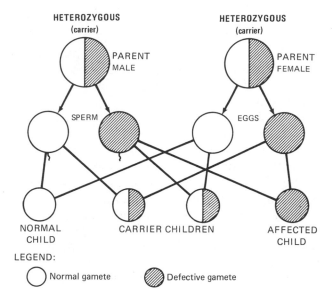

Figure 4-3. Transmission of recessive disorders (25 percent chance for an affected child).

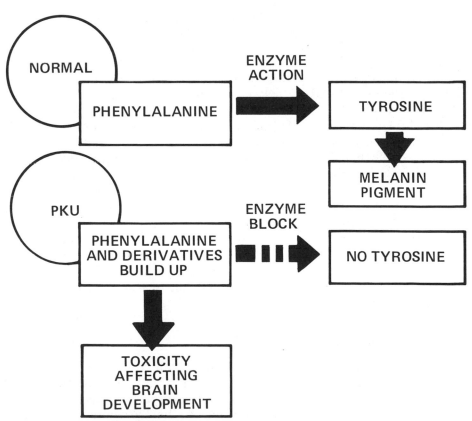

Figure 4-4. Enzyme block in phenylketonuria (PKU).

but the child is very light in color. Production of the pigment melanin is impeded because of inadequate tyrosine, a result of the missing enzyme. The child may manifest disorders of the nervous system such as a lack of balance and may possibly suffer convulsions.

To prevent the serious mental retardation that accompanies PKU, newborn babies are routinely screened for the disease. If it is found, a synthetic diet is prescribed that eliminates phenylalanine. Good results have been achieved with this treatment. The diet is unpleasant, and controversy exists as to the length of time the diet must be maintained. To begin treatment immediately, by excluding phenylalanine during the earliest years of life, seems to be the most critical factor in preventing mental retardation.

Galactosemia is another example of an inborn error of metabolism resulting from autosomal recessive inheritance. The person with this disease lacks the enzyme necessary to convert galactose, a sugar derived from lactose in milk, to glucose. Galactose accumulates in the blood and interferes with development of the brain, liver, and eyes. If untreated, mental retardation develops. The liver becomes enlarged and cirrhotic, and ascites fluid (see Chapter 11) accumulates in the abdominal cavity. Intestinal distress results in vomiting and diarrhea. Early diagnosis and treatment of galactosemia can prevent these signs, and development will then proceed normally. The treatment consists of eliminating lactose from the diet.

Sickle cell anemia, a severe anemia generally confined to blacks, will be described in Chapter 6. The manner of inheritance is best explained in the context of genetic diseases. Sickle cell anemia is an autosomal recessive disorder, in which the hemoglobin is abnormal, resulting in deformed red blood cells. The improperly formed cells become lodged in capillaries and block circulation, causing necrosis and infarcts, death of tissues. The sickle-shaped red blood cells rupture easily, and they are removed from the circulation by the spleen. The depletion of red blood cells results in severe anemia.

The person with sickle cell anemia is homozygous for the trait by inheriting one defective gene from each parent. A person who is heterozygous for sickle cell anemia has both normal and abnormal hemoglobin and possesses the sickle cell trait. The person is mildly anemic, but the one defective gene provides an advantage. The person with sickle cell trait has an immunity against malaria that is significant in tropical climates where malaria abounds.

Sex-linked Inheritance

Diseases of sex-linked inheritance generally result from defective genes on the X chromosome, as the Y chromosome is small and carries very few genes. A recessive gene on the single X chromosome of a male is unmasked, and the trait is expressed. A female may be heterozygous for the gene, having a recessive gene on the one X chromosome but a normal gene on the other X. That female is then a carrier of the disease, and she has a 50% chance of transmitting the gene to half of her sons and daughters. An affected male transmits the disease only to his daughters, as they receive his X chromosome. His sons are unaffected, as the Y chromosome is normal. This is illustrated in Figure 4–5. The abnormalities of **sex-linked inheritance** are generally confined to the male and are transmitted by the female. In a rare case, the female may have the sex-linked disease if she is homozygous for the recessive gene.

■ *Color Blindness.* Color blindness, the inability to distinguish between certain colors, is a disorder of sex-linked inheritance. It is generally confined to males, although it is possible for a female to be color-blind if she receives the recessive gene from each parent, which is rare.

The gene for color blindness is on the X chromosome, but the gene for normal vision is dominant to it. A male with the recessive gene on his one X chromosome will express the trait and be color-blind.

The defect that causes color blindness is apparently in certain specialized receptors of the retina called cones. There are three types of receptors

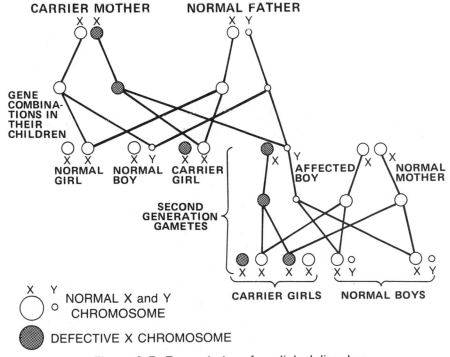

Figure 4-5. Transmission of sex-linked disorders.

that are stimulated by wavelengths of the primary colors: red, green, and blue. Impulses are then sent to the brain and interpreted. The color-blind person is most frequently unable to distinguish reds and greens. There is no correction for color blindness.

Familial Diseases. Some diseases appear in families, but the means of inheritance are not understood. Examples of diseases with a higher incidence in certain families are epilepsy, diabetes, cardiovascular problems, allergies, and familial polyposis (Fig. 4–6). The cause of these diseases does not seem to be a single gene but the effect of several genes working together.

GROSS CHROMOSOMAL ABNORMALITIES

The hereditary diseases that have been described so far result from a defective gene. Abnormalities in the chromosomes, either in their number or structure, cause other disorders. At times, chromosomes fail to separate properly during cell division, causing one daughter cell to be deficient and one to have an extra chromosome. The loss of an autosomal chromosome is

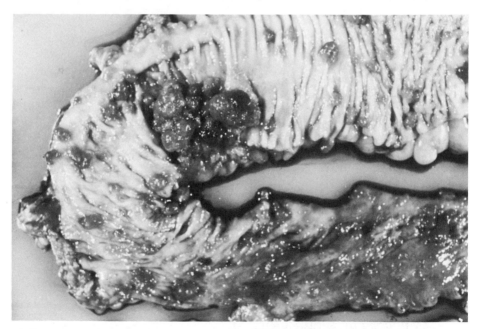

Figure 4-6. Familial polyposis of the colon. (*Courtesy of Dr. David R. Duffell.*)

usually incompatible with life because each autosome contains a large number of essential genes. A fetus affected by this condition is generally aborted. The loss of a sex chromosome or the presence of an extra one is less serious, but many abnormalities accompany the condition.

■ Down's Syndrome (Mongolism)

Down's syndrome is an example of a disorder caused by the presence of an extra autosomal chromosome. The extra chromosome results from **nondisjunction,** the failure of two chromosomes to separate as the gametes—the egg and sperm—are being formed.

The mongoloid child is always mentally retarded. The excessive enzyme production from the extra genes may have a toxic effect on the brain. The child can be taught simple tasks and is generally very affectionate.

The life expectancy of a child with Down's syndrome is relatively short due to complications that accompany the condition. Congenital heart diseases are common, and there is a greater susceptibility to respiratory tract

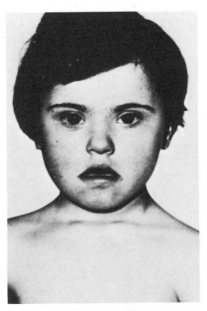 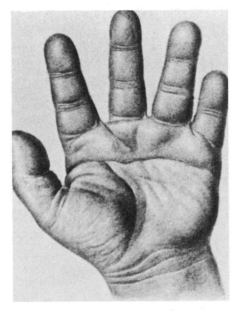

Figure 4-7. Left. Face of a 5-year-old girl with Down's syndrome. Note widely set eyes, underdeveloped bridge of the nose, partially open mouth, and protruding tongue. **Right.** Short, broad hand of a 9-year-old Down's syndrome patient, showing shortened fifth finger and transverse crease across palm. (*From Kosowicz, Atlas of Endocrine Diseases, 1978. Courtesy of The Charles Press.*)

infections, including pneumonia. There is also a higher incidence of leukemia than in a normal child.

The mongoloid child has a very characteristic appearance. The eyes appear slanted due to an extra fold of skin at the upper, medial corner of the eye; the tongue is coarse and often protrudes; and the nose is short and flat. The child is usually of short stature, and the sex organs are under-developed. A straight crease extends across the palm of the hand, and the little finger is often shorter than normal (Fig. 4–7).

The incidence of Down's syndrome is higher in mothers over 35 than in younger women, and the risk increases with age.

■ Turner's Syndrome

One of the sex chromosomes is missing in **Turner's syndrome,** resulting in a karyotype of 45,X0. The patient appears to be female, but the ovaries do not develop; thus, there is no ovulation or menstruation, and the person is sterile. The nipples are widely spaced, the breasts do not develop, and the person is short of stature and has a stocky build. Congenital heart disease, particularly coarctation of the aorta (described in Chapter 7), frequently accompanies Turner's syndrome. Facial deformities are often present. Figure 4–8 shows a patient with Turner's syndrome.

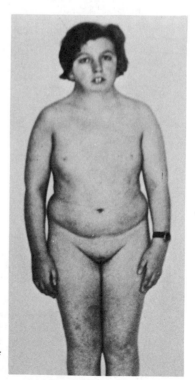

Figure 4-8. A 21-year-old patient with Turner's syndrome. The chest is broad and the nipples are small and pale. Pubic hair is totally lacking. (*From Kosowicz. Atlas of Endocrine Diseases, 1978. Courtesy of The Charles Press.*)

■ Klinefelter's Syndrome

An extra sex chromosome is present in **Klinefelter's syndrome,** and the patient's karyotype is 47,XXY. This person appears to be a male but has small testes that fail to mature and produce no sperm. At puberty, with the development of secondary sex characteristics, the breasts enlarge and a female distribution of hair develops. There is little facial hair, and the general appearance is that of a eunuch. The person is tall (with abnormally long legs), is mentally deficient, and is sterile (Fig. 4–9).

Sex Anomalies

The number of true **hermaphrodites** who have both testes and ovaries is small. Pseudohermaphrodites do develop, and they have either testes or ovaries, usually nonfunctional, but the remainder of the anatomy is mixed. This condition is referred to as sex reversal, in which the chromosomal sex is different from the anatomic sex. Sex reversal occurs during fetal life. The sex glands are neutral during the first few weeks after conception, but the male gonads differentiate at about the sixth week under the influence of masculinizing hormone. In the absence of an adequate amount of this

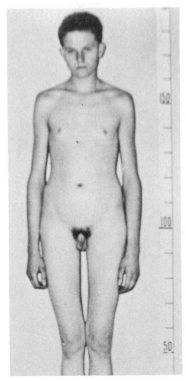

Figure 4-9. A 19-year-old patient with Klinefelter's syndrome. Extremities are excessively long, pubic hair is scanty, and genitals are underdeveloped. Body proportions resemble those of a eunuch. (*From Kosowicz. Atlas of Endocrine Diseases, 1978. Courtesy of The Charles Press.*)

hormone, ovaries develop, and the individual is anatomically female but chromosomally male (XY).

Some cases of pseudohermaphroditism result from excessive production of sex hormones from the adrenal cortex. An affected female develops male secondary sexual characteristics at a very early age. The external genitalia of pseudohermaphrodites resembles that of both males and females. A pseudohermaphrodite is shown in Figure 4–10.

CONGENITAL DISEASES

Congenital diseases are those appearing at birth or shortly after, but they are not caused by genetic or chromosomal abnormalities. Congential defects usually result from some failure in development during the embryonic stage, or first 2 months of pregnancy. Congenital diseases cannot be transmitted to offspring.

Various factors—inadequate oxygen, maternal infection, drugs, malnutrition, and radiation—can interfere with normal development. Rubella, or German measles, contracted by the mother during the first trimester of

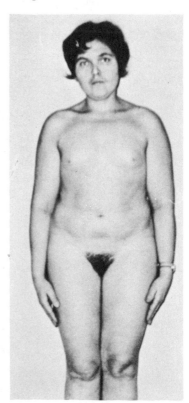

Figure 4-10. A 22-year-old patient with pseudohermaphroditism, reared as a girl because of ambiguous genitalia. Surgery and tissue studies showed the gonads to be testes. [(*From Kosowicz. Atlas of Endocrine Diseases, 1978. Courtesy of The Charles Press.*)

pregnancy, can produce serious birth defects. The rubella virus is able to cross the placental barrier and affect the central nervous system of the embryo, causing mental retardation, blindness, and deafness. Cerebral palsy and hydrocephalus can develop as a result of the viral infection.

Syphilis can be transmitted to a developing fetus and cause multiple anomalies—structural deformities, blindness, deafness, and paralysis; children with congenital syphilis may become insane. Syphilitic infection of a fetus frequently results in spontaneous abortion or a stillbirth. A mother with syphilis should be treated for it before the fifth month of pregnancy to prevent fetal infection. A child born with syphilis should be treated immediately with penicillin, but considerable irreversible damage may have already occurred.

The tragic effect of the drug thalidomide, used during pregnancy many years ago, alerted the public to the danger of drugs to the developing embryo. Babies who had been exposed to thalidomide before birth were born without limbs or had flipperlike appendages.

Many congenital defects result from improper closure of a structure or failure of parts to unite. Congenital heart diseases are discussed in Chapter 7. Spina bifida, an improper union of parts of the vertebral column, is explained in Chapter 15. Congenital defects of the alimentary tract include various types of obstructions. The absence or closure of a normal body opening or tubular structure is called **atresia**. Atresia occurs in various parts of the gastrointestinal tract. The lack of an opening from the esophagus to the stomach is esophageal atresia; it is frequently accompanied by an abnormal opening between the esophagus and the trachea.

Intestinal atresia is a complete obstruction of the intestine, resulting in vomiting, dehydration, scanty stool production, and distention of the abdomen. The bile ducts are blocked in biliary atresia, and the inability to secrete bile into the duodenum causes severe jaundice to develop. The liver and spleen become greatly enlarged. Another congenital obstruction of the intestinal tract is pyloric stenosis, in which the circular sphincter muscle is hypertrophied, closing the opening between the stomach and the duodenum. Symptoms include projectile vomiting, dehydration, constipation, and weight loss. Corrective surgery has been very effective in removing these congenital obstructions of the intestinal tract, just as it has been for congenital heart disease.

SUMMARY

Genetic information is conveyed from parents to their children through the complex activity of the DNA molecule, which duplicates itself when a cell is about to divide. DNA provides a blueprint for protein synthesis in the daughter cells and comprises the genes that are arranged on the chromosomes, with half being received from each parent. Some genes are dominant and are always expressed, whereas others are recessive and require two similar genes for the expression of a trait. One pair of chromosomes, the X and Y chromosomes, determines the sex of the fetus.

Certain diseases are inherited by children just as physical traits are. Some diseases develop if only a single dominant autosomal gene is received. An example of this is Huntington's chorea, a devastating disease of the central nervous system. Other diseases develop only if a recessive gene is received from each parent, as is the case in phenylketonuria. Other diseases are sex-linked, affecting primarily males but being transmitted through females. This is the inheritance pattern in color blindness and hemophilia. Some diseases are found within families but are not attributable to a particular gene. The action of several genes seems to be responsible. Epilepsy, diabetes, and allergies are thought to be caused in this way.

In addition to diseases inherited by specific genes, gross chromosomal abnormalities result in other disorders. Down's syndrome is caused by chromosome 21 being in triplicate (**trisomy 21**). A missing or extra sex chromosome produces sex anomalies and usually mental retardation.

Certain conditions are apparent at birth or soon after, but they are not the result of genetic or chromosomal abnormalities. These are congenital diseases caused by various factors during early development. Certain heart malformations, absence of a natural body opening, or failure of a structure to close are examples of congenital diseases. These diseases are not passed on to offspring.

STUDY QUESTIONS

1. If one parent is heterozygous for a defective dominant gene and the other parent is normal, what percentage of their children have the chance of being affected?
2. Will any of the children in the above case be simply carriers? Why?
3. What is the developmental failure in achondroplasia?
4. If two parents are heterozygous for cystic fibrosis, how many of their children will have the chance of being affected? How many have the chance of being carriers of it? Can any of the children be normal?
5. Explain the abnormality in phenylketonuria (PKU). How is it treated?
6. Why do children with PKU have a light complexion and light hair?
7. How is galactosemia inherited?
8. What is the difference between sickle cell anemia and sickle cell trait?

9. What is the advantage of sickle cell trait?
10. Why is the male generally affected in diseases of sex-linked inheritance?
11. To which of the male's children does he transmit the defective gene? Why?
12. Why are women rarely color blind?
13. Explain the cause of Down's syndrome.
14. What are the signs of Down's syndrome?
15. What is the chromosomal abnormality in Turner's syndrome, and how is the patient affected?
16. Describe the signs at puberty of a patient with Klinefelter's syndrome.
17. Name several factors that can cause congenital birth defects.
18. Why are congenital birth defects generally nontransmissible?

CHAPTER 5

Nutritional Diseases, Obesity, and Alcoholism

Diseases that may be classified as nutritional diseases stem from a wide range of causes. Malnutrition caused by poverty, ignorance, or the unavailability of proper foods comprises one end of the spectrum, whereas excessive intake due to obesity, hypervitaminosis, or alcoholism is at the other extreme.

The concept of malnutrition is generally associated with an inadequate availability of food, but one can suffer nutritional deficiencies in the midst of plenty. Several diseases that will be discussed in this book are actually nutritional diseases in that they deprive the body of essential dietary elements.

Various malfunctionings of the gastrointestinal system (Chapter 10) prevent the use of nutrients in the diet. The absence of gastric, intestinal, and pancreatic enzymes to digest proteins, carbohydrates, and lipids deprives the body of these nutrients. Pancreatitis (Chapter 11), for example, interferes with digestion when the diseased pancreas is unable to function.

Digestive disturbances that cause persistent vomiting or diarrhea also result in malnutrition.

Not only is the digestion of foodstuffs essential for proper nourishment, but the end products of digestion must be absorbed through the intestinal wall. Bile secretion, essential for the absorption of lipids, including the fat-soluble vitamins A, D, E, and K, may be inadequate for such reasons as liver dysfunction, a diseased gallbladder, or obstruction of the bile ducts. The malabsorption syndrome (Chapter 10) causes the loss of essential nutrients in the stools. Pernicious anemia develops in the absence of the gastric intrinsic factor needed for absorption of vitamin B_{12} from the digestive tract. This condition occurs even if vitamin B_{12} is present in the diet.

Impaired blood circulation through the liver due to cirrhosis or severe hepatitis deprives the body of proteins normally synthesized by the liver. The storage of nutrients in the liver is also diminished when the organ is severely damaged. The liver normally stores glucose (as glycogen), vitamins, and iron.

Diabetes mellitus (Chapter 13) is a nutritional disease in which glucose cannot enter the cells to be used in the absence of insulin. Glucose is lost in the urine, and the untreated diabetic metabolizes fat reserves and even tissue protein.

In addition to the diseases already described that cause malnutrition, the failure to eat properly is associated with other problems that will be discussed in this chapter. Vitamin-deficiency diseases that result from an unbalanced diet will be explained along with a disease of psychoneurotic origin in which willful starvation leads to total emaciation and even death.

The effect on the body of excessive food intake that leads to obesity, and of toxicity that results from hypervitaminosis, will be discussed. The medical aspects of alcoholism, many of which are related to malnutrition, will also be explained.

DISEASES OF VITAMIN DEFICIENCIES

The quality of food that one eats, and not the quantity, is essential to good nutrition. A balanced diet includes food from four major groups: (1) dairy products; (2) high protein foods such as meat, poultry, and fish; (3) vegetables and fruits; and (4) cereals and bread. A diet of this type provides vitamins, minerals, and the essential amino acids the body cannot synthesize. A good diet also provides carbohydrates and lipids for energy production. Figure 5–1 shows how the body uses these nutrients.

Vitamins play an essential part in the body's enzyme system, and since vitamins are synthesized by plants rather than by animals, we require fruits and vegetables in our diet. Animals that have ingested plant material also

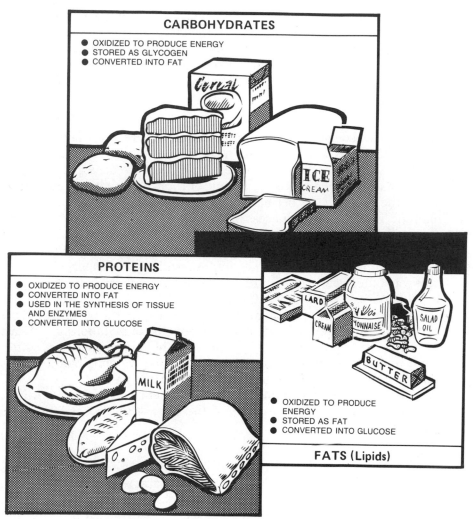

Figure 5-1. Use of carbohydrates, fats, and proteins.

provide a source of vitamins, and some vitamins are synthesized in the digestive tract by bacteria. Vitamin requirements are met by a balanced diet, so vitamin supplements should not be required. A particular disease condition, such as malabsorption syndrome, may require supplemental vitamins, but this is an exception.

Vitamins are divided into two categories: the water-soluble (the B vitamins and vitamin C) and the fat-soluble (vitamins A, D, E, and K). The B vitamins include thiamine, riboflavin, niacin, pantothenic acid, cobalamin (or vitamin B_{12}), and folic acid. The latter two are essential in the formation of red blood cells.

The vitamin deficiency diseases that will be described are relatively rare in the United States, but the symptoms of the diseases show the importance of the various vitamins. Multiple vitamin deficiencies are more common than a single deficiency and result from a diet consisting chiefly of one foodstuff.

■ Beriberi

Beriberi is a disease that is common in China, where the main staple is polished rice that has had the vitamin-containing part removed. **Beriberi** results from a thiamine or vitamin B_1 deficiency. An increased knowledge of the disease has led to thiamine enrichment of foodstuffs, with a subsequent decrease in the incidence of beriberi.

Thiamine is a coenzyme necessary for carbohydrate metabolism, and the lack of this vitamin particularly affects the cardiovascular and nervous systems. Nerve fibers become demyelinated, interfering with the transmission of nerve impulses. "Pins and needles" sensations are experienced, and the limbs become weak and numb. A form of beriberi can develop in chronic alcoholics who do not eat adequately. The effect on the nervous system causes mental confusion, an unsteady walk, and a paralysis of the muscles that move the eyes. Inadequate carbohydrate metabolism in heart muscle results in enlargement of the heart. The myocardium becomes edematous and flabby and unable to function properly, while blood vessels dilate and become permeable, causing widespread edema.

Patients with beriberi respond well to treatment with thiamine, which may be given intravenously. The signs of the disease disappear, but acute brain damage is irreversible.

■ Pellagra

Pellagra is caused by a niacin deficiency and is characterized by dermatitis, diarrhea, and **dementia,** which is the organic loss of intellectual function. Niacin, essential to the enzyme system, is widely distributed in plant and animal food, and pellagra affects only people who have an extremely limited diet, such as one of corn. The dermatitis of pellagra consists of scaly, reddened areas of skin, particularly where it is exposed to the sun or chafed by clothes. The tongue is smooth and sore, and the lips are cracked. Sores develop around the mouth and nose. The patient experiences gastrointestinal disturbances of vomiting and severe diarrhea that compound the problem of vitamin absorption.

The effect of a niacin deficiency on the nervous system is variable, ranging from chronic depression to violent, irrational behavior. Degeneration of neurons in the brain results from the lack of this vitamin. Chronic alcoholics and drug addicts may develop the disease in the absence of adequate nutrition.

The symptoms may be reversed through an improved diet and large doses of vitamin supplements. The diet should include meat, particularly liver, and whole grain cereals. The vitamins may have to be given by injection initially until the digestive disturbances are corrected.

A deficiency in niacin is usually accompanied by a riboflavin deficiency, which occurs with diets consisting primarily of corn, potatoes, and rice. Riboflavin, like niacin, is essential for cellular metabolism. Some of the symptoms of a riboflavin deficiency are similar to those caused by inadequate niacin: lesions on the face around the mouth and nose, a sore tongue, and seborrheic dermatitis—dandruff. The symptoms can be reversed with a balanced diet and supplementary doses of riboflavin and other vitamins. Riboflavin is widely distributed in many foodstuffs but is particularly high in liver, eggs, greens, and enriched cereals.

■ Scurvy

A deficiency in vitamin C (ascorbic acid) causes **scurvy,** a disease that was once associated with long sea voyages, during which the diet of preserved foods left much to be desired. Scurvy can also develop in our time if vitamin C is lacking in the diet. The elderly, who live alone and do not eat properly, and chronic alcoholics, who suffer from malnutrition, can become victims of scurvy. Neglected children often show symptoms of the disease.

A lack of vitamin C prevents proper formation of the cementing substance that holds epithelial cells together. This causes capillary walls to be weak and to rupture easily, resulting in hemorrhage into surrounding tissues. Small back-and-blue spots appear all over the body as a result of the rupture of blood vessels. Anemia may develop over a period of time and manifest itself by weakness, palpitation, and breathing difficulties.

The gums are particularly affected and they bleed easily. The open lesions provide an entry for bacteria, and, as the gum tissue becomes necrotic, the teeth loosen and fall out. Synthesis of collagen, a fibrous protein in connective tissue, is impaired, causing wounds to heal poorly.

A vitamin C deficiency can be prevented by a diet that includes fresh fruits and vegetables, particularly tomatoes, citrus fruits, and greens. The activity of the vitamin is lost by heating and drying. Scurvy can be treated by supplying supplemental doses of vitamin C and by eating a proper diet.

■ Vitamin A Deficiency

Vitamin A is essential for vision because it is an essential component of **rhodopsin,** the pigment that absorbs light in the rods of the retina. A lack of vitamin A results in an inability to see in dim light, a condition known as night blindness.

It is thought that vitamin A contributes to the integrity of mucous membranes—those membranes that line the respiratory, gastrointestinal, and urogenital tracts. In the absence of vitamin A, the membranes become dry and susceptible to cracking, permitting the entrance of infectious organisms. The **conjunctiva,** the membrane that lines the eyelids and covers the eyeball, also becomes dry and cracked, making it a target for infection.

Vitamin A deficiencies are most commonly seen in parts of India and China where the diet is limited. The condition also exists when vitamin A is present in the diet but cannot be used because of malabsorption (Chapter 10).

Vitamin A is derived from a plant pigment, carotene, which is converted into vitamin A by the liver. Dairy products, egg yolks, and vegetables are good sources of vitamin A.

■ Vitamin D Deficiency (Rickets)

Rickets is a bone disease in children in which calcification is impaired, resulting in weak, deformed bones (Chapter 16). Vitamin D is essential for the absorption of calcium from the gastrointestinal tract. Rickets develops when vitamin D is deficient in the diet. The lack of vitamin D in adults results in a softening of the bones, a disease known as osteomalacia (Chapter 16).

Rickets and osteomalacia can be prevented by a diet that includes vitamin D fortified milk. Exposure to sunlight also provides a source of vitamin D, as ultraviolet light converts a substance in the skin (sterol) to vitamin D. Rickets and osteomalacia can be treated by administering vitamin D concentrate and improving the diet, and by exposure to sunlight. Vitamin deficiency diseases are summarized in Figure 5–2.

■ Vitamin K Deficiency

Vitamin K is essential to the blood-clotting mechanism. The liver synthesizes an enzyme, prothrombin, with the aid of vitamin K. This enzyme initiates the chain reaction in the blood coagulation process. In the absence of prothrombin, hemorrhaging occurs.

HYPERVITAMINOSIS

An excess of vitamins, particularly of vitamins A and D, can be harmful because the excess produces a toxicity **(hypervitaminosis).** Children can become very ill after swallowing a large number of vitamin pills, and they can experience gastrointestinal disturbances and drowsiness. A generalized edema develops that even increases intracranial pressure. The affected child is irritable and fails to gain weight. The symptoms are reversible once the toxicity has subsided.

DEFICIENT VITAMIN	DISEASE	MANIFESTATIONS	TREATMENT AND/OR PREVENTION
THIAMINE	BERIBERI	NERVOUS AND CARDIO-VASCULAR DISORDERS	THIAMINE AND THIAMINE-ENRICHED FOODSTUFFS
NIACIN	PELLAGRA	DERMATITIS, DIARRHEA, AND DEMENTIA	NIACIN SUPPLEMENTS, DIET INCLUDING MEAT AND WHOLE GRAIN CEREALS
RIBOFLAVIN		SIMILAR TO NIACIN	BALANCED DIET AND RIBOFLAVIN SUPPLEMENT
VITAMIN C	SCURVY	BLEEDING GUMS AND HEMORRHAGES INTO TISSUES	SUPPLEMENTAL DOSES OF VITAMIN C, CITRUS FRUITS AND GREENS
VITAMIN A	NIGHT BLINDNESS	POOR VISION IN DIM LIGHT; DRY, CRACKED MUCOUS MEMBRANES	DIET INCLUDING DAIRY PRODUCTS, EGG YOLKS, AND VEGETABLES
VITAMIN D	RICKETS, OSTEOMALACIA	WEAK, DEFORMED BONES	VITAMIN D SUPPLEMENTS, VITAMIN D FORTIFIED MILK, AND EXPOSURE TO SUNLIGHT
VITAMIN K		TENDENCY TO HEMORRHAGE	NORMAL DIET

Figure 5-2. Summary of vitamin deficiencies.

Excessive vitamin D causes too much calcium to be absorbed from the gastrointestinal tract. Hypercalcemia results in deposits of calcium in organs such as the kidney, heart, lungs, and the walls of the stomach. The digestive system is affected, and excessive thirst and polyuria develop. Some of the damage to the tissues may be irreversible.

MINERAL DEFICIENCIES

Minerals are only required in minute amounts, but a lack of them has serious consequences. An inadequate level of calcium prevents proper bone formation and maintenance, as described in Chapter 16. A calcium deficiency also interferes with the blood-clotting mechanism. One type of anemia develops in the absence of the iron needed to form hemoglobin. One type of goiter results from insufficient iodine.

Potassium may be adequate in the diet but missing from the body under certain conditions. An excessive secretion of aldosterone causes a loss of potassium through the kidneys. A prolonged loss of fluid through vomiting or diarrhea removes potassium, as will the action of certain diuretics. The muscles are weak in a potassium deficiency and the heart muscle is particularly affected.

Sodium is usually adequate in the diet but may be lacking in Addison's disease (Chapter 13), in which aldosterone is not secreted by the adrenal cortex. Sodium is essential for the transmission of nerve impulses and muscle contraction. The principal functions of minerals are summarized in Figure 5–3.

■ PROTEIN-CALORIE MALNUTRITION

Millions of young children in developing countries suffer from a disease called **kwashiorkor** that is caused by a protein deficiency. The disease develops as a child is taken off breast milk when a second baby is born. The first child begins to eat a diet of starchy food only, such as polished rice. The lack of protein interferes with development, and the child is affected mentally and physically. The skin of African children suffering from kwashiorkor is hypopigmented, and their hair is thin and light in color. The liver becomes infiltrated with fat and ceases to function properly. This causes ascites (Chapter 11), and the abdomen distends greatly; the child is anemic and lacks energy. The pancreas and intestinal mucosa are affected, preventing proper digestion.

The child has poor resistance to infection, as the thymus gland and lymphoid tissues, sites of antibody production, atrophy. Microorganisms enter the body through skin lesions and damaged mucous membranes of the gastrointestinal tract. The child will die if not treated and usually requires treatment in a hospital, where the diet can be corrected and antibiotics administered as needed.

Adults can suffer from this severe protein–calorie malnutrition, but the causes are different. Cancer and serious intestinal diseases prevent the adequate use of nutrients. A psychoneurotic disease, anorexia nervosa, described next, can cause malnutrition so severe that death results. Chronic alcoholism is also often accompanied by serious malnutrition.

■ ANOREXIA NERVOSA

Anorexia nervosa is a disease of psychoneurotic origin in which the aversion to food leads to emaciation and malnutrition. Anorexia nervosa is most

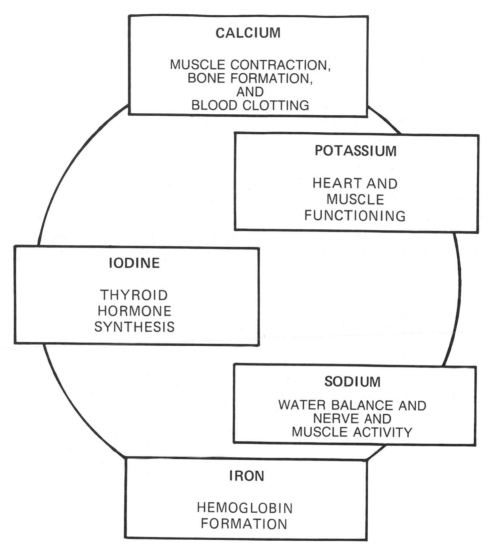

Figure 5-3. Minerals and their principal functions.

common in teen-age girls, and the incidence of the disease has greatly increased in recent years. The disease is rare in males and older age groups. The desire to be thin and the patient's misconception of her own body size underlie the onset of the disease. The girl may have been socially normal before the initial dieting or may have shown some social maladjustments.

The anorexia nervosa patient actually starves herself, yet denies that she is not eating adequately. Personality changes are noticeable as she becomes irritable, full of anxiety, and depressed. She may become hostile toward her parents who encourage her to eat and to see a doctor, and family relationships become strained.

Anorexia nervosa is not an accurate name for this disease. *Anorexia* means loss of appetite, but the patient with this disease experiences hunger and may be obsessed with food. She may elaborately prepare food for others but not for herself. Counting calories and weighing food becomes ritualistic. She often prepares her food—consisting primarily of fruits, vegetables, and cheese—when she is alone and sure that no one is giving her extra calories. At least she does not suffer from a vitamin deficiency, but she avoids all carbohydrates.

Hunger may cause occasional orgies of overeating, and the patient then induces vomiting and uses laxatives excessively. She exercises strenuously, increasing the weight loss. The girl becomes absolutely emaciated in appearance. Her face is gaunt with protruding bones, yet she denies that she is thin and even perceives herself as fat. An anorexia nervosa patient is seen in Figure 5–4.

Amenorrhea always accompanies anorexia nervosa. The ovaries stop producing estrogen and gonadotropins are not secreted by the anterior pituitary. The absence of menstruation occurs early in the disease, so it is not considered a result of malnutrition. A possible hypothalamic disturbance is indicated in which releasing factors for the gonadotropins are not being secreted. In rare cases of males with anorexia nervosa, the levels of gonadotropic hormones and testosterone are also decreased.

The patient with anorexia nervosa rejects the suggestion to see a physician. If the person can be persuaded to be examined, the findings include low blood pressure, decreased heart rate, and anemia. Dehydration caused by the induced vomiting and excessive use of laxatives results in a depletion of potassium. This deficiency causes muscular weakness and heart abnormalities. A lowered resistance due to malnutrition makes the patient susceptible to infections.

Treatment is directed toward correcting the malnutrition and the abnormal psychological state. Hospitalization is usually required to assure close observation of eating and bathroom habits. The patient may resist eating the required diet, fearing that she will become fat. The therapist must assure the patient that the weight she gains will help to make her more attractive and improve her health. Cooperation between the patient and therapist is essential to recovery.

The psychological problems that underlie the disease must be uncovered and proper psychotherapy given. The condition of anorexia nervosa is extremely serious. The patient can actually starve herself to death, and her depressed state may make her suicidal. Even after an apparent recovery, close supervision is required as relapses of the disease are common and the mortality rate is quite high.

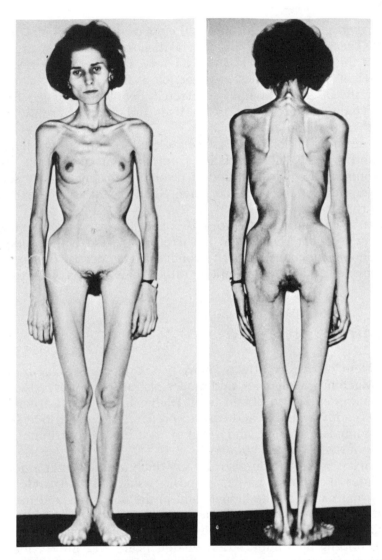

Figure 5-4. A 19-year-old patient with anorexia nervosa showing emaciation and premature aging. Note protruding bones, muscle atrophy, and sunken abdomen. Patient is about 5′ 6″ tall and weighs 66 pounds. (*From Kosowicz. Atlas of Endocrine Diseases, 1978. Courtesy of The Charles Press.*)

■ Bulimia

Bulimia, a gorge–purge syndrome, is the opposite of, yet similar to, anorexia nervosa. Teenage girls and women in their early twenties are the usual victims of this condition. As in anorexia nervosa, the goal of the patient is to avoid weight gain. Bulimics may be of average weight or obese, and therefore the disease may not be detected. Food-eating binges followed by induced vomiting and the use of laxatives and diuretics are the manifestations of this condition.

The detrimental long-term effects include tooth decay, constant sore throat, and swollen salivary glands from the abnormal acidity of the induced vomiting. Dehydration and electrolyte imbalance cause serious disturbances, and liver damage is common. Sudden death from heart failure or stomach rupture is possible.

Bulimia, like anorexia nervosa, is linked to a psychoneurotic condition such as depression. The patient is therefore treated with antidepressants and psychological counseling. The condition may persist through much of the bulimics's life, and management, rather than cure, is often the ultimate goal.

■ OBESITY

The problem of obesity affects many people in our mechanized, modern society. Machines, appliances, and modes of transportation reduce the need for expending energy to obtain food. High-calorie foods attractively packaged are readily available and easy to prepare. Life styles that include TV snacks, eating late at night, and a diet of "fast foods" contribute to the high incidence of obesity in the country.

Obesity is a nutritional disorder in which an abnormal amount of fat accumulates in adipose tissue. Adipose tissue is found under the skin, around organs such as the kidney, and in the omentum and mesentery of the peritoneal cavity. Adipose tissue acts as a reserve energy supply and as an insulating material against body heat loss. An excess of fat tissue is harmful, putting an undue strain on the heart and interfering with the contraction of muscles.

The distribution of fat varies in males and females and may be genetically determined. Men accumulate fat in the upper trunk and not in the arms and legs, but women store fat in the lower trunk and in the arms and legs. Women also have more subcutaneous fat than men, which is probably an effect of the female sex hormones. Estrogen given in high dosage in birth control pills, for example, often causes a weight gain.

Obesity develops when an excess of calories is consumed for the energy expended by a person. Too much food or too little exercise causes the deposition of fat. The rate of fat synthesis is faster than the mobilization of fat to active muscles for the production of energy.

A person is considered obese if his or her weight is 15 to 20 percent more than the ideal weight given in standard life insurance height–weight tables. These tables give the proper weight ranges for men and women of light, medium, and heavy frames. A person is overweight if the upper limit of the appropriate range is exceeded.

Causes of Obesity

Obesity generally results from overeating high-calorie foods—carbohydrates and fats—and from insufficient exercise. Genetic factors are probably involved, as obese children tend to have parents who are overweight. Obesity that develops in children is due to the formation of an increased number of adipose cells, the number of which may be genetically determined.

Culture and environment also play a part in the obesity of children. Excessive intake of food may be encouraged, and, too often, good behavior is rewarded with foods such as cookies and candy. This overfeeding of children sets a regulatory system of the hypothalamus at a level that will maintain the habit of overeating.

The central nervous system regulates food intake. An area of the hypothalamus contains the "satiety center," which has an inhibiting effect on the "feeding center." The satiety center senses when enough food has been eaten and it inhibits the feeding center from stimulating further food intake. Eating should be directed toward relieving genuine hunger. The obese person tends to eat because food is available or looks attractive.

Adult-onset obesity results from an enlargement of already existing adipose cells rather than from an increase in their number. The number of adipose cells formed in childhood is irreversible, and for this reason a child's diet should be carefully controlled to prevent excessive weight gain throughout life. Rarely is obesity due to a hypoactive thyroid, a popular misconception. Excessive water retention is not a cause of obesity. Adipose cells, which are filled with fat, contain very little water.

Psychological factors can cause obesity if a person's reaction to stress often precipitate a desire for food as a means of satisfaction.

Diseases Aggravated by Obesity

Excessive weight poses many problems, both psychologic and physical. The obese person feels unattractive and may become withdrawn. Children who are obese have difficulty participating in sports, are often teased about their weight, and are hurt by their peers.

Cardiovascular problems accompany obesity, and the death rate due to these ailments is significantly higher among the obese than among those who are not. Atherosclerosis develops as a result of the high level of serum lipids. Excessive fat deposits in heart muscle interfere with its contractions, the heart is overworked as it pumps blood through the extensive vascularity of the adipose tissue, and the left ventricle enlarges. Hypertension is often a complication of obesity.

Respiratory difficulties of hypoventilation with carbon dioxide retention occur when the chest wall cannot be moved adequately. Fat deposits interfere with contraction of the diaphragm and the other respiratory muscles. Inadequate oxygenation of the brain results in lethargy or somnolence.

Osteoarthritis, a degenerative joint disease, is aggravated by excessive weight. As will be explained in Chapter 16, osteoarthritis affects primarily weight-bearing joints: the knees, lower spine, and joints of the big toe. Flat feet also worsen due to obesity.

Varicose veins frequently develop in the obese, as the excessive adipose tissue interferes with the return of blood from the legs. Diaphragmatic hernias and gallbladder disease are also more common in overweight people.

Maturity-onset diabetes occurs far more often in those who are obese than in those who are not. A habit of excessive carbohydrate intake over-taxes the beta cells, the insulin-producing cells of the pancreas, and they cease functioning. One of the most serious complications of diabetes is atherosclerosis, to which obese people are already prone.

The liver is an important organ for the metabolism of fat, but when fat is in excess, metabolic disturbances occur, and fat accumulates in the liver. The fatty infiltration severely injures the liver cells, so they are no longer able to function. This condition is known as "fatty liver" and occurs in chronic alcoholism as well as in obesity. The complications of obesity are summarized in Figure 5–5.

Diagnosis and Treatment of Obesity

Comparison of a person's weight with the standard height–weight tables, mentioned previously, is the best way to diagnose obesity. Another technique is to measure the thickness of subcutaneous fat with an instrument called a skin-fold caliper. The percentage of body fat can then be determined using a special chart.

Obesity is treated with diet, exercise programs, and drugs, but the most efficient method is diet. Weight loss is a slow, painful process and requires great effort. The loss of one to three pounds per week is considered ideal. An obese patient may lose weight successfully at the beginning of a diet and then reach a plateau, at which time no weight is lost and even a slight gain may occur. Although this is normal, it is very discouraging to the patient, who then may stop dieting.

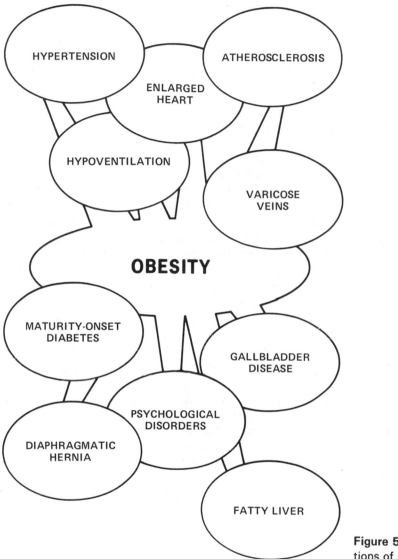

Figure 5-5. Complications of obesity.

Appetite depressants, **amphetamines** and related compounds, may be prescribed at the beginning of a diet regimen while the patient is establishing new eating habits. The use of amphetamines must be carefully controlled to prevent side effects. These drugs can cause excessive nervousness, restlessness, insomnia, dry mouth, and constipation.

A good diet should be balanced nutritionally and include protein, some unsaturated fat, and enough carbohydrate to provide glucose to the cells and to minimize the feeling of hunger. Vitamins and minerals should be provided through a balanced diet. Mild reduction in the use of table salt will prevent excessive retention of water. The patient must learn to change eating habits and to train the appetite so that weight will not be regained once the strict diet is completed.

Reduction diets that take into account the patient's size, sex, physical activity, and desired speed of weight loss are the most satisfactory. Women usually lose weight on a diet of 500 to 1000 calories per day and men lose on a diet of 1500 to 2000 calories.

Fad diets or crash diets are rarely successful and may even be harmful by causing malnutrition or metabolic disturbances. These diets do not help the obese person to change eating habits or train the appetite. Weight lost on fad diets is generally regained. The adipose cells are not destroyed with weight loss, but only shrink in size and refill easily with fat when the diet is stopped. An exercise program should accompany the reducing diet. The strenuousness of the exercise depends on the physical condition of the person. Great exertion is required to burn up calories, but even a regular program of walking can increase muscle tone.

Obesity is easier to prevent than to overcome. By establishing proper eating habits in childhood, an excessive number of adipose cells will not be formed if the diet is nutritionally high but calorically low. Control of diet is particularly important if a child has a genetic tendency toward obesity.

Excessive weight gain occurs often during certain periods of childhood, infancy, early school age, and puberty. In women, pregnancy and the menopause are times when weight is easily gained, and special care should be taken to avoid excessive caloric intake. The avoidance of sugar in the form of pastries and soft drinks, and fat in cream, fried foods, gravy, and salad dressing will limit caloric intake and subsequent adipose tissue development. Alcohol is also very high in calories—100 calories per ounce—and has no nutritional value.

Weight reduction in the overweight person dramatically improves the physical ailments associated with obesity. Blood pressure is reduced, the level of circulating lipids that cause atherosclerosis is lowered, and the distress of osteoarthritis is lessened. Diabetes is more easily controlled when excessive weight is lost. The self-image of the obese person who successfully loses weight is greatly improved, and the psychological change makes the effort worthwhile.

■ ALCOHOLISM

Alcoholism is a serious disease with far-reaching consequences. It disrupts marriages, adversely affects children, and threatens job security. Physical damage to the alcoholic is extensive, affecting the nervous system, the cardiovascular system, and the gastrointestinal tract particularly. The American Medical Association supports the following definition of alcoholism: "Alcoholism is an illness characterized by significant impairment that is directly associated with persistent and excessive use of alcohol. Impairment may involve physiological, psychological, or social dysfunction.

The alcoholic is totally dependent on the drug, alcohol, and centers life around it, making sure of an adequate supply and opportunity to drink. The use of other drugs with alcohol frequently compounds the problem. Most authorities agree that there is no single cause of alcoholism but that a combination of factors contribute to its onset and progression. There is no conclusive evidence that it is caused by a genetic factor.

Many psychological problems have been proposed as the cause of alcoholism: emotional disturbances during childhood, a feeling of insecurity, hostility, depression, and countless others. While any of these factors may play a part in the complex etiology of alcoholism, none is considered the sole cause.

Sociological setting may be a factor in the development of the disease. In some circles, heavy drinking is considered a socially sanctioned behavior. Parties are not considered complete without alcohol, and often the host or hostess will encourage the guests to have "one more drink" when they have already had too much. The effects of alcohol on the nervous system include a feeling of relaxation and a release from anxieties, tension, and fears. As this experience is repeated through heavy drinking, alcohol becomes the habitual response to the problems of life.

Effects of Excessive Alcohol on the Nervous System

Alcohol is a depressant on the central nervous system. Large quantities of alcohol interfere with the transmission of nerve impulses in the brain and affect coordination, speech, and judgment. A very high concentration of alcohol in the blood can even suppress the respiratory, cardiac, and vasomotor centers of the brain, causing shock and death.

The effect of alcohol on the central nervous system depends on the amount and the time span in which it was consumed. Alcohol is rapidly absorbed from the gastrointestinal tract into the blood. Some is absorbed from the stomach, but most alcohol absorption is from the duodenum. Drinking "on an empty stomach" is not only irritating to the gastric mucosa, but the alcohol is more rapidly absorbed by the blood when there is nothing in the duodenum to delay gastric emptying.

Alcohol is carried to the liver through the portal vein and is then circulated through the body. Most metabolism and detoxification of alcohol actually occurs in the liver, but the rate of the reaction is limited. Enzymes convert alcohol to acetaldehyde and other fragments that are burned to produce energy.

The effect of excessive alcohol ingestion wears off when it has been metabolized. This causes a period of nerve excitability, a release from the depressive effect, that accounts for the "morning-after" tremors. The effectiveness of another drink in overcoming the shakiness leads to a physical dependence on alcohol that becomes stronger as alcoholism progresses.

Signs and Symptoms of Alcoholism

Alcoholism can have an insidious and gradual onset. The alcoholic generally experiences feelings of guilt and denies that drinking has become a problem. He or she begins to drink surreptitiously, drinks early in the day, and gulps down drinks when the opportunity arises. Periods of intoxication become regular and more serious, and blackouts are common, with periods of complete amnesia. Behavior becomes irresponsible, resulting in arrest for drunken driving, frequent absenteeism from work, and family problems. The alcoholic resents any discussion about drinking and generally resists treatment.

A physician may suspect alcoholism in a patient whose face is flushed and who shows a tremor about the mouth and tongue. Coarse tremors of the hands are observed, the patient may appear nervous and complain of digestive or motor disturbances. Further examination of the patient reveals other complications of alcohol abuse.

Complications of Alcoholism

Long-term abuse of alcohol takes its toll on the digestive system, the cardiovascular system, and the brain. Malnutrition often accompanies alcoholism depriving the patient of essential nutrients for cellular activity.

Effects of Alcoholism on the Digestive System. Alcohol in excess is an irritant to the gastric mucosa, causing erosion and ulceration of the tissue. Gastritis is often a complication of alcoholism, as will be explained in Chapter 10. Ulceration that occurs due to the irritating effect of alcohol, particularly on an empty stomach, can lead to serious hemorrhaging. Some alcoholics experience nausea and vomiting in the morning after heavy drinking and are able to suppress the symptoms with another drink. This enables them to continue drinking during that day, and the cycle repeats itself.

Liver ailments caused by alcoholism are discussed in Chapter 11. Excessive alcohol has a toxic effect on the liver cells, causing tissue destruction and fibrosis. Alcoholic hepatitis and cirrhosis interfere with essential functions of the liver. Blood-clotting disturbances result from the inability of the liver to synthesize plasma proteins essential to coagulation, and hemorrhages in the gastrointestinal and urogenital tracts are common. Severe **ecchymoses**—hemorrhagic spots—develop in the skin and mucous membranes. **Epistaxis,** or bleeding from the nose, also results from the deficiency of proteins essential to clotting. Esophageal varices, described in Chapter 8, are a complication of cirrhosis and may lead to a fatal hemorrhage.

Feminization of the male cirrhosis patient results from a hormonal imbalance. The nonfunctioning liver is unable to inactivate estrogen secreted by the adrenal cortex, and the hyperestrogenism that develops causes enlargement of the breasts (gynecomastia) and testicular atrophy. Pubic and axillary hair becomes sparse.

The treatment of cirrhosis includes the absolute restriction of alcohol and the consumption of a nutritious diet. A reduction of salt intake may eliminate some water retention and relieve the ascites (Chapter 11). If the cirrhosis is extremely advanced, the arrest of further liver destruction is the only hopeful prognosis. Death can result from infections because of the limited immunity caused by liver failure or from thrombus formation in the congested portal vein. Hemorrhages of esophageal varices can also be fatal.

Hepatic coma develops in the final stages of advanced liver disease. This is caused by an accumulation of ammonia in the blood, which has a toxic effect on the brain. The ammonia accumulates when the liver is unable to detoxify it and form urea, the normal breakdown product of protein metabolism. The hepatic coma patient has periods of stupor or coma and manifests neurologic abnormalities. The flapping of outstretched arms is characteristic of the uncontrolled muscular contractions.

Oxygen or a combination of oxygen and carbon dioxide, the stimulus for the respiratory center of the brain, must be administered. Airways must be cleared using mechanical aids. If the patient is in shock, intravenous fluids or blood transfusions are required.

Pancreatitis, although it has other causes, is often related to chronic alcoholism (Chapter 11). The disease destroys the pancreas through enzymes that are abnormally released into the tissue. The patient generally experiences nausea, vomiting, and severe pain. As the pancreas becomes more and more necrotic, the likelihood of hemorrhaging increases. Treatment includes a nonirritating diet with no fat or alcohol.

Effects of Alcoholism on the Cardiovascular System. Chronic alcoholism leads to progressive cardiac failure. Alcohol reduces the force of heart muscle contractions and an **arrhythmia,** a deviation from the normal rhythm of the heart beat, develops. The heart enlarges, and thrombi frequently form in the coronary arteries. Fatty infiltration of the heart muscle generally occurs. If cirrhosis accompanies the alcoholism, circulation is impaired further as congestion develops in the veins. A severely damaged liver interferes with blood flow through the portal vein, causing a back pressure in the vessels emptying into it.

Effects of Alcoholism on the Central Nervous System. Long-term excessive consumption of alcohol affects the central nervous system, causing a condition known as the organic brain syndrome. Its manifestations include impaired judgment, poor powers of concentration, and memory lapses. The symptoms progress with continued drinking, but they may be reversed with abstinence.

Wernicke's encephalopathy is a brain disease often associated with chronic alcoholism, although it may have other causes such as thiamine deficiency. Wernicke's disease is a medical emergency in which the patient becomes mentally confused and disoriented and may suffer delirium tremens. Eye movements are abnormal and double vision may be experienced. **Nystagmus**—involuntary, rapid movement of the eyeball—is characteristic of the disease. The muscular coordination necessary for standing and walking is impaired. Treatment includes a highly nutritious diet and vitamin B supplements, particularly thiamine. If prompt treatment is administered, the symptoms can be reversed.

Delirium tremens, DTs, is a medical emergency caused by heavy drinking over a long period of time and may occur after withdrawal from heavy alcohol intake. The symptoms include delirium with illusions and vivid hallucinations that are terrifying to the patient. The patient is extremely restless and shakes uncontrollably. The metabolic rate is increased, causing excessive sweating.

The patient with delirium tremens requires hospitalization in a quiet restful atmosphere. Attendants should show a calm, reassuring manner and observe the patient carefully to prevent self-injury. A comprehensive medical examination is essential to determine if there are any other complications such as signs of heart failure or pneumonia. The patient is very susceptible to respiratory tract infections because of lowered resistance.

Fluid, electrolyte, and nutritional balance must be maintained, and this may require intravenous feeding. Sedation may be required, but it must be administered with caution to prevent overdosage. When the patient is able to take food, the diet should be high in protein and carbohydrates but low in fat and include vitamin B supplements. The complications of chronic alcoholism are summarized in Figure 5–6.

Alcohol and Pregnancy

There is an increasing awareness of how a mother's excessive consumption of alcohol during pregnancy affects the developing fetus. Alcohol diffuses into the bloodstream of the fetus through the placenta, just as nutrients and oxygen do. Because of its small size, the fetus is significantly affected by the alcohol and is likely to be born with physical and mental defects. The earliest weeks of pregnancy are the most critical for development and the most dangerous time for the mother to drink excessively.

Babies of alcoholic mothers are frequently born with **fetal alcohol syndrome.** Mental retardation is the most serious component of the syndrome, but physical growth before and after birth is also retarded. Heads

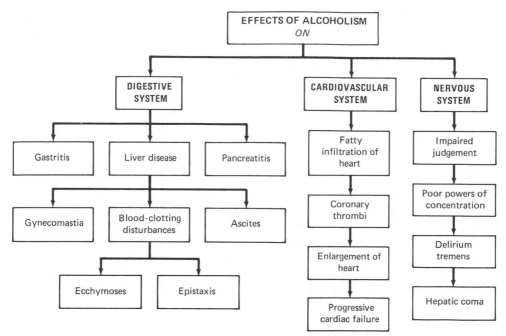

Figure 5-6. Complications of chronic alcoholism.

tend to be smaller than those of normal babies, and limb and joint abnormalities are common. A characteristic facial appearance, particularly of the mouth and eyes, develops. The eye slits are small, the nose is short and pugged, and the jaws are underdeveloped. The babies are often born suffering withdrawal symptoms, manifested by stiffness and irritability. Fetal alcohol syndrome is most likely to occur if the mother has had a drinking problem for 5 to 10 years.

Treatment of Alcoholism

Alcoholism is a treatable chronic disorder that is best controlled by early intervention and continuing attention. The treatment is directed toward enabling the alcohol-dependent patient to deal with problems and environment without using alcohol.

The best treatment for a particular alcoholic patient depends on the person. The patient may deny having a drinking problem and resist treatment for a time, but with the help of a physician, family member, employer, or friends, he or she may come to realize the need for assistance. Once the drinking problem has been recognized and the patient is willing to be treated, numerous facilities and resources are available.

Alcoholics Anonymous has been extremely effective for countless people and is very widespread geographically in its operation. Alcoholism Information Centers are listed in telephone books and offer valuable suggestions. Many programs are offered for alcoholics by church organizations, the Veterans Administration, employers, and local community organizations.

The mental and physical health of the alcoholic patient determines the most appropriate type of treatment. A personal physician, a psychotherapist, group therapy, or behavior-modification programs are among the options. The emphasis is always directed toward rehabilitation.

Admission to a general or psychiatric hospital is often required for serious alcoholism problems. Comprehensive alcohol treatment centers are also available where the physical and mental problems of the alcoholic can be treated. Delirium tremens and hepatic coma are medical emergencies requiring hospitalization.

Other facilities include detoxification centers for the acutely intoxicated, who once would have been put in jail. Half-way houses or recovery houses are helpful for the alcoholic who is adjusting to coping with life without alcohol. Relapses occur, but as with any chronic illness, they should not indicate that the treatment has failed. The alcoholic who achieves control of the disease sees life in a new light and believes that the struggle was worth it.

SUMMARY

Malnutrition develops from a wide variety of causes: the unavailability of required nutrients, diseases that prevent use of ingested food, chronic alcoholism, eating unbalanced meals, and psychoneurotic disorders. Multiple vitamin deficiencies result from diets that consist primarily of a single staple such as rice or corn. Vitamins are essential parts of cellular enzyme systems and must be obtained from fruits and vegetables because the body cannot synthesize them. Animals that have ingested plant material also provide a source of vitamins. Various diseases develop as a result of specific vitamin deficiencies.

A nutritional disease that is becoming quite common among young girls in this country is anorexia nervosa, in which the patient starves herself to the point of emaciation and even death. Psychological problems underlie the disease, and the girl has a misconception about her own body size, envisioning herself as fat when, in fact, she is extremely thin.

Another problem related to food intake is obesity. Excessive eating and inadequate exercise are generally the cause of the problem. Obesity is a serious condition that adversely affects the cardiovascular and respiratory systems and may lead to maturity-onset diabetes mellitus. Gallbladder disease and osteoarthritis are also aggravated by obesity.

The excessive consumption of alcohol over a prolonged period of time seriously impairs body functioning. Chronic alcoholism can lead to many diseases of the digestive system—gastritis, pancreatitis, cirrhosis of the liver—and is frequently accompanied by malnutrition. The cardiovascular system is affected together with the central nervous system. Manifestations of the effect of alcohol on the brain are impaired judgment, poor powers of concentration, and memory lapses. The medical emergencies, hepatic coma and delirium tremens, result from long-term alcohol abuse.

Treatment for the nutritional diseases discussed in this chapter is a balanced diet with adequate vitamin supplementation. Treatment for obesity includes diet, exercise, and, often, psychological counseling or group therapy. Alcoholism is treated medically and psychologically in a variety of ways, all of which are directed toward rehabilitation of the patient physically, mentally, and socially.

STUDY QUESTIONS

1. Explain three causes of malnutrition that are not related to a food shortage.
2. What are the effects of beriberi? What is the cause?
3. What is the cause of pellagra? How does the disease manifest itself?
4. What are the symptoms of scurvy? How can it be prevented?
5. What are the effects of a vitamin A deficiency?
6. Explain the relationship between vitamin D and the development of rickets.
7. What is the effect of excessive vitamin D intake?
8. What is the significance of vitamin K?
9. How does kwashiorkor affect children? What is its cause?
10. Why is anorexia nervosa a disease of psychoneurotic origin? How is it treated?
11. How is bulimia related to anorexia nervosa? How do they differ?
12. When is a person considered (a) obese, (b) overweight?
13. Explain several complications of obesity.
14. Give two reasons why obesity should be prevented in children.
15. What is the difference between the development of obesity in children and in adults?
16. How does obesity affect the cardiovascular system?
17. Why is an obese person more prone to develop maturity-onset diabetes?
18. What is the danger in fad diets? Why are they generally not successful?

19. How does excessive consumption of alcohol affect the nervous system?
20. Give two reasons why alcohol should not be consumed on an empty stomach.
21. What are some signs that may lead a physician to suspect alcoholism?
22. What are the effects of chronic alcoholism on the digestive system?
23. Explain the numerous complications of a liver severely damaged by cirrhosis.
24. What causes hepatic coma? How is it manifested?
25. Describe the symptoms of delirium tremens. How is it treated?
26. What are the symptoms of fetal alcohol syndrome?

PART II

Diseases of
the Systems

CHAPTER 6

Diseases of the Blood

Our life depends on an adequate blood supply to all body tissues. Blood distributes oxygen, nutrients, salts, and hormones to the cells, and carries away the waste products of cellular metabolism. Blood provides a line of defense against infection, toxic substances, and foreign antigens.

Red bone marrow and lymph nodes are the blood-forming tissues of the body. Erythrocytes, or red blood cells, and platelets are made in red bone marrow. Leukocytes, or white blood cells, are made in both red marrow and lymph tissue. These formed elements comprise about 45 percent of the blood, and plasma, the remaining 55 percent. The ratio of formed elements, mostly red cells, to whole blood is called the **hematocrit.**

Erythrocytes normally number about 5 million mm^3 of blood in males, and about 4.5 million/mm^3 of blood in females. Red blood cells are biconcave in shape and when mature possess no nucleus. The **hemoglobin** contained within the red cells is responsible for carrying oxygen throughout the body. The amount of hemoglobin is normally about 16 **grams per 100 milliliters** (g/dl) of blood in males, about 14 g/dl of blood in females.

The process of red cell formation is called **erythropoiesis.** This takes place in the red marrow of flat bones such as the sternum, hip bones, ribs, and skull bones. A hormone, **erythropoietin,** synthesized principally by the kidney stimulates this cell development. As they mature, erythrocytes go through several stages before entering the circulation. They begin as large, nucleated, primitive cells called **proerythroblasts** and at this stage possess no hemoglobin. The proerythroblasts multiply, but daughter cells, called **normoblasts,** are small. The normoblasts contain a nucleus, but it begins to shrink as the cytoplasm fills with hemoglobin synthesized by the endoplasmic reticulum. The nucleus is eventually digested and absorbed, and the cell is then called a **reticulocyte.** When the reticulum is lost, the cells become mature erythrocytes ready to circulate. Figure 6–1 illustrates red cell formation. Maturation of erythrocytes is more a degenerative process than one of differentiation, which makes these cells unique. Understanding this developmental pattern is important. Certain serious blood conditions are evident when immature red cells, normoblasts, or reticulocytes, are found in the circulation. Examples of these conditions will be discussed.

THE ANEMIAS

One of the most common blood diseases is anemia. Although there are many kinds of anemia and as many causes, there is one common denominator: a reduction in the amount of oxygen-carrying hemoglobin. **Anemia** can result from a loss of red blood cells due to prolonged bleeding or rupture of the cells, which is called hemolysis. Anemia can also be caused by the improper formation of new red blood cells. This can be the result of poorly functioning bone marrow or an iron or vitamin deficiency. Erythrocytes are unusual cells because they do not possess a nucleus and therefore cannot divide to form new cells. The life span of red blood cells is about 120 days, and new cells must constantly replace those that die.

Certain symptoms are common to all anemias. The anemic person is generally pale, and the mucous membrane of the mouth is light in color, as is the nail bed. This lack of normal color is due to hemoglobin deficiency. Fatigue and muscular weakness accompany the disease because of the inadequate oxygen supply to the cells and tissues. The anemic person experiences **dyspnea,** or shortness of breath. To meet the need for more oxygen, the respiration rate is quickened and the patient experiences palpitations of the heart as it attempts to pump more blood to the tissues.

The anemias may be classified in several ways. They will be considered here on the basis of their causes. It is important for the physician to diagnose the cause of a patient's anemia, for this is what must be treated. The iron prescribed appropriately for one type of anemia is ineffective, even harmful, for another type.

■ Pernicious Anemia

Pernicious anemia is a blood disease in which the red blood cells are few in number, although each cell contains the normal amount of hemoglobin. In this disease the body is unable to use certain elements in the diet that are essential for proper blood cell formation. Two factors are necessary for erythrocytes to mature: an **intrinsic factor** found in normal gastric juice and

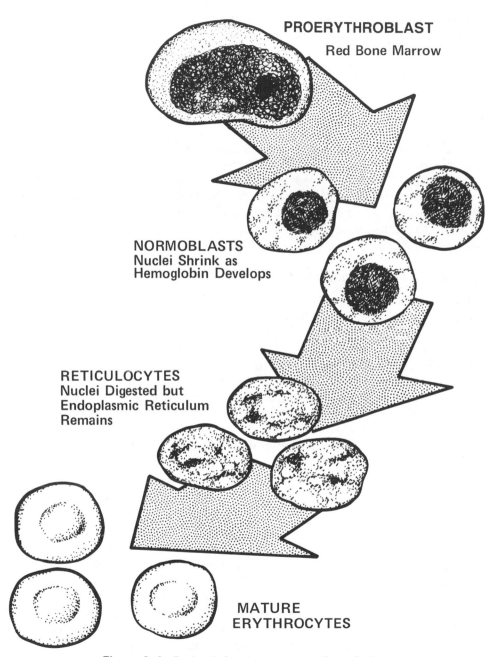

PROERYTHROBLAST

Red Bone Marrow

NORMOBLASTS
Nuclei Shrink as
Hemoglobin Develops

RETICULOCYTES
Nuclei Digested but
Endoplasmic Reticulum
Remains

**MATURE
ERYTHROCYTES**

Figure 6-1. Red cell development—erythropoiesis.

an **extrinsic factor,** vitamin B_{12}. The intrinsic factor acts as a carrier for vitamin B_{12}, enabling the vitamin to be absorbed from the small intestine and into the blood. Vitamin B_{12} is essential to erythrocyte development. The intrinsic factor is not secreted in pernicious anemia. In its absence, vitamin B_{12} cannot be absorbed even if it is present in the diet, and red cells cannot develop properly. This causes the anemia. The red cell count falls significantly and many immature forms of erythrocytes—normoblasts and reticulocytes—are found.

The signs of pernicious anemia are a low red cell count, low hematrocit, and absence of the intrinsic factor. Hydrochloric acid normally found in the stomach is also absent. Digestive disturbances occur, and the tongue appears sore with a smooth, glazed look. The lack of vitamin B_{12} also causes disturbances in the nervous system such as numbness and tingling sensations in the hands and feet. Pernicious anemia responds well to vitamin B_{12} given by injection.

■ Hypochromic Anemia

In hypochromic anemia the number of red cells is adequate but the amount of hemoglobin per cell is reduced. The word **hypochromic** means lighter than normal color. Since it is hemoglobin united with oxygen that gives red cells their color, this deficiency causes the cells to appear pale and washed-out. Hypochromic anemia is an iron-deficiency anemia. It can result from chronic blood loss from an ulcer, a malignant lesion, or menorrhagia (excessive bleeding during menstruation). A diet deficient in iron can also cause this type of anemia. Hypochromic anemia frequently develops after a pregnancy. The mother's iron supply has been depleted through red blood cell development in the fetus. This anemia responds well to treatment with large doses of iron.

■ Hemolytic Anemia

Certain anemias are due to the rupturing of red blood cells and are classed as hemolytic anemias. With the hemolysis of the cells, hemoglobin is released into the plasma. The hemoglobin itself breaks down, yielding another colored pigment, **bilirubin,** which is normally detoxified by the liver and converted into bile. This pigment is orange, and as it accumulates in the plasma, it causes a **jaundiced**—yellow or orange—appearance in the tissues. Some hemolytic anemias are acquired through an environmental factor, whereas others are hereditary; a gene for imperfect red cell formation is transmitted.

Sickle cell anemia is an example of an inherited red cell deficiency and is generally confined to blacks (see Chapter 4). Neither the hemoglobin molecule nor the cell itself can form properly. The cells are crescent- or sickle-shaped (see Fig. 6–2) and tend to rupture. The rapid destruction of erythrocytes stimulates production of new red cells, but at a rate faster than

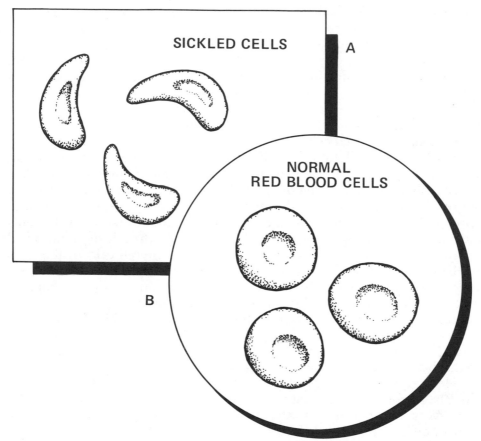

Figure 6-2. Sickled red blood cells (A) compared with normal red blood cells (B).

they can mature. As a result, many reticulocytes and nucleated red cells enter the circulation.

The symptoms of sickle cell anemia include jaundice of the sclera (the white of the eye); pain in the arms, legs, abdomen; and recurrent fever. In a crisis period, headache, paralysis, and convulsions can develop from a cerebral blood clot that forms as a result of the abnormally viscous blood. There is no effective treatment for sickle cell anemia. Only the symptoms can be treated.

Spheroidal or spherocytic anemia results from cell formation that is spherical rather than biconcave. The abnormal shape of the cell makes it fragile and susceptible to rupture. A characteristic symptom of this disease is jaundice caused by the release of hemoglobin. The spleen becomes enlarged due to an accumulation of red cells, many of which are immature.

The immature cells result from hyperactivity of the bone marrow as it attempts to compensate for the red cell destruction. The spleen is often removed (splenectomy) to prevent the misshapen cells from becoming trapped in the spleen and rupturing. The splenectomy renders the patient very susceptible to infection since the defense provided by the spleen has been lost.

Hemolytic anemias can be acquired. An allergic reaction to drugs such as the sulfonamides may cause this condition. The malarial parasite also causes hemolysis of red cells and severe anemia.

Erythroblastosis fetalis, hemolytic anemia of the newborn, can result when the mother is Rh⁻ and the fetus has Rh⁺ blood inherited from the father. Although the fetal and maternal circulations are separate, fetal blood can reach the mother's blood through ruptures in the placenta occurring at delivery. The mother then becomes sensitized to the Rh factor of the fetus and makes antibodies against it. If these antibodies reach the fetal blood through the placenta in subsequent pregnancies, the red cells of the fetus will be hemolyzed. The destruction of the cells stimulates rapid production and release of new cells before they mature. Therefore, many erythroblasts appear in the fetal blood. The name **erythroblastosis** means an abnormal increase, *osis*, of erythroblasts, immature cells. The severity of this disease ranges from mild anemia with jaundice to death of the fetus. The first child is usually not affected, but in subsequent pregnancies the possibility of erythroblastosis increases. Rh incompatibility is illustrated in Figure 6–3.

Medical science has developed a technique to prevent this condition. The Rh⁻ mother is given a vaccine of Rh immune globulin within 24 hours of delivery or aborting an Rh⁺ infant. The vaccine prevents antibody production against the Rh factor. This treatment is effective only if the mother is not already immune to the Rh factor; that is, she has had no previous Rh⁺ pregnancies. Blood testing to determine if Rh incompatibility exists is an essential part of prenatal care.

■ Aplastic Anemia

If the bone marrow fails to function, another type of anemia, **aplastic** anemia, results. The bone marrow stops producing erythrocytes, leukocytes, and platelets. The patient then is not only anemic but cannot fight infection, a leukocytic function, and has a bleeding tendency due to platelet depletion. Exposure to excessive radiation, certain drugs, and industrial poisons can cause the bone marrow to stop functioning. This is a very serious condition, and regular blood transfusions are generally necessary.

■ Secondary Anemia

If anemia is the result of another disease, it is referred to as secondary anemia. It generally accompanies chronic kidney disease, leukemia, and

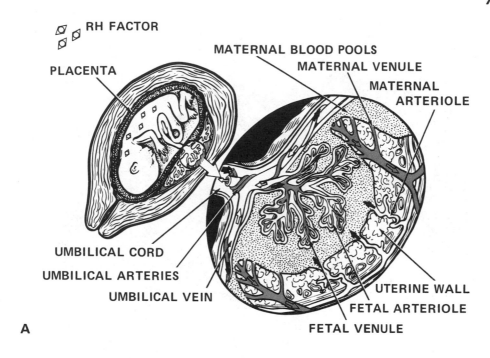

RH FACTOR

PLACENTA

MATERNAL BLOOD POOLS
MATERNAL VENULE
MATERNAL ARTERIOLE

UMBILICAL CORD

UMBILICAL ARTERIES

UMBILICAL VEIN

UTERINE WALL
FETAL ARTERIOLE

FETAL VENULE

A

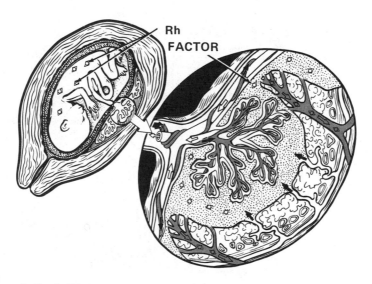

Rh FACTOR

B

Figure 6-3. A. Rh incompatibility: Rh⁺ fetus of Rh⁻ mother. **B.** Sensitization of mother: Rh factor enters mother's blood through ruptures in placenta at time of delivery. *(cont.)*

Rh
FACTOR

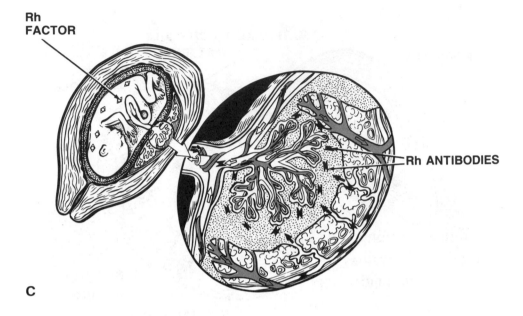

Rh ANTIBODIES

C

Rh FACTOR

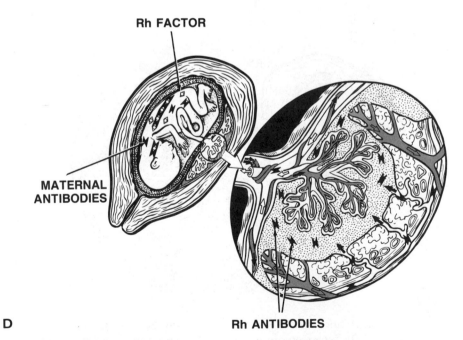

MATERNAL
ANTIBODIES

D

Rh ANTIBODIES

Figure 6-3. C. Subsequent pregnancy: mother sensitized to Rh factor
makes antibodies against it. **D.** Maternal antibodies enter fetal circulation:
antibodies destroy fetal Rh$^+$ red cells causing severe anemia.

cancer. In this anemia the number of cells is near normal but the amount of hemoglobin is low. The best treatment is the administration of iron. The types of anemia and their causes are summarized in Figure 6-4.

EXCESSIVE RED BLOOD CELLS

■ Primary Polycythemia

The effects of a red blood cell deficiency have been considered. What about an excessive RBC count? This condition is known as polycythemia, and it too has detrimental effects. Hyperactivity of red bone marrow causes polycythemia. In polycythemia the erythrocytes can number 7 to 11 million/mm^3 of blood. The hematocrit of a person with polycythemia may be as high as 70 to 80 percent compared to the normal of 45 percent. The elevated cell count increases blood volume; this raises the blood pressure, placing an increased workload on the heart. Blood flow is reduced due to increased viscosity and a tendency to clot. Polycythemia results from **hyper-**

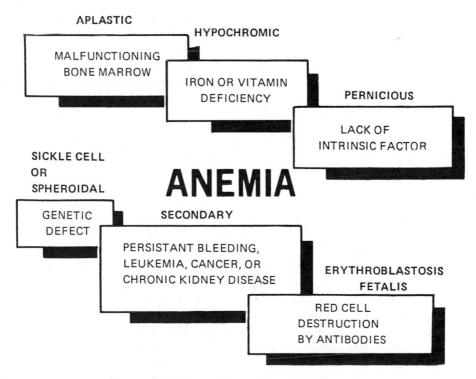

APLASTIC

HYPOCHROMIC

MALFUNCTIONING
BONE MARROW

IRON OR VITAMIN
DEFICIENCY

PERNICIOUS

LACK OF
INTRINSIC FACTOR

SICKLE CELL
OR
SPHEROIDAL

ANEMIA

GENETIC
DEFECT

SECONDARY

PERSISTANT BLEEDING,
LEUKEMIA, CANCER, OR
CHRONIC KIDNEY DISEASE

ERYTHROBLASTOSIS
FETALIS

RED CELL
DESTRUCTION
BY ANTIBODIES

Figure 6-4. Types of anemia and their causes.

activity of the bone marrow, perhaps due to a tumorous condition. The excessive number of red cells gives the skin a purplish appearance. Mucous membranes are extremely red, and the eyes appear bloodshot. The spleen, a reservoir for erythrocytes, is always enlarged. Leukocytes and platelets, also produced in the bone marrow, show elevated counts. This is important for diagnostic purposes. Treatment is aimed at reducing the red cell and the blood volume. Periodic bloodletting (phlebotomy) is used to reduce the volume and radiation therapy to decrease red cell production.

■ Secondary Polycythemia

The body often compensates for an inadequate oxygen supply by producing an excessive number of erythrocytes. This can occur when no disease condition exists. Natives of very high altitudes have elevated red cell counts because of the low oxygen content in the air. Trained athletes often have high red cell counts because their muscles have an increased need for oxygen. This compensatory mechanism is called **erythrocytosis** or secondary polycythemia.

In certain diseases of the circulatory and respiratory systems, secondary polycythemia can also occur. It frequently accompanies congenital heart diseases, congestive heart failure, and emphysema. These diseases will be discussed later.

One factor distinguishes secondary polycythemia, or erythrocytosis, from primary polycythemia. In erythrocytosis only the red cell count is elevated, but in polycythemia all blood cell types produced in the bone marrow are affected.

BLEEDING DISEASES

■ Hemophilia

The mechanism for control of bleeding is defective in some people. Hemophilia is a blood disease that results from this inability to clot. It is strictly a hereditary disease, generally affects only males, and is transmitted by females (see Chapter 4). The hemophiliac can experience prolonged and severe bleeding from even a minor cut or injury. Internal bleeding occurs, often into the joints, causing intense pain and injury. This inability to clot blood is due to the lack of a plasma protein required in the chain reaction of coagulation. Blood platelets, essential in the clotting mechanism, are normal in the hemophiliac. Treatment includes transfusions of whole blood or plasma and the administration of clotting protein concentrates.

◼ Purpura (Thrombocytopenia)

A deficiency in the number of platelets causes spontaneous hemorrhages in the skin (Fig. 6–5), mucous membranes of the mouth, and internal organs. Small, flat, red spots called petechiae, appear, or larger hemorrhagic areas, **ecchymoses,** may develop. Gastrointestinal and urogenital hemorrhages, as well as severe nosebleeds, may also occur. The disease is known as **purpura,** or **thrombocytopenia.** Thrombocyte is another name for platelet, and the suffix, *penia,* means a scarcity.

The disease may result from impaired platelet production or from an allergic response to drugs. Thrombocytopenia may also be idiopathic, that is, of unknown origin. In the latter case, the patient may have a history of bleeding after injury or minor surgery such as a tooth extraction. The condition is referred to as **ITP,** for **idiopathic thrombocytopenia purpura.**

Corticosteroids are generally administered. If the hemorrhagic condition is chronic, the spleen is often removed, as it is a major site of platelet destruction.

DISEASES OF WHITE BLOOD CELLS AND BLOOD-FORMING TISSUE

◼ Leukemia

Many people refer to leukemia as cancer of the blood, which is not strictly accurate. Leukemia is cancer of the tissues that form white blood cells, the

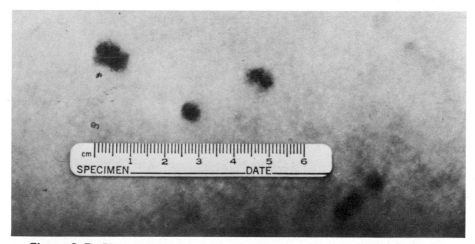

Figure 6–5. Photograph of ecchymotic hemorrhages in the skin. (*Courtesy of Dr. David R. Duffell.*)

bone marrow, or lymph tissue. The leukocyte count is extremely elevated from the normal range of 7000 to 9000/mm ^{3} of blood to 200,000 to 1 million/mm^3 of blood.

The symptoms are fever, swollen lymph nodes, and joint pain. Anemia with its manifestations of weakness, shortness of breath, and heart **palpitation** accompanies the leukemia. The red cells cannot develop properly in the malignant bone marrow. Organs where blood is stored, the spleen and liver, become greatly enlarged with the infiltration of white cells.

The cancerous tissues grow at a rapid rate, using up the body's nutrients. White cells are produced faster than they mature, so they are unable to fight infection normally. The patient becomes highly susceptible to infection and must be protected from exposure to bacteria. As the number of leukocytes increases, the number of platelets decreases; this interferes with the blood-clotting mechanism, causing a tendency to hemorrhage.

The two kinds of leukemia are named on the basis of the site of the malignancy. If the cancer is in the bone marrow it is called **myelogenic** or **myelocytic** leukemia. The primitive white cells in this tissue are called myelocytes. In myelogenic leukemia it is granulocytes that are greatly increased, whereas the red blood cell and platelet production are decreased.

The other type of leukemia is **lymphatic** or **lymphocytic,** cancer of the lymph nodes. The lymphocytes in this case are the only white cells that are increased, but they become disproportionately high in number.

The cause of leukemia is unknown. It may be due to a virus, or exposure to radiation may be a factor. A high incidence of leukemia has been found in people exposed to fallout from atom bombs. Heredity may also play a part.

Leukemia can be chronic or acute. Acute lymphocytic leukemia is the more common form in children. It has an abrupt onset and progresses rapidly. Acute myelogenous leukemia is more common in adults. Chronic leukemias have a prolonged course and may be either lymphocytic or myelogenous.

Progress is being made in controlling the diseases and even curing it. Blood transfusions help meet the body's needs. Chemotherapy is usually indicated. In this approach, chemical substances (**antineoplastic agents**) are used to inhibit growth of the cancerous tissue. Radiation is sometimes used to reduce swollen lymph nodes, and the spleen is often removed when it becomes enlarged. Removal of the spleen reduces red cell and platelet destruction. Experimental work on bone marrow transplants offers some hope for control of the disease.

■ Malignant Lymphomas

Lymphomas include several types of malignancies of lymphoid and reticulo-endothelial tissue. The origin of the disease is thought to be a virus that interferes with normal lymphocyte production. Patients have a significantly impaired immune system.

Lymphomas have been classified based on the cell type involved and include lymphocytic lymphoma, histiocytic lymphoma, and Hodgkin's disease. Lymphocytic lymphoma is very similar to chronic lymphocytic leukemia. It affects the elderly and runs a prolonged course. In histiocytic lymphoma the cells are poorly differentiated. The disease has a low cure rate.

Hodgkin's disease, of which there are several forms, is the most common type of lymphoma. Diagnosis is made on the presence of a characteristic cell found in lymphoid tissue. Hodgkin's disease is thought to be of viral or infectious origin. It manifests itself as a painless swelling in one lymph node, fever, and weight loss. The disease may progress affecting other lymph tissue and organs. The malignancy responds well to radiation and chemotherapy if it is localized in one or two areas. The disease is characterized by long periods of remission, and the cure rate is good if treated early. One form of Hodgkin's disease affects primarily young adults and more often men than women.

■ Mononucleosis

Many children and young adults experience infectious mononucleosis. The symptoms are rather vague—mild fever, fatigue, sore throat, and swollen lymph nodes. Blood tests show an elevated white cell count with an abnormally high percentage of atypical lymphocytes that resemble monocytes. Mononucleosis results from a viral infection of the upper respiratory tract. Diagnosis is based on the presence of antibodies to the virus. Viral diseases do not respond to antibiotics and therefore are not effective in treating mononucleosis. The symptoms can be treated: bedrest for the fatigue, aspirin for the fever, and gargles for the sore throat.

Mononucleosis is not a particularly contagious disease. It may be transmitted by kissing and is sometimes called the "kissing disease." Because it often affects young adults it is also referred to as the "college disease."

SUMMARY

The principal diseases of the blood considered have been those involving erythrocytes, leukocytes, and platelets. Each of these formed elements of the blood has a specific function. If any is insufficient in number, improperly formed, or immature, that function cannot be adequately performed. In distinguishing the various anemias, the symptoms were related to their cause, and the best treatment for each was explained. The inability to clot blood and prevent hemorrhaging was seen in hemophilia and purpura. In one a protein factor in plasma was lacking, and in the other platelets were too few in number. A malignancy of blood-forming tissues causes leukemia. Its complications of anemia, susceptibility to infection, and a tendency to hemorrhage were considered.

STUDY QUESTIONS

1. What is the relationship between erythrocyte development and diseases of the blood?
2. How do the characteristic symptoms of anemia relate to the disease?
3. Contrast pernicious anemia and hypochromic anemia as to red cell counts and the amount of hemoglobin per cell.
4. Why is vitamin B_{12}, taken orally, ineffective for treating pernicious anemia?
5. Which type of anemia frequently follows a pregnancy? Why?
6. What class of anemias causes jaundice? Why?
7. How would you distinguish polycythemia from erythrocytosis?
8. What is the deficiency in hemophilia?
9. Explain the condition of ITP (idiopathic thrombocytopenia purpura).
10. In what diseases is a splenectomy sometimes performed? Why is this done?
11. Why is anemia a complication of leukemia?
12. Why is the leukemia patient extremely susceptible to infection?
13. What is thought to cause Hodgkin's disease?

CHAPTER 7

Diseases of the Heart

STRUCTURE AND FUNCTION OF THE HEART

No one questions the importance of a well-functioning heart. It is the pump that keeps blood flowing to all the cells and tissues of the body.

The heart consists of four chambers: a right and left atrium and a right and left ventricle. The walls of these chambers are cardiac muscle, or myocardium. Lining these chambers is a smooth delicate membrane, the endocardium, that is continuous with the lining of the blood vessels. The heart is enclosed in a double membranous sac, the pericardium. Figure 7–1 shows these tissues of the heart, any of which can become diseased.

A partition, or septum, separates the right and left sides of the heart. Between the atria and the ventricles are valves that assure a one-way blood flow. These are the atrioventricular valves, or AV valves. The valves are delicate but very strong and are continuous with the endocardium. The valve between the left atrium and left ventricle has two flaps, or cusps, that meet when the valve is closed. This is the bicuspid or mitral valve. The valve between the right atrium and right ventricle has three cusps and is called the tricuspid valve. Figure 7–2 shows these valves in the closed position. Valves are frequently damaged by rheumatic fever and endocarditis, diseases that will be explained.

At the entrance to the great vessels leaving the heart, the aorta and pulmonary artery, is another set of valves called the semilunar valves. The

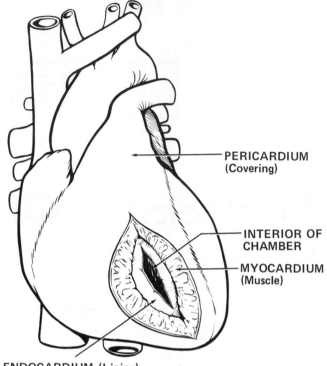

PERICARDIUM
(Covering)

INTERIOR OF
CHAMBER

MYOCARDIUM
(Muscle)

Figure 7-1. Tissues of
the heart.

ENDOCARDIUM (Lining)

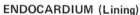

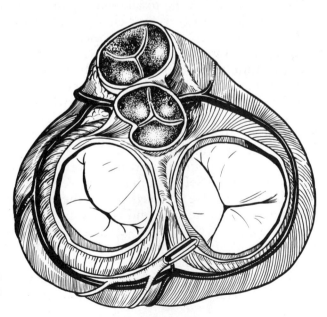

Figure 7-2. Heart valves in
closed position viewed from
top.

functions of all the valves is to prevent the backflow of blood. The atria are the receiving chambers for blood returning from the body and the lungs. The ventricles serve as pumps sending blood throughout the body and to the lungs.

The ventricles alternately contract and relax. When the ventricles are contracting, the atria are relaxing and filling with blood. This filling period is

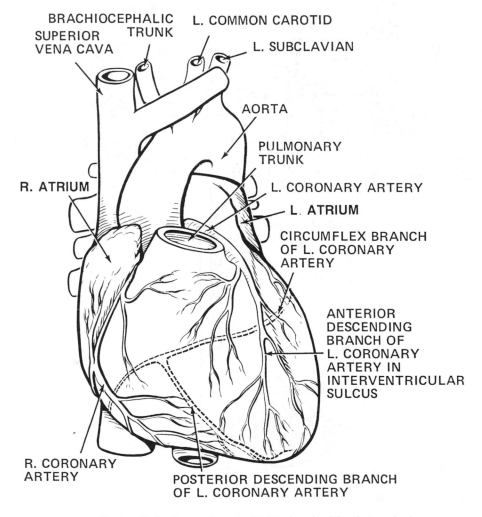

Figure 7-3. Coronary arteries and major blood vessels.

the **diastole,** or the diastolic phase, of the atria. The atria then contract and the ventricles relax and fill in their diastolic phase. The contracting phase of each is the **systole,** or systolic phase.

The heart muscle itself needs a good blood supply, which is provided by the coronary arteries that course over the surface of the heart (Fig. 7–3).

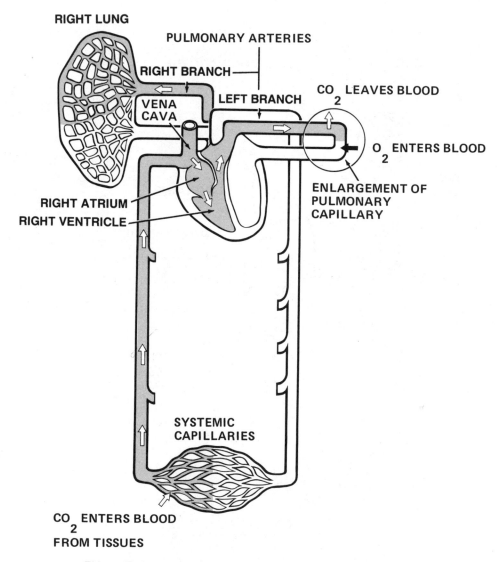

Figure 7-4. Venous return to heart and blood flow to lungs.

These are the small vessels that frequently become blocked, causing a heart attack.

An understanding of the blood flow pattern through the heart and lungs will make the various diseases of the heart more meaningful. Valve defects, septal defects, heart attacks, and more will be considered in the light of the disease's interference with heart action.

THE RELATIONSHIP BETWEEN HEART AND LUNGS

Blood that has circulated throughout the body has given up most of its oxygen and has picked up waste products of cellular metabolism, particularly carbon dioxide. This blood enters the right atrium from the vena cavae and flows through the tricuspid valve to the right ventricle. It is then pumped into the pulmonary artery, which branches to the right and left lung. Figure 7–4 shows this path of blood flow.

At the lungs, carbon dioxide is given off and a fresh supply of oxygen is acquired by the hemoglobin. The oxygenated blood enters the left atrium through pulmonary veins and flows through the mitral valve to the left ventricle. From here the blood is pumped into the aorta, which distributes it to all parts of the body. Figure 7–5 shows the return of oxygenated blood to the left side of the heart.

INFLUENCE OF THE AUTONOMIC NERVOUS SYSTEM

Unlike other muscle, cardiac muscle can contract continuously and rhythmically without nervous stimulation. A small patch of tissue in the right atrial wall initiates the beat, and the impulse for contraction spreads over the atria and ventricles. This specialized patch of tissue, the sinoatrial node, is called the **pacemaker.** A bundle of fibers, known as the bundle of His, conducts the impulse from the atria to the ventricles and terminates in the Purkinje fibers. This conduction system is illustrated in Figure 7–6.

Although the heart muscle is not dependent on nerve stimulation for contraction, it is influenced by nerves of the autonomic nervous system for its rate of beating, the pulse rate. Two sets of nerves work antagonistically to each other, one slowing the heart, the other accelerating it. The vagus nerve slows heart action by means of a chemical it transmits, acetylcholine. This vagus nerve action is important because it prevents the heart from overworking by slowing it down during rest and sleep. The cardiac accelerator nerve of the sympathetic portion of the autonomic nervous system speeds up the action of the heart during periods of stress, strenuous physical activity, and excitement, when the body needs a greater blood flow. The sympathetic system triggers (or stimulates) the release of epinephrine

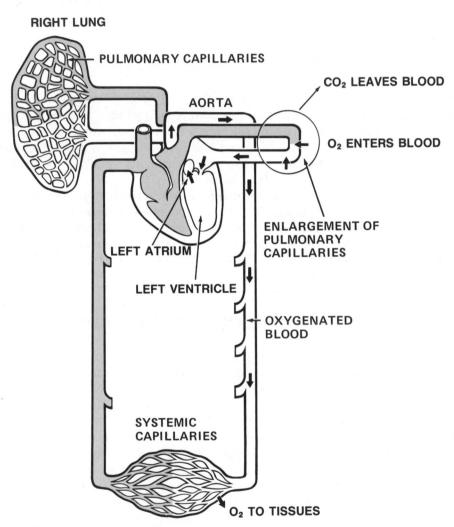

Figure 7-5. Return of oxygenated blood to heart and entry into aorta.

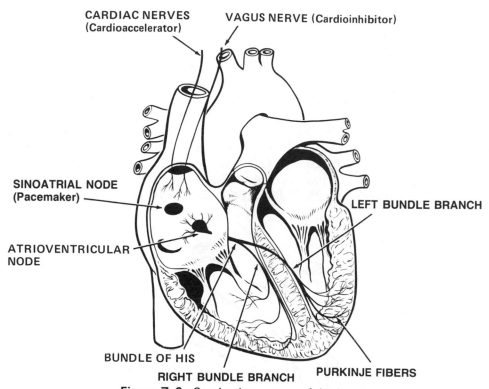

Figure 7-6. Conducting system of the heart.

into the blood stream. As this reaches the pacemaker of the heart, the speed of contraction is increased.

DISEASES OF THE HEART

■ Coronary Artery Disease

The importance of the coronary arteries in supplying oxygenated blood to the myocardium, the heart muscle, has already been mentioned. Unfortunately, these small vessels can become blocked (occluded). This results when a blood clot forms on the inner wall of a coronary artery, causing a **coronary thrombosis;** or from narrowing of the lumen, the opening within the vessel.

The narrowing of the lumen is due to deposits of fatty material on the inner arterial wall. This is the condition of atherosclerosis. More will be said about this disease later. Figure 7–7A illustrates possible means of occlusion or blockage. **Ischemia,** a deficiency of blood supply to the heart, is the leading cause of death in the United States.

If the lumen of the coronary artery narrows slowly, some heart muscle cells die and are replaced by scar tissue. When an area of the myocardium is suddenly deprived of blood due to occlusion of the coronary artery, that tissue dies. The area of dead muscle is called an infarct. This is a true heart attack, and the condition is referred to as a **myocardial infarction.** Severe chest pains generally accompany the attack, but the pain may be referred to the neck or left arm.

The prognosis for the patient with a myocardial infarction depends on many factors. The speed with which medical attention is given is very important. A certified rescuer in CPR (cardiopulmonary resuscitation) can be of great assistance while waiting for an emergency care unit to arrive. Figure 7–7B shows a myocardial infarction with perforation.

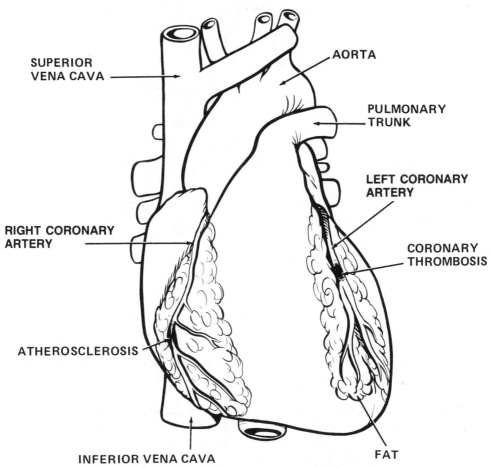

Figure 7-7. A. Blockage of coronary arteries.

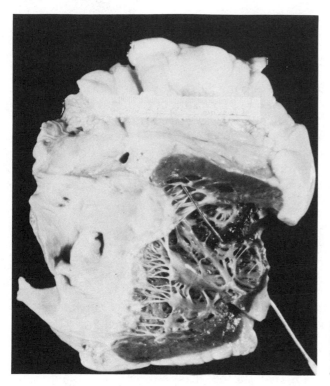

Figure 7-7. B. Myocardial infarction with perforation of heart. (*Courtesy of Dr. David R. Duffell.*)

The size of the coronary artery that is occluded and the extent of heart muscle damage, which is indicated by the level of certain blood enzymes, are also factors in the prognosis. The greater the area affected, the poorer the prognosis will be. If blood from a surrounding area channels into the damaged tissue, recovery will be better. This establishment of new blood vessels is called **collateral circulation.**

The damaged area can repair itself with scar tissue, but it will never serve as heart muscle again. There will be a tendency for blood clots to form or for a weakened area to rupture. Rest is needed for the repair period, but after this period, controlled exercise is advised to maintain circulation. In today's society the predisposing causes of coronary artery disease are generally well known: obesity, hypertension, smoking, a sedentary life style, and a high-cholesterol diet.

Angina pectoris is caused by a temporary oxygen insufficiency. The patient experiences severe chest pains, which may radiate to the neck, jaw, and left arm. There is a feeling of tightness or suffocation. Attacks of angina may follow strenuous exercise, a heavy meal, exposure to severe cold, or emotional stress. Nitroglycerin is generally administered for angina to dilate the coronary arteries, permitting adequate blood flow. A person who experiences recurring attacks of angina should control exercise carefully.

■ Hypertensive Heart Disease

This condition is caused by long-standing high blood pressure known as hypertension. The heart is overworked as it continues to pump against great resistance. The resistance is narrow blood vessels that result from hypertension. The **hypertensive heart** is an enlarged heart. The left ventricle, which does the most work, hypertrophies in an attempt to meet its demands for pumping action. The ventricle finally **dilates,** the chamber enlarges, and it becomes exhausted, unable to pump adequately, and fails.

■ Cor Pulmonale

Cor pulmonale is a serious heart condition in which the right side of the heart fails as a result of chronic lung disease. Pulmonary hypertension develops as the lung blood vessels become diseased, impairing blood flow to the lungs. This hypertension overworks the right ventricle, causing it to dilate and hypertrophy. Treatment is aimed at relieving the causative lung disease by administration of bronchodilaters and the use of a ventilator.

■ Congestive Heart Failure

Congestive heart failure means that the heart is pumping inadequately to meet the needs of the body. Pressure builds within the pulmonary or systemic veins, leading to distention and edema as fluid oozes into the adjacent tissues.

■ Congenital Heart Disease

The tremendous accomplishments in open heart surgery have drastically reduced the mortality rate of children born with heart defects. Most of the **congenital** abnormalities are in the septum that separates the right and left side of the heart. An opening in this septum allows a mixing of unoxygenated and oxygenated blood that causes the heart to overwork.

Septal defects may be large or small, with the smaller defects causing no problem. An example of a small septal defect is failure of the foramen ovale to close after birth. The **foramen ovale** is a small opening that allows blood from the right side of the heart to enter the left directly, bypassing the nonfunctional fetal lungs. Failure of this opening to close is the most common but least serious septal defect.

The septal defect may be in the wall between the two atria or between the ventricles and it may be large (Fig. 7–8). Because blood pressure is higher on the left side than on the right side of the heart, blood is generally shunted through the opening in a left-to-right direction. This factor alone would not

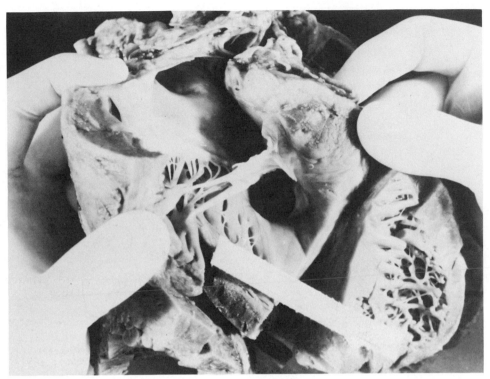

Figure 7-8. Large ventricular septal defect. (*Courtesy of Dr. David R. Duffell.*)

be significant concerning oxygenation of the blood. Blood from the left side is already oxygenated, and blood from the right side is on its way to the lungs, but the right side of the heart is overworked. It receives blood as usual from the vena cava but also from the left side of the heart. To accommodate this blood volume the right side dilates. Because it is required to pump more blood to the lungs, the right ventricle enlarges (hypertrophies). The left ventricle is overworked if a ventricular septal defect is large. Blood is shunted to the right ventricle, yet the left ventricle must pump enough blood into the aorta. This ventricle can become exhausted and fail.

Cyanosis, a blue color in the tissues, does not occur if the shunt of blood through the septal defect remains left to right. If the pressure becomes greater in the right ventricle than in the left, the shunt reverses and cyanosis does occur. The unoxygenated blood from the right side of the heart enters the general circulation. The blue color is due to unoxygenated hemoglobin. Figure 7-9 illustrates the routine shunt and that which causes cyanosis.

Tetralogy of Fallot is one of the most serious of the congenital defects

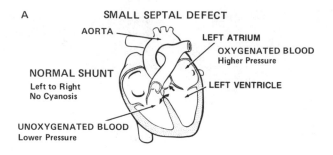

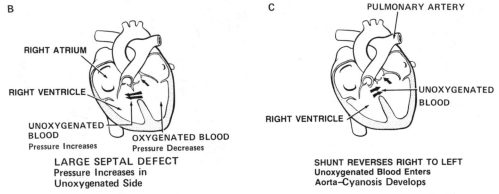

Figure 7-9. Effect of septal defects. **A.** Normal shunt—no cyanosis. **B.** Increased pressure in right ventricle. **C.** Shunt reverses—cyanosis develops.

and consists of four (*tetra*) abnormalities. The victim of this condition is the true "blue baby"; it is born cyanotic, with all the tissues a definite blue. Cyanosis is due to poorly oxygenated blood. The union of oxygen with hemoglobin gives normal arterial blood its bright red color.

The first cause of the cyanosis is pulmonary stenosis. Remember, a valve leads into the pulmonary artery. **Stenosis** of a valve means that the opening is too small. Because of the narrow opening, an inadequate amount of blood reaches the lungs to be oxygenated. All body tissues suffer from this lack of oxygen.

Second, accompanying the pulmonary stenosis is a large ventricular septal defect, the seriousness of which has already been discussed. Third, a misplaced aorta overrides the ventricular septum. Normally, only oxygenated blood from the left ventricle enters the aorta, but in this case the right ventricle also feeds into the aorta, permitting the mixing of oxygenated and unoxygenated blood. Last, because of the increased strain on the right ventricle attempting to pump through a stenotic valve, the ventricle hypertrophies.

In addition to cyanosis, other symptoms accompany the disease. There is secondary polycythemia, a disease described in Chapter 6, as a compensatory mechanism. The inadequate oxygen supply stimulates erythropoiesis, and an excessive number of red blood cells are formed.

The fingers are clubbed and fingernails curled in this condition. This is caused by poor oxygenation of tissues at the fingertips. The child experiences **dyspnea** following any exertion, even crying. The child may assume a squatting position after exercise, which provides some relief from the breathlessness. Surgery can be performed quite successfully. It is essen-

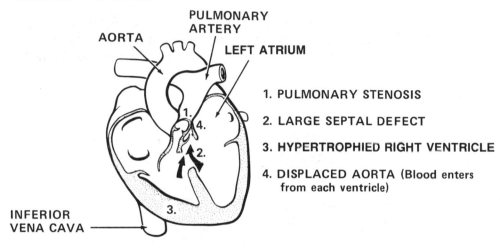

TETRALOGY OF FALLOT

AORTA

PULMONARY ARTERY

LEFT ATRIUM

1. PULMONARY STENOSIS

2. LARGE SEPTAL DEFECT

3. HYPERTROPHIED RIGHT VENTRICLE

4. DISPLACED AORTA (Blood enters from each ventricle)

INFERIOR VENA CAVA

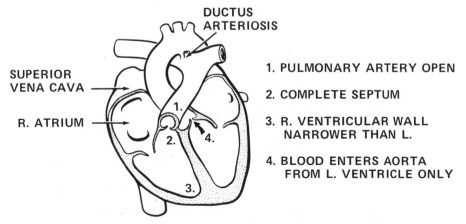

NORMAL ANATOMY OF HEART

DUCTUS ARTERIOSIS

SUPERIOR VENA CAVA

R. ATRIUM

1. PULMONARY ARTERY OPEN

2. COMPLETE SEPTUM

3. R. VENTRICULAR WALL NARROWER THAN L.

4. BLOOD ENTERS AORTA FROM L. VENTRICLE ONLY

Figure 7-10. Tetralogy of Fallot **(top)** compared to normal anatomy **(bottom).**

tial to bypass the narrow opening to the lungs. Figure 7–10 shows the four abnormalities in the tetralogy of Fallot.

Patent ductus arteriosis is a common congenital disease. The ductus arteriosis is a fetal blood vessel connecting the pulmonary artery and the aorta, shunting the blood from the nonfunctional lungs. Figure 7–11 shows this vessel diagrammatically. Soon after birth it normally closes, but if it remains open (patent), blood flows from the aorta to the pulmonary artery, where pressure is lower. This blood is oxygenated, so there is no cyanosis. One danger is bacterial infection at the site of the lesion. This is a common problem with all congenital heart defects. The open ductus can be corrected surgically by dividing the connection between the pulmonary artery and the aorta.

Coarctation of the aorta is a narrowing, or stricture, of the artery that provides blood to the entire body. The stricture occurs beyond the branching of blood vessels to the head and arms, so the blood supply to the upper

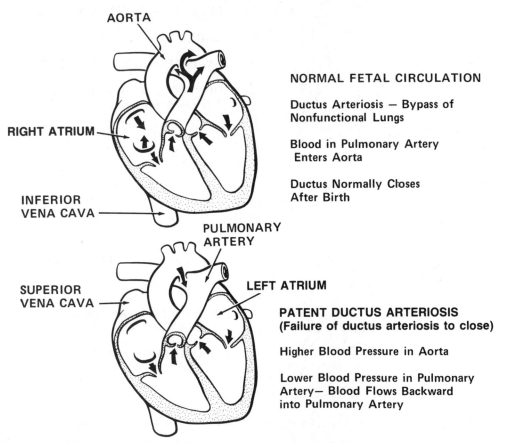

Figure 7-11. Patent ductus arteriosis.

part of the body is adequate. Little blood, however, flows through the constricted area to the abdomen and legs. Blood pressure is very low in the legs but is high in the arms. Many collateral blood vessels develop to compensate for this poor blood supply. This is comparable to the collateral circulation that develops after a myocardial infarction. The coarctation can be corrected surgically by cutting out (excising) the narrow segment and sewing the good ends of the aorta together. Coarctation of the aorta is pictured in Figure 7–12A as compared with the normal branching of the aorta (Fig. 7–12B).

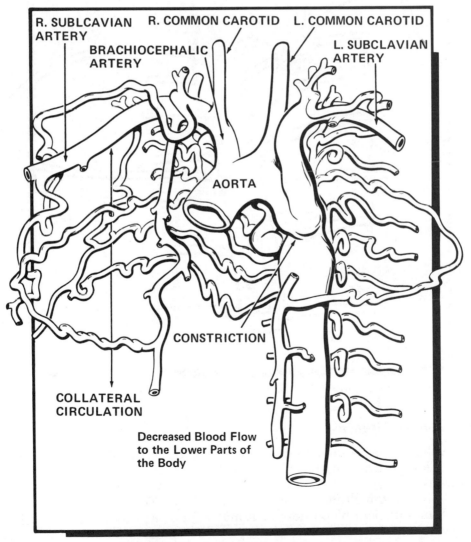

R. SUBLCAVIAN ARTERY
R. COMMON CAROTID
L. COMMON CAROTID
BRACHIOCEPHALIC ARTERY
L. SUBCLAVIAN ARTERY
AORTA
CONSTRICTION
COLLATERAL CIRCULATION
Decreased Blood Flow to the Lower Parts of the Body

Figure 7-12. A. Coarctation of the aorta.

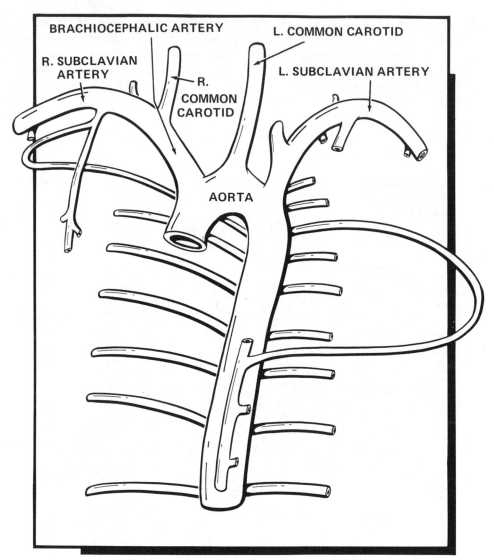

Figure 7-12. B. Normal branching of the aorta.

■ Valvular Diseases

The valves assure a unidirectional flow of blood through the heart. Closed, they allow a heart chamber to fill with blood; open, they let blood flow forward.

Valves can malfunction in one of two ways. The opening may be too small for sufficient blood flow, or it may be too large to prevent backflow, **valvular insufficiency.** Valve defects cause heart murmurs with characteristic sounds that indicate the nature of the defect. If a valve problem is particularly serious, it can be corrected surgically by reconstruction or replacement. Some of the various valve defects and the effect they have on the heart are considered below.

In mitral stenosis the mitral valve opening is too small. The cusps that form the valve, normally flexible flaps, become rigid and fuse together. A deep funnel-shaped valve is formed, and much pressure is required to force enough blood through the narrow opening. Mitral stenosis often follows rheumatic fever. It is more common in women than in men. Rheumatic heart disease will be described in the next section.

What about the effect on the heart? The chambers that contain blood that must pass through this valve become greatly dilated. Keeping in mind the blood flow path through the heart, one can see that the left atrium and right side of the heart would be affected. This is illustrated in Figure 7-13. The left atrium also becomes hypertrophied because of overwork in pumping blood through the stenotic valve.

One of the complications of any valve defect is the tendency for a thrombus, a clot, to form in the affected area. As blood flows over the

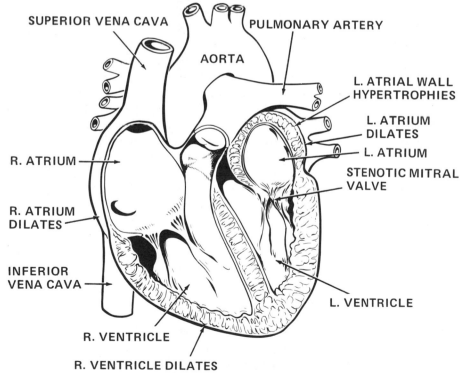

Figure 7-13. Effect of mitral stenosis on the heart.

malfunctioning valve, clotting elements of the blood are deposited. If the thrombus becomes detached, it will travel as an embolism and possibly occlude a blood vessel to the brain, kidney, or other vital organ.

The damming up of blood behind the stenotic mitral valve causes a congestion in the veins. The veins, attempting to empty into the right atrium, do so with difficulty. The veins in the neck stand out prominently. As the congestion builds in the veins, fluid from the blood leaks out into the tissue spaces, causing edema.

Poor circulation causes cyanosis because an inadequate amount of oxygen is reaching the tissues. The backup of blood and congestion cause the heart to become exhausted, and congestive heart failure can result.

Mitral insufficiency, or incompetence, means that the opening in the mitral valve is too large and cannot close completely. This can occur if the cusps become hardened, sclerotic, and retract. Another cause is the failure of specialized muscles called papillary muscles in the ventricle. These are attached to the underside of the cusps by means of little cords and normally prevent the cusps from swinging up into the atria when the ventricles contract. If the papillary muscles fail to contract, the cusps open toward the atria under the force of ventricular blood.

Aortic stenosis, the narrowing of the valve leading into the aorta, occurs more often in men than in women and most frequently in men over 50. It may result from rheumatic fever but not as frequently as does mitral stenosis. Sometimes it is a congenital defect or it may occur with hardening of the arteries. The cusps become rigid and adhere together. Masses of hard, calcified material are deposited giving a warty appearance to the valve. Because the left ventricle of the heart must pump through this valve into the aorta, this chamber hypertrophies greatly through overwork. This condition is shown in Figure 7–14. An inadequate amount of blood may be pumped into the aorta to meet the requirements of the body. An insufficient blood supply to the brian can cause **syncope** (fainting). This valve defect, like others, can be corrected surgically.

In aortic insufficiency the valve does not close properly. During diastole, blood flows back into the left ventricle from the aorta. This condition of the valve can result from an inflammation within the heart, **endocarditis.** It may also be due to a dilated aorta, where the ring around the valve is too large. Because of the backflow of blood, the left ventricle becomes greatly dilated. The left ventricle also hypertrophies because of overwork.

■ Rheumatic Heart Disease

Rheumatic heart disease is a peculiar disease that results from a streptococcal infection, although the organisms are no longer present when the disease presents itself. Rheumatic fever develops from a throat or ear infection caused by **Group A hemolytic streptococci.** The symptoms are fever, in-

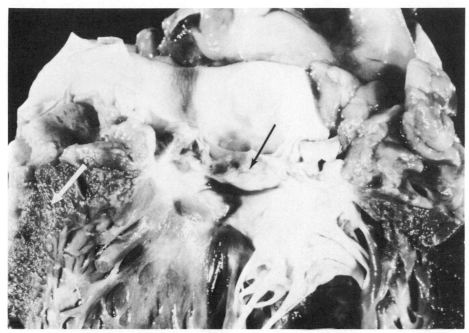

Figure 7-14. Calcified aortic stenosis (black arrow). Left ventricle is greatly hypertrophied (white arrow). (*Courtesy of Dr. David R. Duffell.*)

flamed and painful joints, and sometimes a rash. There is a latent period of a few weeks between the infection and the development of rheumatic fever. The disease usually strikes children or very young adults.

Rheumatic fever is an **autoimmune disease.** It results from a reaction between streptococcal antigens and the patient's own antibodies against them. All parts of the heart may be affected, but most frequently it is the mitral valve that is damaged. The exact mechanism that causes the valve lesion is not known. There seems to be an attraction of the antigen–antibody complex for the mitral valve. The aortic semilunar valve is also affected at times.

The valves become inflamed as a result of the infection, and clotting elements are deposited by blood flowing over the valves. Small nodular structures called **vegetations** form along the edge of the cusps (Fig. 7–15). The normally delicate cusps thicken and adhere to each other. Later, fibrous tissue develops, which has a tendency to contract.

If the adhesions of the cusps seriously narrow, the valve opening the mitral valve becomes stenotic. The effects of mitral stenosis are described in this chapter (see Valvular Diseases). An inadequate amount of blood flows from the left atrium to the left ventricle. **Stasis,** or slowed blood flow, frequently causes thrombus formation.

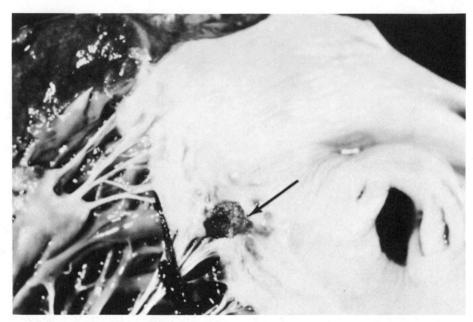

Figure 7-15. Vegetations on mitral valve (arrow). (*Courtesy of Dr. David R. Duffell.*)

It is possible for the cusps to retract to the extent that they fail to meet and the valve cannot close. The mitral valve is then insufficient, or incompetent. There is a backflow of blood, regurgitation, from the left ventricle to the left atrium. Fortunately, rheumatic fever is not as common today as it once was, the decline being due to the widespread use of antibiotics in treating streptococcal infections.

■ Infectious Endocarditis

Infectious endocarditis is a disease that was once considered fatal but that now responds well to antibiotics if treated early. The endocardium is the inner lining of the chambers of the heart and covers the valves. Endocarditis is an inflammation of this lining caused by a **nonhemolytic streptococci.** These organisms can enter the bloodstream from an infected tooth, a skin infection, urinary tract infection, or other infections. Frequently this inflammation occurs on a rheumatic fever lesion, an already damaged valve, or on a congenital heart defect. Various routes of bacterial invasion are illustrated in Figure 7–16.

The nodules or vegetations that form in endocarditis are larger than those of rheumatic fever. They are also **friable,** tending to break apart easily and enter the bloodstream. The vegetations are filled with bacteria, unlike

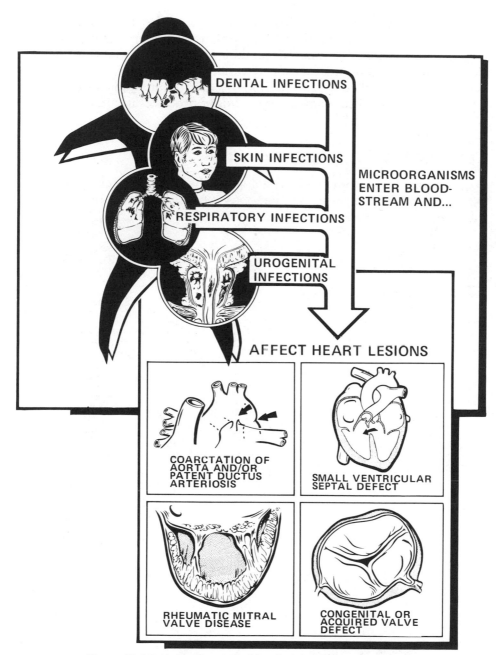

DENTAL INFECTIONS

SKIN INFECTIONS

RESPIRATORY INFECTIONS

UROGENITAL INFECTIONS

MICROORGANISMS ENTER BLOOD-STREAM AND...

AFFECT HEART LESIONS

COARCTATION OF AORTA AND/OR PATENT DUCTUS ARTERIOSIS

SMALL VENTRICULAR SEPTAL DEFECT

RHEUMATIC MITRAL VALVE DISEASE

CONGENITAL OR ACQUIRED VALVE DEFECT

Figure 7-16. Infections resulting in bacterial endocarditis.

rheumatic fever vegetations. Typical lesions of endocarditis are shown in Figure 7–17. As fragments of the vegetations break apart, they enter the bloodstream to form emboli. The emboli can travel to the brain, kidney, lung, or other vital organs, causing a variety of symptoms. The emboli can lodge in small blood vessels of the skin or other organs and cause the blood vessels to rupture. These small hemorrhages produce tiny red spots called petechiae.

ABNORMALITIES OF HEART ACTION

In reviewing the anatomy and physiology of the heart, a specialized patch of tissue, the pacemaker, was mentioned as establishing heart rate. Normally, the impulse for contraction then spreads over the atria and is conducted to

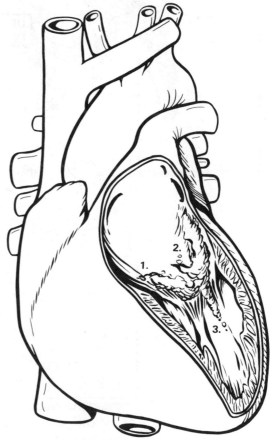

Figure 7-17. Bacterial endocarditis.

1. Vegetations cover mitral valve
2. Extend to atrial wall and on to
3. Cords which support valve

the ventricles through a conduction bundle. This conduction system can fail. If the impulse does not spread from the atria to the ventricles, the pulse is drastically reduced, and this failure in passage of the impulse is known as heart block. Heart block can result from scar tissue interfering with the conduction bundle. In this case, it may be necessary to implant an electric pacemaker if the block is complete.

At times, the impulse for contraction spreads over the atria in an uncoordinated fashion. Because the heart muscle fibers are not working as a unit, atrial contraction is uncoordinated and ineffective. This is known as **atrial fibrillation.** As a result of the uncoordinated contraction of the atria, the ventricles receive irregular input. They also begin to beat faster, but again in an uncoordinated and less efficient fashion. A medication, digitalis, can be administered to slow the condition of the impulse through the bundle of His to the ventricles. This allows the ventricles to fill properly before contraction.

Ventricular fibrillation is far more serious than atrial fibrillation. If the impulse for contraction spreads over the ventricles irregularly, they will twitch rather than contract. They fail to pump blood, and this can lead to **cardiac arrest,** the sudden stoppage of heart action. Immediate attempts at **resuscitation** must be made or death will ensue. Permanent damage to other organs, particularly the brain, results when an inadequate blood supply reaches them. A machine called a **defibrillator** is used when available, which gives electrical shocks to the heart enabling it to re-establish its normal beat.

Heart beat rhythm may become irregular and is known as **cardiac arrythmia.** Beats may be skipped or come in prematurely.

The heart rate may increase significantly, which is called **tachycardia.** An abnormally slow pulse rate is termed **bradycardia.**

Modern medicine provides many techniques for diagnosing and treating heart problems. **Auscultation**—listening through a stethoscope for abnormal sounds—and the electrocardiogram provide valuable information regarding heart condition. The electrocardiogram is a means of recording heart contractions, their rate, strength, and rhythm. It can detect heart block, an enlarged heart, and areas damaged by a myocardial infarction.

Another very valuable procedure is **cardiac catheterization.** By means of a long, fine catheter passed through a blood vessel, samples of blood can be taken from each chamber and analyzed for oxygen content. Pressure in the various chambers can also be measured. These findings can indicate valve disorders, various deformities, and other malfunctions. Figure 7–18 illustrates this procedure.

X-rays of the heart and great vessels, the aorta and pulmonary artery, can be taken by means of **angiocardiography.** In this procedure, an opaque dye is administered into one of the blood vessels or into the heart. A blockage is indicated by an area in which the dye fails to penetrate. Coronary bypass surgery may be indicated by this procedure.

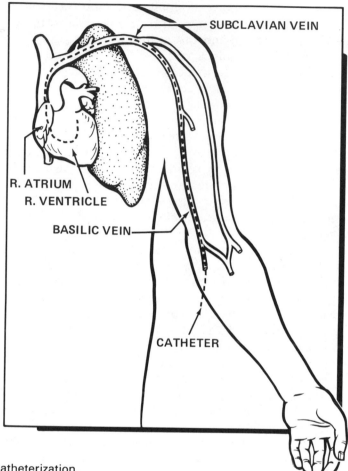

Figure 7-18. Cardiac catheterization.

SUMMARY

After reviewing the normal structure and function of the heart, heart diseases were considered. Some heart diseases, such as myocardial infarction and angina pectoris, cause severe chest pain or referred pain in the arm or neck. Dyspnea is a common symptom of many heart diseases. The lack of oxygen in the tissues stimulates the respiratory center, and the patient experiences difficulty in breathing or shortness of breath. Fainting or loss of consciousness occurs when the brain is deprived of an adequate blood supply.

All of the tissues and organs are affected by poor circulation. Cyanosis occurs when blood is not properly oxygenated. Fluid accumulates in the tissues, causing edema, when veins become congested. Heart murmurs are caused by malfunctioning valves. The abnormal sounds result from blood being forced through a stenotic valve or being regurgitated through an insufficient valve. The various congenital heart diseases were considered. It was noted that a congenital defect is frequently the site of a bacterial infection.

The advantage of such diagnostic procedures as the electrocardiogram, cardiac catheterization, and angiocardiography were discussed. Advances in open heart surgery have made it possible to correct congenital heart defects, replace valves, and implant electric pacemakers. The use of antibiotics has reduced the danger of endocarditis and the frequency of rheumatic heart disease.

STUDY QUESTIONS

1. Name two ways in which the coronary arteries can become occluded.
2. What is the most significant difference between a myocardial infarction and an attack of angina pectoris?
3. Why is a hypertensive heart an enlarged heart?
4. What is the relationship between the lungs and heart in cor pulmonale?
5. What are the four congenital defects in the tetralogy of Fallot? Explain the accompanying cyanosis.
6. What is patent ductus arteriosis? Is cyanosis a symptom of this disease? Why?
7. Explain the difference in blood pressure in the arms and legs resulting from coarctation of the aorta.
8. Why is a right-to-left shunt more serious than a left-to-right shunt?
9. Describe the dilation and hypertrophy in a heart with mitral stenosis. What is the difference between hypertrophy and dilation?
10. Name two complications that can result from a valve defect.
11. Describe the appearance of the valve in aortic stenosis. Which chamber of the heart hypertrophies? What is the greatest danger with this valve defect?
12. Contrast the causes of rheumatic heart disease and infectious endocarditis. How do the lesions differ?
13. What is meant by heart block? What can cause it? How is the pulse affected?
14. Name the conditions in which nitroglycerin and digitalis may be used.
15. Why is ventricular fibrillation more serious than atrial fibrillation?
16. What information can be gained from (a) an electrocardiogram, (b) cardiac catheterization, and (c) angiocardiography?

CHAPTER 8

Diseases of the Blood Vessels

The importance of a well-functioning heart acting as a pump to provide blood to all parts of the body has been discussed. Another factor is essential to this distribution of blood, and this is healthy blood vessels. These vessels can become hard **(sclerotic)** or **occluded** (closed).

DISEASES OF THE ARTERIES

■ Arteriosclerosis

Arteriosclerosis, hardening of the arteries, is a degenerative condition that affects most people to some extent in the process of aging. There is a diffuse thickening of the inner lining, the **intima,** of the blood vessels. The vessels become brittle and are susceptible to rupture.

■ Atherosclerosis

One form of arteriosclerosis that is extremely serious, and frequently the cause of death, is **atherosclerosis.** Fatty deposits called **plaques** develop in the intima, narrowing the opening, or lumen, of the blood vessel, in some instances completely occluding it. This lipid material consists mostly of cholesterol. The aorta and its branches can be affected as seen in Figure 8–1 but so can small arteries such as the coronary and cerebral arteries. Occlusion of these vessels interferes with blood flow to the heart muscle, causing a myocardial infarction, and to the brain, causing a stroke or

113

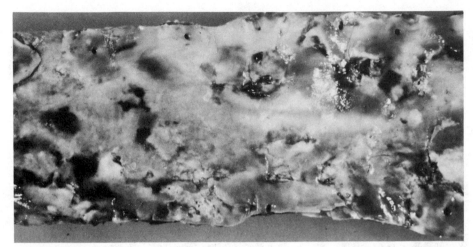

Figure 8-1. Atherosclerosis of the aorta. Inner surface should be smooth. (*Courtesy of Dr. David R. Duffell*).

cerebral vascular accident. Lack of blood to any organ is called **ischemia** and promotes tissue damage. Figure 8–2 shows the build up of lipids and narrowing of the lumen.

The cause of atherosclerosis is not completely known, but it does have a hereditary basis. Atherosclerosis is a common complication of diabetes, also a disease with a hereditary tendency. A low-cholesterol diet and regular exercise should reduce the risk of developing atherosclerosis.

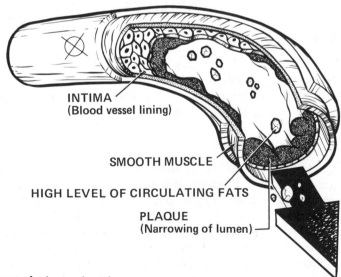

INTIMA
(Blood vessel lining)

SMOOTH MUSCLE

HIGH LEVEL OF CIRCULATING FATS

PLAQUE
(Narrowing of lumen)

Figure 8-2. Development of atherosclerosis.

■ Thrombosis and Embolism

One of the body's protective devices is the blood-clotting mechanism. When there is injury to tissues and blood vessels, excessive bleeding is prevented as the blood starts to clot. This same mechanism can function within the intact blood vessels, and this intravascular clotting produces a thrombus.

Several factors lead to **thrombosis,** the forming of blood clots. Clots tend to form where blood flow is slower. Since blood flows more slowly in veins than in arteries, veins are the more common site of thrombus formation. Clots are also likely to form where there is turbulence in the bloodstream, as there is over the heart valves. A diseased valve is a likely site for a clot formation.

Platelets, which normally initiate the blood clotting mechanism, are deposited on the inner wall of a blood vessel or on a heart valve. Normally, these surfaces are very smooth, and platelets do not adhere. But when they are injured or diseased, the platelets stick and the clot begins to form. Atherosclerosis and rheumatic heart disease are predisposing causes of thrombus formation. Thrombosis in an atherosclerotic aorta is seen in Figure 8–3. Clots frequently form in coronary and cerebral arteries and in the legs when circulation is poor. Figure 8–4 illustrates thrombus formation. Changes in the blood itself can cause thrombosis. The blood may become too viscous or the platelet count may be excessively high.

Anticoagulants such as heparin and dicumarol may be administered to prevent intravascular clotting. These medications can interfere with the person's normal ability to stop bleeding, and a small injury or cut may prove serious.

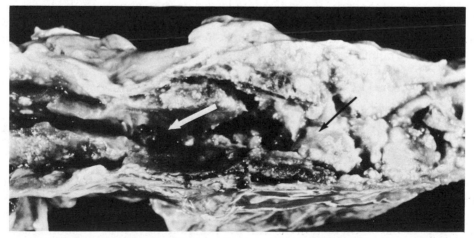

Figure 8–3. Thrombus (white arrow) in an atherosclerotic aorta. Black arrow indicates plaque. (*Courtesy of Dr. David R. Duffell.*)

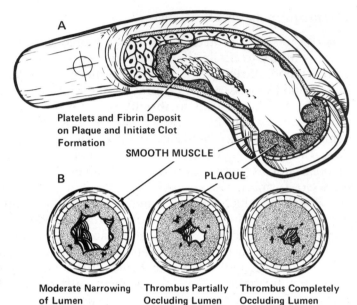

Figure 8-4. Thrombus formation in an athero-sclerotic vessel. Depicted are the initial clot formation **(A)** and the varying degrees of occlusion **(B)**.

The thrombus may retract and allow blood to flow, or it may permanently occlude the vessel. The thrombus can become detached and travel in the bloodstream as an embolus. Infected tissue around the thrombus can cause this detachment as can sudden movement.

Let us imagine a thrombus in a leg vein and follow its course as it travels as an **embolism.** Veins become larger as they approach the heart, so the clot travels easily to the heart. Vessels become smaller as they leave the heart; the embolus can then get stuck in a pulmonary artery and even occlude it. A pulmonary embolus is illustrated in Figure 8–5.

When rheumatic heart disease was considered, the damaged mitral valve was named as a potential site for thrombus formation. A clot formed on this valve can break loose and enter the aorta. It then may travel to the brain, kidney, or some other organ. Figure 8–6 shows an embolus traveling to the brain through the carotid artery.

An embolism may contain infected material from pyogenic bacteria and is then called a **septic embolism.** This sometimes results from a lack of sterile technique during labor and delivery or an abortion. Substances other than blood can comprise an embolism. Air introduced into a vein during surgery producing air bubbles, fat globules, and groups of cancer cells can all travel in the blood as emboli with the potential of closing a blood vessel.

Lack of blood due to a closed blood vessel causes tissue death, an infarct. Bacteria can enter the **necrotic,** dead, tissue and cause gangrene. If

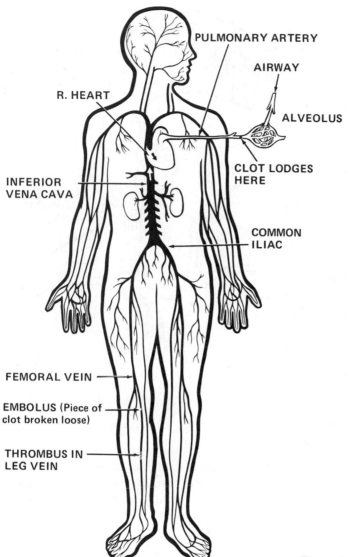

PULMONARY ARTERY

AIRWAY

R. HEART

ALVEOLUS

CLOT LODGES
HERE

INFERIOR
VENA CAVA

COMMON
ILIAC

FEMORAL VEIN

EMBOLUS (Piece of
clot broken loose)

THROMBUS IN
LEG VEIN

Figure 8-5. Pulmonary embolism.

this occurs in the foot, a greenish color develops that turns to black, and the condition spreads up the leg.

■ Aneurysms

A weakening in the wall of a blood vessel due to disease, a congenital defect, or physical injury can cause a localized dilation or saclike formation known as an **aneurysm.** Aneurysms may produce no symptoms and may only be

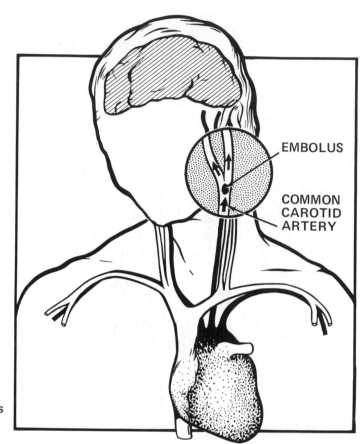

Figure 8-6. Embolus traveling to the brain.

detected on an x-ray taken for another purpose. The danger of an aneurysm is its tendency to increase in size and rupture, resulting in a hemorrhage, possibly in a vital organ such as the heart or brain. An abdominal aortic aneurysm is seen in Figure 8–7. Atherosclerosis is a common cause of aneurysm formation.

Surgical procedures have been very successful in repairing blood vessels affected by aneurysm formation. The diseased area of the vessel is removed and replaced with a plastic graft or segment of another blood vessel. This procedure reduces the risk of hemorrhage and thrombus formation.

DISEASES OF THE VEINS

Vein structure is different from that of arteries. Veins have thinner walls than arteries with less elastic and smooth muscle tissue in the walls and tend to collapse when empty. Many veins, particularly the veins of the leg, have valves that aid in the return of blood to the heart when it moves against gravity.

■ Phlebitis

Phlebitis is an inflammation of a vein, usually in the leg. Veins are both superficial and deep. It is only when the deep veins are affected that the condition is considered potentially serious. Several factors may cause phlebitis: injury, general infection, poor circulation, and obesity to name a few.

The greatest danger in the deep veins is thrombus formation, and the condition is then called **thrombophlebitis.** If a vein becomes occluded by a clot, edema develops. The blood cannot return properly to the heart, the veins become congested with blood, and fluid seeps out into the tissues. It is important that the clot does not become dislodged and travel as an embolism. Anticoagulants may be administered to prevent further clot formation, and antibiotics, to prevent infection. Surgery is sometimes required to remove the thrombus.

■ Varicose Veins

Varicose veins generally develop in the superficial veins of the leg. The veins become swollen, painful, and appear knotty under the skin. The condition is caused by stagnation of blood in the veins that can result from several factors.

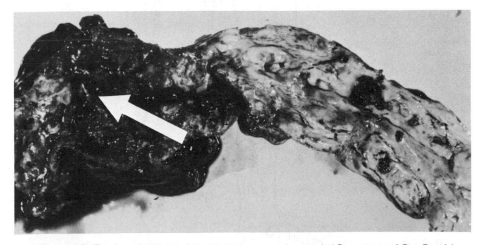

Figure 8-7. An abdominal aortic aneurysm (arrow). (*Courtesy of Dr. David R. Duffell.*)

Development of varicose veins can be an occupational hazard for someone who stands or sits still for long periods of time. Normally the action of the leg muscles helps move the blood upward from one valve to the next. In the absence of this "milking action" of the muscles, the blood exerts a pressure on the closed valves and thin walls of the veins. The veins then dilate to the extent that the valves are no longer competent. The blood then collects, becomes stagnant, and the veins become more swollen.

Pregnancy or a tumor in the uterus can also cause varicose veins. The return flow of blood from the legs encounters resistance and a back pressure of blood results, breaking down more and more valves. Heredity often plays a part in the development of varicose veins. Figure 8–8 illustrates normal veins and the flow of blood upward through the valves and varicose veins where the valves have become incompetent. Ulcers tend to develop because of poor circulation. The slowing blood flow (stasis) often causes infection. The distended veins can rupture, causing hemorrhage into the surrounding tissues.

Treatment varies with the severity of the symptoms. At times an elastic bandage or stocking is adequate to give veins support. A surgical procedure called "stripping the veins" is very successful. The superficial veins are tied off, ligated, and removed. A collateral circulation to the deep veins takes over.

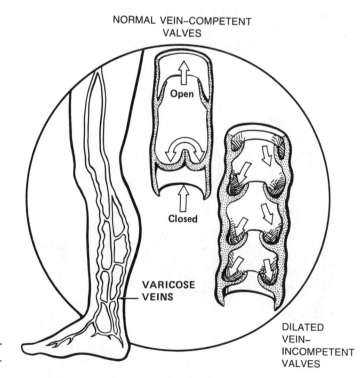

Figure 8-8. Development of varicose veins.

Hemorrhoids are varicose veins of the rectum and cause pain, itching, and bleeding. Like varicose veins in the leg, hemorrhoids can develop from pressure on the veins. Straining due to constipation, pressure on the veins from a pregnant uterus, or a tumor may promote their development.

Esophageal varices, or varicose veins of the esophagus, frequently accompany cirrhosis of the liver. They result from pressure that develops within the veins as they try to empty. Because of blocked blood vessels within the damaged liver, there is a back up of blood and general congestion. A fatal hemorrhage from these varices can occur.

■ HYPERTENSION

Hypertension, or high blood pressure, is a condition most people are familiar with to some extent. Called the "silent killer," it is the leading cause of strokes and congestive heart failure. Warnings of the factors that can aggravate this disease are well publicized: smoking, obesity, excessive salt and lipid intake, and lack of exercise. The exact cause of hypertension is not known. It is thought to be a hereditary disease, but the site of the defective mechanism is not clear.

What determines blood pressure? It is a function of cardiac output, the amount of blood pumped per minute by the heart, and the resistance the blood meets from the walls of the blood vessels, total peripheral resistance. Hypertension results from persistent arterial resistance as atherosclerosis.

A blood pressure reading has two parts, corresponding to the two phases of heart activity: the **systolic pressure** and **diastolic pressure.** A normal adult has an average arterial pressure of 120 **millimeters of mercury** over 80 **millimeters of mercury** (120/80 mm Hg). The 120 mm Hg, or systolic pressure, is the highest pressure in the arteries due to the force of contraction of the heart. The 80 mm Hg, or diastolic pressure, is the pressure in the arteries when the ventricles are relaxing and filling.

Control Mechanisms

In the normal person, several mechanisms function to control blood pressure. Changing from a reclining to a standing position temporarily decreases blood flow to the head. Reflexes within the nervous system bring about constriction of blood vessels, increase peripheral resistance, and blood pressure to the head increases.

After a severe hemorrhage, blood pressure decreases and, again, a nerve reflex constricts blood vessels and pressure is elevated. On the other hand, if blood pressure is excessively high, specialized nerve receptors sense this and cause dilation of the arterioles of the kidney. This stimulates increased blood flow through the kidney and increased urine formation.

With the loss of fluid, the blood volume is reduced, which decreases blood pressure. The kidneys are highly responsive to changes in blood pressure. When pressure is high, large quantities of water and salt are lost in the urine. When blood pressure is low, salt and water, and therefore blood volume, are retained.

Another means of reducing blood pressure, by reducing blood volume, is the **capillary fluid shift mechanism.** The pressure within the capillaries is higher than that of the tissue fluid outside. The high pressure within forces fluid through the walls of the capillaries into the tissue spaces, thus reducing blood volume and pressure.

Hypertension and Kidney Disease

There is a close relationship between hypertension and kidney disease. Hypertension can contribute to kidney disease, and kidney disease can contribute to hypertension. Decreased function of the kidneys leads to water and salt retention, causing increased blood volume and elevated blood pressure levels. Long-standing hypertension causes arteriosclerosis of the renal artery that reduces blood flow to the kidneys and damages them.

Primary and Secondary Hypertension

A distinction is made between primary and secondary hypertension. **Primary** or essential **hypertension** is also called idiopathic, meaning that the cause is unknown. The hypertension may have a gradual onset and continue for a long time, or it may be malignant, with a sudden onset, and run its course very quickly. The latter type is quite rare but will end in death if not treated.

Secondary hypertension is high blood pressure that results from another disease. It may be a complication of malfunctioning kidneys or a tumor of the adrenal gland, the gland that regulates salt retention.

Effects of Hypertension

High blood pressure over a long period of time has several adverse effects on the body. It overworks the heart, causing the left ventricle to greatly enlarge, but the blood vessels to the hypertrophied heart muscle do not correspondingly increase. This means an inadequate blood supply going through the heart, and the patient is likely to experience attacks of angina pectoris (see Chapter 7). High blood pressure affects all the arteries of the body, including the coronary arteries. The risk of a coronary occlusion is very great.

All of the blood vessels become hard (sclerotic), and this is a frequent cause of thrombus formation. Weakened blood vessels can rupture and bleed due to the high pressure within, causing local tissue damage in the brain, kidney, or other organ.

Treatment of Hypertension

Medications, many of which are diuretics, are very effective in reducing blood pressure by reducing blood volume through the kidneys. Because salt holds water within the body, restricting salt intake lessens body fluids and blood volume. Exercise improves circulation, decreasing the progress of arteriosclerosis. This means less **peripheral resistance** to increase blood pressure. Hypertension overworks the heart and damages the arteries, causing them to become sclerotic. The converse is also true; sclerotic arteries cause hypertension by increasing peripheral resistance.

■ SHOCK

Shock is a vascular change resulting from assault or injury to the body. Any condition that reduces the heart's ability to pump effectively or decreases venous return can cause shock. **Hypovolemic shock** results from fluid volume loss after severe hemorrhage or loss of plasma in burn patients. **Neurogenic shock** is due to generalized vasodilation, resulting from decreased vasomotor tone. The reduced blood pressure causes poor venous return to the heart and hence poor cardiac output. The decreased vasomotor tone may be due to spinal anesthesia, spinal cord injury, or certain drugs. **Anaphylactic shock** accompanies a severe antigen–antibody reaction such as occurs in an incompatible blood transfusion. The types of shock are summarized in Figure 8–9.

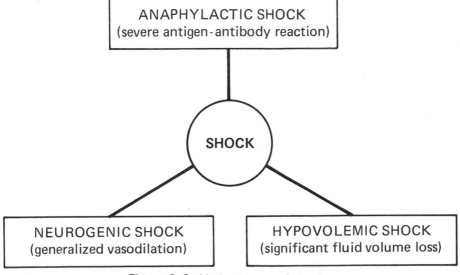

Figure 8-9. Various types of shock.

SUMMARY

Healthy blood vessels are essential to adequate distribution of blood to all the tissues of the body. The condition of arteriosclerosis makes vessels susceptible to rupture and the roughened inner lining a site for clot formation. In atherosclerosis the fatty deposits that build up in the intima of the arteries narrow the lumen, greatly reducing blood flow. These lipid plaques can actually occlude the opening.

Although clotting within blood vessels does not normally occur, certain factors can promote it. Rough or diseased surfaces provide a site for thrombus formation. The clot may become detached and travel as an embolism, possibly lodging and blocking a critical artery. Veins may become congested with blood and distended to the extent that the valves cannot function. The stagnation of blood causes the infection and ulceration associated with varicose veins.

STUDY QUESTIONS

1. Atherosclerosis is a form of arteriosclerosis. What is the characteristic lesion of atherosclerosis?
2. What is the danger of atherosclerosis? What vessels can it affect?
3. Distinguish between a thrombus and an embolus.
4. Name some conditions that lead to thrombosis.
5. Where might an embolus from (a) a leg thrombus and (b) the mitral valve lodge?
6. In which specific blood vessels is phlebitis most serious?
7. Name three factors that can influence development of varicose veins.
8. Explain the manner in which varicose veins develop.
9. What condition is called the "silent killer"?
10. Hypertension is a hereditary disease. Name four factors that might help reduce its development.
11. How are the kidneys important in regulating blood pressure?
12. What are some adverse effects of hypertension?

CHAPTER 9

Diseases of the Excretory System

FUNCTIONS OF THE KIDNEYS

The kidneys are very interesting and complex organs. Not only do the kidneys remove waste products from the body, but they concentrate them by conserving body fluids. The kidneys play an essential role in maintaining **electrolyte** (salt) **balance,** a factor essential to normal nerve and muscle physiology. The proper balance of salts like sodium, potassium, and calcium is required for normal heart activity.

Another kidney function is to help maintain the correct pH, or acid–base balance, of blood and body fluids. The body tolerates a very limited pH range of 7.35 to 7.45. If the pH of blood is lower than this, the blood is too acidic, and a condition called **acidosis** develops. The effect of acidosis will be discussed with diabetes mellitus because it is a complication of this disease. If the pH of blood is higher than 7.45 the blood is too alkaline, and the condition is called **alkalosis.** Death can result from either of these extremes. The kidneys help regulate body pH by excreting an acid urine when blood and body fluids are too acidic, and an alkaline urine when the pH is abnormally high. The kidneys also produce a hormone, erythropoietin, that stimulates red blood cell production. When kidneys become diseased, the hormone is not secreted and severe anemia develops. Specialized cells within the arterioles leading to the functional kidney area comprise the **juxtaglomerular apparatus.** These cells secrete **renin,** which is converted to angiotensin, an enzyme to help elevate blood pressure.

The Nephron

The functional unit of the kidney is the **nephron.** There are about a million nephrons in each kidney. It is the work of these minute structures to filter waste products from the blood, to reabsorb water and nutrients such as glucose and amino acids from the tubular fluid, and to secrete excess substances from the body fluids.

Each nephron consists of a **Bowman's capsule,** a proximal convoluted tubule, loop of Henle, and a distal convoluted tubule that leads to a collecting tubule. Urine is formed in the nephron. Figure 9–1 illustrates the parts of the nephron. As the various kidney diseases are considered, the effect of the malfunction of these parts will become clear.

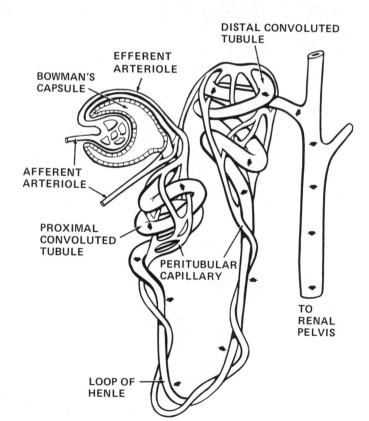

Figure 9-1. A nephron—the kidney's functional unit—shown with the capillary network.

Formation of Urine

Blood to be filtered is carried to a tuft of capillaries called the **glomerulus,** which is situated inside Bowman's capsule. These capillary walls are very thin. Their surface area is large, and the blood pressure within them is higher than the pressure in Bowman's capsule. These factors cause the filtration of fluid into Bowman's capsule. This fluid is initial urine and is equivalent to protein-free plasma. In a healthy nephron, neither protein nor red blood cells pass through the filter into Bowman's capsule.

In the proximal convoluted tubule, most of the nutrients and a large amount of water are reabsorbed and taken back into blood capillaries surrounding the tubules. Salts, particularly sodium and chloride, are selectively reabsorbed according to the body's needs. Water is also reabsorbed with the salts.

The nitrogen-containing waste products of protein metabolism, urea and creatinine, pass on through the tubules to be excreted in the urine. Substances that are in excess in the body fluids, such as hydrogen ions if the fluid is too acidic, are secreted into the distal tubules to be excreted.

Two hormones play a very important role in the regulation of salt and water reabsorption. They are aldosterone, secreted by the adrenal glands, and antidiuretic hormone, secreted by the posterior pituitary gland. More will be said of these hormones when the diseases of the endocrine glands are discussed (Chapter 13).

Final urine from all the collecting ducts empties into the renal pelvis, the juncture between the kidneys and the **ureters.** It then moves down the ureters to be stored in the urinary bladder, which empties to the outside through a single tube called the **urethra.** Figure 9–2 illustrates the urinary system.

An obstruction along this path can set the stage for infection. The obstruction may be a kidney stone; an enlarged prostate gland, the male gland which surrounds the urethra; or a tumor. Any blockage causes stasis and a diminished flow of urine, and bacteria thrive in the stagnant fluid.

DISEASES OF THE KIDNEY

■ Glomerulonephritis

■ *Acute Glomerulonephritis.* Acute **glomerulonephritis** is a common disease primarily affecting children and young adults. It usually results from a previous streptococcal infection: strep throat, scarlet fever, or rheumatic fever. The symptoms are chills and fever, loss of appetite, and a general feeling of weakness. There may be edema, or puffiness, particularly in the face and ankles. A urinalysis shows **albuminuria,** the presence of the plasma protein albumin in the urine. **Hematuria,** blood in the urine, is also com-

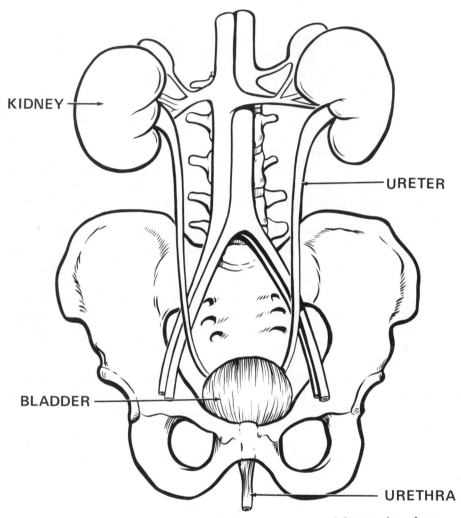

Figure 9-2. The urinary system. (*From A Programmed Approach to Anatomy and Physiology—the Urinary System, 1972. Courtesy of Robert J. Brady Co.*)

monly found. **Casts,** which are molds of kidney tubules consisting of coagulated protein and blood, are present. The signs and symptoms of acute glomerulonephritis are presented in Figure 9–3.

The presence of blood, albumin, and casts in the urine indicates that the glomeruli are diseased. Glomerulonephritis is a degenerative inflammation of the glomeruli. It is nonsuppurative, that is, no pus formation is associated with it, nor are any bacteria found.

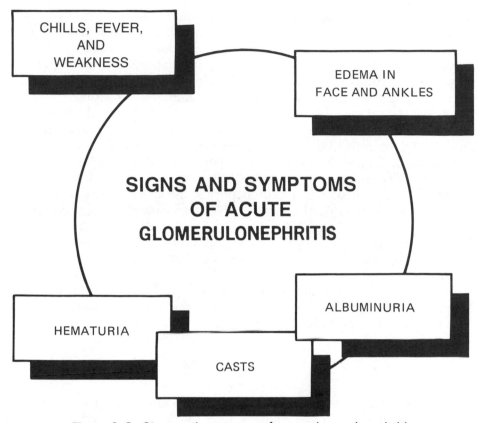

Figure 9-3. Signs and symptoms of acute glomerulonephritis.

Glomerulonephritis is a type of allergic disease caused by an antigen–antibody reaction. One to 4 weeks before the onset of the kidney inflammation, the strep infection triggers antibody production against the strep antigen. The antigen–antibody complexes become trapped in the glomeruli, blocking them and causing the inflammatory response. Numerous neutrophils crowd into the inflamed loops of the glomeruli, and blood flow to the nephrons is reduced. Less filtration into Bowman's capsule occurs, and less urine is formed.

Many glomeruli degenerate along with the nephrons they serve. This causes a shrinking of the kidney tissue. The remaining glomeruli become extremely permeable, allowing albumin and red blood cells to enter the nephrons and appear in the urine.

The prognosis for acute glomerulonephritis is generally good. Normal kidney function is restored after a period of time. Repeated attacks of acute glomerulonephritis can lead to the chronic condition.

■ *Chronic Glomerulonephritis.* Chronic glomerulonephritis may persist for many years with periods of remission and exacerbation. Hypertension generally accompanies this disease. The relationship between high blood pressure and kidney disease was discussed in Chapter 8. As more and more glomeruli are destroyed, the work of filtering the blood is accomplished by the remaining ones. Elevated blood pressure makes this possible.

A significant test to determine the extent of kidney function is to measure the specific gravity of a urine specimen. **Specific gravity** indicates the amount of dissolved substances in a sample compared with distilled water. Distilled water has a specific gravity of 1.000. The normal range for specific gravity of urine is 1.015 to 1.025, with variations throughout the day.

In advanced chronic glomerulonephritis, the specific gravity is low and fixed. This indicates that the kidney tubules are unable to concentrate the urine.

After a long period of this disease, the kidneys shrink severely and are referred to as granular contracted kidneys. They gradually atrophy, dry up, and cease functioning.

Uremia, a toxic condition of the blood, is the end result of kidney failure. Waste products not excreted by the kidney accumulate to a poisonous level in the blood.

RENAL FAILURE

Several factors can cause the renal system, or kidneys, to stop functioning. Lack of blood flow to the kidneys due to severe hemorrhage, various poisons, and severe kidney diseases are some causes of renal failure. The kidneys are unable to clear the blood of **urea** and **creatinine,** which are nitrogen-containing waste products of protein metabolism. As the level of **blood urea nitrogen (BUN)** and creatinine increases, a toxicity develops that affects the entire body. The accumulation of nitrogen-containing substances in the blood is called **azotemia.** The condition is known as uremia.

■ Acute Renal Failure

Acute renal failure is a condition that develops suddenly and that can usually be treated successfully. The cause is often decreased blood flow to the kidneys resulting from surgical shock, shock after an incompatible blood transfusion, or severe dehydration. Kidney disease or trauma can also cause renal failure.

There is a sudden drop in urine volume, or **oliguria,** or even a total stoppage of urine production known as **anuria.** The patient experiences headache and gastrointestinal distress. The breath has the odor of ammonia due to accumulation in the blood of nitrogen-containing substances. An excess of potassium, hyperkalemia, causes muscle weakness and can slow the heart to the point of cardiac arrest.

If proper treatment is administered the prognosis is good. The condition causing the kidney failure must be corrected, and restoration of the patient's blood volume to normal is very important. Fluid intake should be restricted, allowing the kidneys to rest and the nephrons to regenerate. A dialysis machine, an artificial kidney, may be used temporarily to clear the patient's blood of toxic substances.

■ Chronic Renal Failure

Chronic renal failure is a very serious disease generally ending in death. The condition develops slowly; there is no sudden drop in urinary output as there is in acute renal failure. Chronic renal failure can be the result of long-standing kidney disease such as chronic glomerulonephritis, hypertension, or diabetic nephropathy, a kidney disease resulting from diabetes mellitus.

The poisonous substances accumulate in the blood with adverse effects on all the systems. Urea is converted to ammonia, which acts as an irritant in the gastrointestinal tract to produce nausea, vomiting, and diarrhea. The nervous system is affected; vision becomes dim, mental ability is decreased, and convulsions or coma may ensue. Manifestations of chronic renal failure are summarized in Figure 9–4.

Dialysis—the artificial cleansing of the blood—may be used, but in advanced chronic renal failure it is not very successful. Although kidney transplants involve many problems, great success has been achieved in recent years. Improved antirejection medications with fewer side effects have contributed significantly to the success of transplants.

■ PYELONEPHRITIS

Pyelonephritis is a suppurative inflammation of the kidney and renal pelvis, the expanded upper end of the ureter. It is caused by pyogenic bacteria, pus-forming bacteria. *Escherichia coli,* streptococci, and staphylococci are examples of such bacteria. Interstitial tissue, the kidney tissue between the tubules, is the site of the inflammation.

The infection may be an ascending one that originates in the lower urinary tract, possibly the bladder, and spreads up into the kidneys. It may be a descending infection carried by the bloodstream or lymph. Figure 9–5 shows the possible routes of infection. Any obstruction of the urinary tract—a congenital defect, a kidney stone, or an enlarged prostate gland—paves the way for an infection due to stagnation of the urine.

Abscesses frequently form and rupture. Pus can then enter the renal

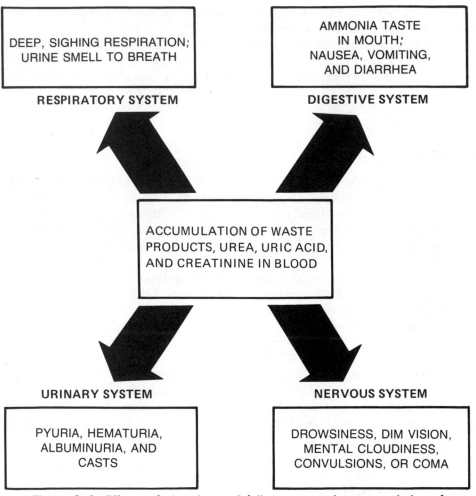

Figure 9-4. Effects of chronic renal failure—azotemia, accumulation of nitrogen-containing compounds in the blood.

pelvis and appears in the urine. This condition is called **pyuria.** The abscesses can fuse until the whole kidney is filled with pus. Renal failure occurs and uremia develops.

If the infection is less severe, healing can occur, but scar tissue will form. Fibrous scar tissue tends to contract, and as it does, the kidney shrinks and becomes a granular contracted kidney.

The symptoms of pyelonephritis are chills, high fever, and sudden back pain that spreads over the abdomen. Painful urination, **dysuria,** is experienced. Microscopic examination of the urine reveals numerous pus cells

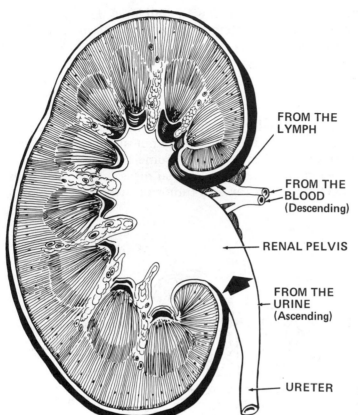

FROM THE
LYMPH

FROM THE
BLOOD
(Descending)

RENAL PELVIS

FROM THE
URINE
(Ascending)

URETER

Figure 9-5. Routes of infection for pyelonephritis.

and bacteria. Hematuria is also common. Antibiotics are prescribed to counteract the infection.

■ PYELITIS

Pyelitis is an inflammation of the renal pelvis, the juncture between the ureter and the kidney. Pyelitis, like pyelonephritis, is caused by *E. coli* or other pyogenic bacteria. It can result from a bladder infection, or the organism can be carried by the blood.

Pyelitis occurs commonly in young children, particularly girls. The urethra in females is shorter than that of males. Microorganisms from fecal material can enter from the outside and travel easily to the bladder. The infection can then spread up to the ureter to the renal pelvis. Painful urination as well as frequency and urgency are common symptoms of pyelitis. A urinalysis will reveal numerous pus cells.

This disease responds well to treatment with antibiotics. Early diagnosis and treatment are important in preventing the spread of the infection into the kidney tissue and, thus, in pyelonephritis.

■ RENAL CARCINOMA

Carcinoma of the kidney, also called **hypernephroma,** causes enlargement of the kidney and destroys the organ. The tumor may not manifest itself for a long time. Painless hematuria will eventually become the chief symptom. When the tumor has become large, and abdominal mass may be felt. This mass could then be detected on an x-ray as a tumor of the kidney.

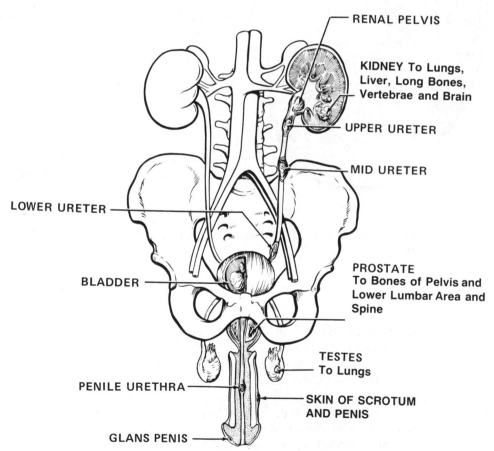

Figure 9-6. Sites of tumors and metastases in the male urogenital system, with surrounding lymph nodes affected at each site.

Metastasis to other organs often occurs before the presence of the kidney tumor is known. The malignancy frequently spreads to the lungs, the liver, bones, and the brain. Sites of metastasis from the male urogenital tract are illustrated in Figure 9–6.

Late symptoms include pain, loss of appetite, weight loss, anemia, and an elevated white blood cell count. Surgical removal is the best treatment.

A malignant tumor of the kidney that develops in very young children is **Wilms' tumor.** The tumor grows very fast and spreads through the blood and lymph vessels. The symptoms are the same as those described in renal carcinoma of an adult. Prognosis for this fast-growing cancer has improved in recent years.

■ KIDNEY STONES

Urinary calculi, kidney stones, may be present and cause no symptoms until they become lodged in the ureter. The stones then cause intense pain that radiates from the kidney area to the groin.

Calculi are formed when certain salts in the urine form a precipitate, that is, come out of solution, and grow in size. Small stones are often passed spontaneously in the urine, but larger stones may require surgery. A stone may become so large that it fills the renal pelvis completely, blocking the flow of urine. A stone of this type, named for its shape, is the staghorn calculus illustrated in Figure 9–7. A kidney containing numerous small calculi is also shown. Calcium excess often leads to stone formation. Hyperactive

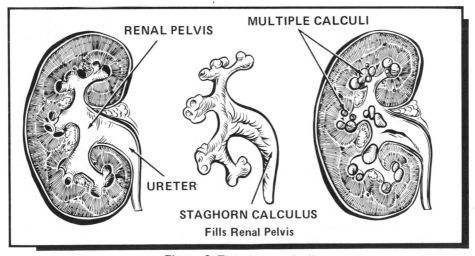

Figure 9–7. Urinary calculi.

parathyroid glands can cause the excess of circulating calcium, thus promoting urinary calculi formation.

Stones can also form in the urinary bladder. The presence of stones causes urinary tract infections as they frequently obstruct the flow of urine. The converse is also true; urinary tract infections can lead to stone formation.

Urinary calculi are sometimes partially dissolved by medication and then passed in the urine. **Lithotripsy,** the crushing of kidney stones, is now the preferable procedure to remove them, replacing the need for surgery. Laser beams have been effectively used in crushing stones, either with the patient immersed in a tank of water, a procedure called **hydrolithotripsy** or performed out of water, **nephrotripsy.** In the newest technique, the patient is immersed in a tank of water to which acoustic shock waves from a lithotripter are admitted. These shock waves shatter the hard stones into sand-sized particles that are eliminated through the urine. Drugs that prevent new stones from forming are a significant advance in treating urinary calculi, as some patients tend to develop stones repeatedly.

■ HYDRONEPHROSIS

As a result of urinary calculi, a tumor, an enlarged prostate gland, congenital defect, or other obstruction of the renal pelvis, the kidney can become extremely dilated with urine. This condition is called **hydronephrosis.** The ureters above the obstruction are dilated from the pressure of urine that is unable to bypass the obstruction and are called **hydroureters.** Figure 9–8 shows this dilated condition.

The degree of pain accompanying hydronephrosis depends on the nature of the blockage. Hematuria is generally present. If an infection develops because of the stagnation of urine, pyuria may be detected. Fever would then be a symptom too. Figure 9–9 depicts hydronephrosis of the kidney.

■ TUBERCULOSIS OF THE KIDNEY

Tuberculosis can develop in the kidney as a secondary site of infection. It usually begins in the lung, but the organism that causes tuberculosis, the tubercle bacillus, can be carried to the kidney in the bloodstream.

The lesion is similar to that of tuberculosis in the lungs. Tissue is broken down and cavities form, destroying the kidney. The necrotic tissue enters the ureter and is discharged in the urine. The tuberculous infection can then spread along the urinary tract.

Due to the breakdown of tissue, pus and blood are present in the urine. The tubercle bacilli are also found. If tuberculous lesions form in the

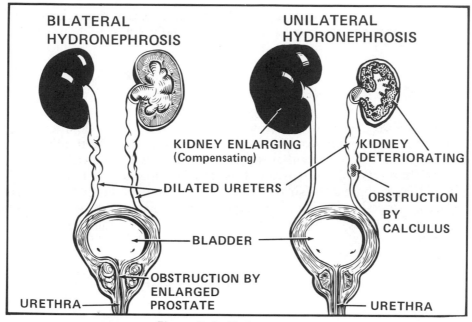

BILATERAL
HYDRONEPHROSIS

UNILATERAL
HYDRONEPHROSIS

KIDNEY ENLARGING
(Compensating)

KIDNEY
DETERIORATING

DILATED URETERS

OBSTRUCTION
BY
CALCULUS

BLADDER

OBSTRUCTION BY
ENLARGED
PROSTATE

URETHRA

URETHRA

Figure 9-8. Hydronephrosis.

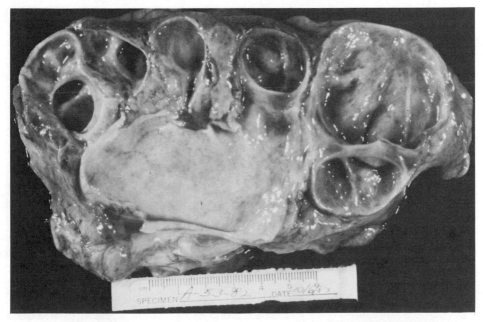

Figure 9-9. Hydronephrosis. (*Courtesy of Dr. David R. Duffell.*)

bladder wall, urination becomes painful. The bladder is a muscular sac and contractions irritate the lesion. Uremia is the end result if both kidneys are affected.

■ POLYCYSTIC KIDNEY

Polycystic kidney is a congenital anomaly, an error in development. Both kidneys are usually involved in this hereditary disease. The multiple cysts are dilated kidney tubules that do not open into the renal pelvis as they should. The cysts enlarge, fuse, and usually become infected. As the cysts enlarge they compress the surrounding kidney tissue. Figure 9–10 illustrates the polycystic kidney of an adult. Hypertension develops as a result of this long-standing kidney disease. The kidneys eventually fail, and death is caused by uremia.

DISEASES OF THE URINARY BLADDER AND URETHRA

■ Cystitis

Cystitis is an inflammation of the urinary bladder. It is more common in women than in men due to their shorter urethra. The chief causative agent

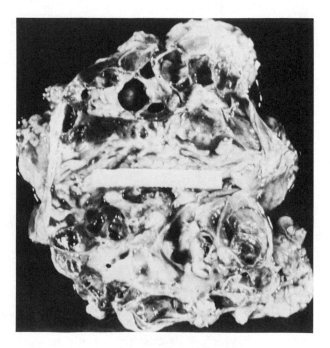

Figure 9-10. A cut view of polycystic kidney. (*Courtesy of Dr. David R. Duffell.*)

is one present in fecal material, *Escherichia coli,* which can reach the urinary opening and travel upward to the bladder. Cystitis can also develop from sexual intercourse when infecting organisms around the vaginal opening spread to the urinary opening.

The symptoms are urinary frequency, urgency, and a burning sensation during urination. Microscopic examination of the urine reveals bacteria, pus, and casts. As in any inflammation, leukocytes are present.

■ Carcinoma of the Bladder

Certain chemicals used in industry have been linked to carcinoma of the urinary bladder. The tumor may grow, sending fingerlike projections into the lumen of the bladder. These tumors can be seen with a **cystoscope** and removed, but they tend to recur. A more invasive pattern of growth develops where the tumor infiltrates the bladder wall. Surgery is then required to remove the malignant section (Figure 9–11).

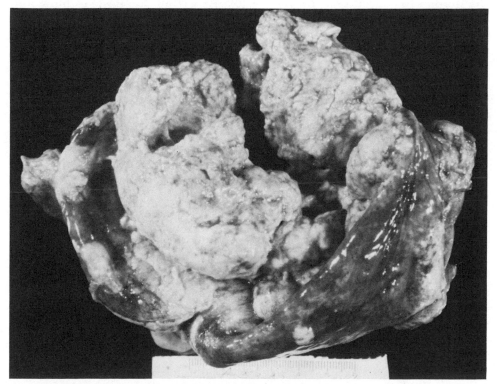

Figure 9-11. Advanced carcinoma of the bladder. (*Courtesy of Dr. David R. Duffell.*)

■ Urethritis

Any part of the urinary tract can become inflamed, and the urethra is no exception. This inflammation is called **urethritis.** In males the infecting organism is usually a gonococcus, although other bacteria, viruses, or chemicals can cause this disease. The symptoms of urethritis include a discharge of pus from the urethra, an itching sensation at the opening of the urethra, and a burning sensation during urination. In females urethritis frequently accompanies cystitis. An obstruction at the urinary opening is sometimes responsible for the inflammation in women.

ABNORMAL CONDITIONS OF THE URINE

Urine is normally yellow or amber, but hematuria (blood in the urine) can darken the color to a reddish brown. The degree of color depends on the amount of water the urine contains. Urine is pale in the case of diabetics, whose water output is large. In long-standing kidney diseases, the ability of the tubules to concentrate the urine is lost. As a result the urine is dilute and pale. Specific gravity is low in this case.

The pH of urine has a broad range. The ability of the kidneys to excrete an acid or an alkaline urine is a mechanism for maintaining the narrow range of pH tolerated by the blood. Urine specimens should be examined when fresh. They tend to become alkaline on standing due to bacterial contamination. Urine from a cystitic patient tends to be alkaline for the same reason.

Albuminuria indicates inflammation of the urinary tract, particularly of the gomeruli. The inflammation increases the permeability of blood vessels, allowing the protein, albumin, to enter the nephrons and appear in the urine. This loss reduces the level of protein in the blood, causing the condition called **hypoproteinemia.**

The presence of sugar (glucose) in the urine usually indicates diabetes mellitus. This is not a disease of the kidneys but of the endocrine glands of the pancreas. Diabetes over a period of time does affect the kidneys adversely.

Hematuria may be obvious to the naked eye or require microscopic determination. Any serious disease of the urinary tract may give this symptom: glomerulonephritis, kidney stones, tuberculosis, cystitis, or tumors. If the passage of urine is accompanied by pain, a stone or tuberculosis may be the cause. Painless hematuria indicates the possibility of a malignant tumor in the urinary system.

Pyuria results from a suppurative inflammation caused by pyogenic bacteria. Pus causes the urine to appear cloudy. Microscopic examination of the urine reveals numerous pus cells, or polymorphs, engaged in fighting the infection. Diseases such as pyelonephritis, pyelitis, tuberculosis, and cystitis show pus in the urine.

Casts are cylindrical rods, molds of kidney tubules. They consist of coagulated protein, a substance not normally present in kidney tubules. Casts can include various kinds of blood cells, as well as epithelial cells from the lining of the urinary tract. Casts always indicate inflammation.

Microscopic examination determines the presence or absence of bacteria. Bacteria are found in tuberculosis of the kidney, pyelonephritis, and frequently, cystitis. For microscopic examinations a urine sample may be removed from the bladder by catheterization to ensure that no external contamination occurs.

DIAGNOSTIC TESTS

Kidney disease symptoms such as pain, dysuria (painful urination), blood or pus in the urine, or edema indicate that specific diagnostic tests should be performed. Edema is caused by the loss of protein from the blood, resulting in hypoproteinemia. Normally these blood proteins have a water-holding power within the blood vessels. With their depletion, fluid moves out of the capillaries and into the tissues, causing swelling or puffiness.

A cystoscopic examination enables the physician to view the inside of the bladder and urethra. The cystoscope is a long, lighted instrument resembling a hollow tube. Tumors, stones, or inflammations may be identified with this device. Using an additional instrument, small tumors may be removed or biopsied. Stones in the bladder can be crushed and removed.

The **intravenous pyelogram (IVP)** allows the visualization of the urinary system by means of contrast dyes injected into the veins followed by x-ray examination. When these dyes concentrate in the urinary system, it is possible to note tumors, obstructions, or other deformities.

SUMMARY

The importance of kidney function was reviewed to show the seriousness of kidney disease. Although acute glomerulonephritis generally has a good prognosis, repeated attacks can lead to chronic glomerulonephritis. This chronic disease, possibly persisting for many years, is one that often ends with kidney failure. Kidney failure can be acute due to a newly developed condition. If the cause of the kidney failure is treated, renal function is restored to normal. Chronic renal failure does not respond to treatment and generally ends with uremia. Pyelonephritis is a destructive, suppurative inflammation of the kidney. Abscesses usually form and pus appears in the urine. If not treated, renal failure results. Various other urinary tract infections were considered: cystitis, pyelitis, and urethritis. These infections frequently follow some obstruction of the flow of urine. Urinary calculi, tumors, and congenital anomalies can cause such blockages. Symptoms of kidney disease may include pain, painful urination, and blood or pus in the urine. Edema is also a symptom of certain kidney diseases. An abnormal mass may be felt when a tumor of the kidney or bladder is large. This is a late sign of malignancy, and metastases have probably already occurred. Interpretations of abnormal conditions of the urine were also discussed along with certain diagnostic procedures.

STUDY QUESTIONS

1. Name three functions of the kidney.
2. Explain the formation of urine in terms of (a) filtration, (b) reabsorption, and (c) secretion.
3. What is the relationship between a streptococcal infection and glomerulonephritis?
4. Name the abnormal findings in the urine of an acute glomerulonephritic patient.
5. Why is the specific gravity of urine low and fixed in a patient with chronic glomerulonephritis?
6. What are some causes of (a) acute renal failure and (b) chronic renal failure?
7. Explain the possible routes of entry of the infecting organisms in pyelonephritis.
8. Why is pus found in the urine in pyelonephritis and not in acute glomerulonephritis?
9. What is the difference between pyelitis and pyelonephritis?
10. What is the greatest danger in renal carcinoma?
11. Explain the complications after kidney stone formation.
12. What is lithotripsy?
13. What abnormal substances appear in the urine of a patient with tuberculosis of the kidney?
14. Which of the kidney diseases studied is hereditary?
15. Why is cystitis more common in women than in men?
16. Name five conditions that may be present in a urine specimen indicating kidney disease.

CHAPTER 10

Diseases of the Digestive System

Food would be of no value to us if it were not broken down into units small enough to be absorbed out of the gastrointestinal tract and into the bloodstream. The digestive system accomplishes this by breaking down carbohydrates to glucose and other simple sugars, proteins to amino acids, and lipids or fats to fatty acids and glycerides. Once these small units are absorbed by the blood, they are distributed to all the cells and tissues of the body. It is only in the cells that these units are metabolized—that is used for production of energy—and converted into other material needed by the cells.

THE DIGESTIVE PROCESS

Digestion begins in the mouth with chewing, the mechanical breakdown of food. Salivation, the secretion of saliva, moistens the food and provides an enzyme for initial digestion of starch. The food is then swallowed and passes through the pharynx, or throat, and into the esophagus.

The moistened food moves down the esophagus to the stomach, where the digestion of proteins, large complex molecules, begins. A sphincter muscle at the juncture of the esophagus and stomach prevents regurgitation. The stomach secretes gastric juice that contains enzymes—biological catalysts—that act on protein. Gastric juice also contains hydrochloric acid, which activates these enzymes. The high acidity of gastric contents would be very irritating to the stomach lining if the lining were not protected by a thick covering of mucus. A great deal of moistening and mixing occurs within the stomach.

The next part of the gastrointestinal tract is the small intestine. The entrance to this intestine is guarded by a sphincter muscle, the **pyloric sphincter.** This sphincter is closed until it receives nerve and hormonal signals to relax and open. The moistened food, referred to as chyme at this stage, is propelled along its course by rhythmical smooth muscle contractions called **peristalsis.**

The greatest amount of digestion occurs in the first part of the small intestine, the duodenum. Intestinal juice contains mucus and is rich in enzymes. Here digestive substances from other organs enter by means of ducts. The pancreas secretes enzymes for the digestion of protein, lipid, and carbohydrate. It also secretes an alkaline solution for the neutralization of acid carried into the small intestine from the stomach. This pancreatic juice enters the duodenum through the pancreatic duct.

Bile, secreted by the liver and stored in the gallbladder, enters the duodenum through the common bile duct. Bile is not an enzyme but an emulsifier, a substance that allows the mixing of fat and water much like the action of soap. The action of bile enables the lipid enzymes to digest fat into small, absorbable units.

When digestion is complete, the nutrients are absorbed into blood capillaries and lymph vessels in the intestinal wall. The inner surface of the small intestine is arranged to provide the greatest amount of surface area possible for digestion and absorption. This mucosal surface contains numerous fingerlike projections called villi, each of which contains blood capillaries and lymph vessels for absorption (Figure 10–1).

Material not digested passes into the large intestine, or colon. The first part of the colon is a blind sac, the cecum. The appendix, a nonfunctional structure is attached to this sac. Water and minerals are absorbed from the large intestine, and the remaining matter is excreted as feces. Figure 10–2 illustrates the complete digestive tract.

Diseases of the gastrointestinal tract are caused by a variety of factors. Tumors or malformations can produce obstructions, the mucous membrane lining can become ulcerated, and cells can fail to function in their secretory or absorptive action.

In this chapter the diseases of each part of the digestive tract will be described. These include diseases of the mouth, esophagus, stomach, and small and large intestines. In the next chapter, diseases of the accessory organs of digestion—the pancreas, liver, and gallbladder—will be covered.

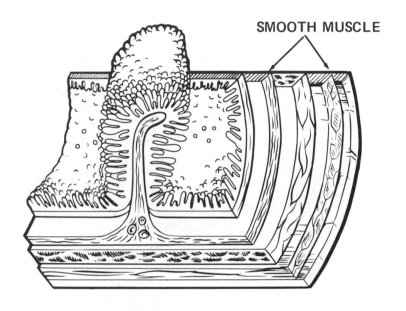

SMOOTH MUSCLE

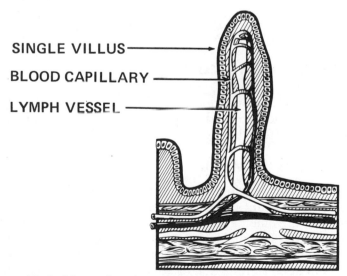

SINGLE VILLUS

BLOOD CAPILLARY

LYMPH VESSEL

Figure 10-1. Mucosal surface of the small intestine.

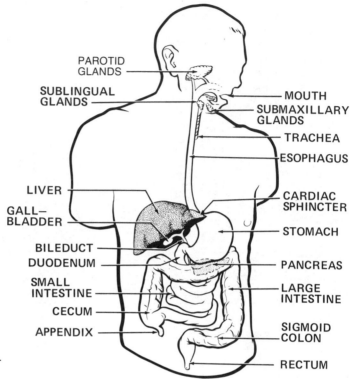

Figure 10-2. The digestive tract.

DISEASES OF THE MOUTH

It would be impossible in a book this size to cover oral pathology, diseases of the teeth and gums, adequately. This study will be limited to the diseases that directly affect the digestive system.

■ Cancer of the Mouth

Neoplasms can develop in any part of the mouth: gums, cheeks, or palate. A common malignant tumor is carcinoma of the lip. It occurs more often in men than in women and generally affects the lower lip. It may be related to pipe smoking. This malignancy may develop from a chronic lesion, a sore or crack that does not heal. It is a type of cancer that responds well to treatment such as radiation or surgery. If it is not treated, it will spread.

A malignant tumor can develop on the tongue, usually at the edge. Carcinoma of the tongue may be caused by a chronic irritation from a tooth or denture. This cancer spreads rapidly and is more difficult to treat than cancer of the lip.

DIAGNOSTIC PROCEDURES FOR THE DIGESTIVE TRACT

A combination of procedures enables the physician to view the inside of the digestive tract. To make the digestive tract stand out on an x-ray film or fluoroscope, the patient swallows a barium mixture before the examination. **Barium** is opaque to x-rays, so the rays do not pass through it. The silhouette produced shows tumors, malformations, or other obstructions that may be present. Motion pictures can even be taken of the movement of barium through the gastrointestinal tract. These pictures can show abnormalities of smooth muscle action or improperly functioning sphincters.

Certain lesions of the inner wall of the digestive tract do not show up on x-ray examination. To view this inner surface an instrument called an **endoscope** is used. It is a hollow tube with a lens and light system. There is an endoscope designed specially for each part of the digestive tract. It is possible with this technique to take a biopsy of a suspected malignant lesion.

DISEASES OF THE ESOPHAGUS

The **esophagoscope** is the endoscope used to view the inside of the esophagus. It may be used in combination with a microscopic study of the cells of the esophagus. Malignant tumors tend to shed cells, as was mentioned in Chapter 3. Washings from the esophagus can be examined for the presence of cancer cells.

■ Cancer of the Esophagus

A malignant tumor of the esophagus narrows the lumen causing the principal symptom, difficulty in swallowing, or **dysphagia.** The obstruction causes vomiting, and the patient may experience a bad taste in his or her mouth or bad breath. There is accompanying weight loss because of the inability to eat.

The carcinoma spreads into adjacent organs and to remote sites through the lymph vessels. It frequently metastasizes before it is detected. Prognosis for cancer of the esophagus is poor.

■ Esophageal Varices

Varicose veins sometimes develop in the esophagus and are called esophageal varices. They result from pressure within the veins. This pressure develops when venous return to the liver is obstructed. The veins appear very dilated and knotty. Esophageal varices are frequently a complication of cirrhosis of the liver. The destruction of liver tissue interferes with drainage of the portal vein. Congestion then builds within the veins, and those of the esophagus are unable to empty. The most serious danger in esophageal varices is that of hemorrhage.

◼ Esophagitis

The most common cause of esophagitis, inflammation of the esophagus, is a **reflux**—a back flow of the acid contents of the stomach. This is caused by an incompetent **cardiac sphincter.** The acid of the stomach is an irritant to the lining of the esophagus and stimulates an inflammatory response. The various causes of **esophagitis** are illustrated in Figure 10–3.

The patient experiences burning chest pains, which can resemble the pain of heart disease. The pain may follow eating or drinking, and some vomiting of blood **(hematemesis)** may occur.

Treatment includes a nonirritating diet and antacids. Frequent small meals are recommended. Alcohol is an irritant to the inflamed mucosal lining and should be avoided.

◼ Hiatal Hernia

A hernia is the protrusion of part of an organ through a muscular wall or body opening. A **hiatal hernia** is the protrusion of part of the stomach through the diaphragm at the point where the esophagus joins the stomach. Figure 10–4 shows this condition.

The patient experiences indigestion and heartburn after eating and may feel short of breath. Avoidance of irritants such as spicy foods and caffeine and frequent small meals may be adequate treatment. If the patient is obese, weight loss is recommended. Various kinds of supports can some-

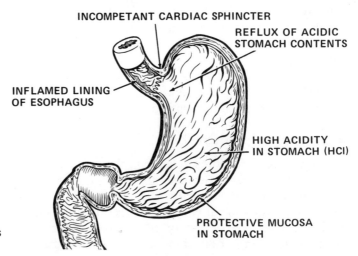

Figure 10-3. Various causes of esophagitis.

INCOMPETANT CARDIAC SPHINCTER

REFLUX OF ACIDIC STOMACH CONTENTS

INFLAMED LINING OF ESOPHAGUS

HIGH ACIDITY IN STOMACH (HCl)

PROTECTIVE MUCOSA IN STOMACH

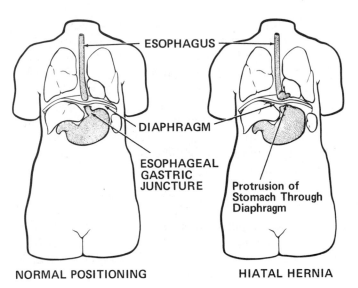

ESOPHAGUS

DIAPHRAGM

ESOPHAGEAL
GASTRIC
JUNCTURE

Protrusion of
Stomach Through
Diaphragm

NORMAL POSITIONING   HIATAL HERNIA

Figure 10-4. Hiatal hernia.

times be worn to hold the organs in place. Surgery is often required to correct the defect.

DISEASES OF THE STOMACH

When a person experiences indigestion (**dyspepsia**), abdominal pain, or bleeding from the digestive tract, it is difficult to know the exact cause. Many gastrointestinal disorders have similar symptoms. Due to the arrangement of the abdominal nerves, there is sometimes referred pain. This pain is felt in one area but is caused in another.

Many excellent diagnostic procedures are available for abnormalities of the digestive system. In addition to barium x-ray films and fluoroscopy, which show the contour of the gastrointestinal tract, the endoscope is used to view the inside of the organs. The specific endoscope for the stomach is the **gastroscope.**

Washings from the stomach may reveal cancer cells. This procedure can distinguish between a malignant and benign ulcer. Malignant tumors frequently ulcerate. Analysis of gastric juice, obtained by means of a stomach tube, reveals abnormalities of various secretions. Excessive secretion or the lack of secretion are very significant diagnostically.

■ Gastritis

Acute **gastritis** is an inflammation of the stomach. It is caused by some agent that acts as an irritant, such as aspirin or excessive coffee, tobacco, or alcohol, or by an infection. Vomiting of blood frequently occurs as the principal symptom. **Gastroscopy** is extremely valuable in diagnosing this disease. A camera may be attached to the gastroscope and the entire inner stomach photographed. Gastritis cannot be seen on an x-ray, but it can be viewed well with this technique.

If bleeding of the mucous membrane is observed by gastroscopy, it can sometimes be stopped with the use of ice water, which constricts the small blood vessels. Acute alcoholism is a major cause of hemorrhagic gastritis. Alcohol stimulates acid secretion, which irritates the mucosa. If the bleeding cannot be controlled, surgery may be required.

■ Chronic Atrophic Gastritis

Lack of intrinsic factor as a cause of pernicious anemia was described in Chapter 6. In the absence of intrinsic factor, vitamin B_{12} cannot be absorbed. In cancer of the stomach neither intrinsic factor nor hydrochloric acid is secreted. This inability of the **mucosal** lining of the stomach to secrete its normal juices is due to chronic atrophic gastritis. Little can be done to treat the disease as the name, **atrophic** (wasting), suggests. It is a degenerative condition. Irritants such as alcohol, aspirin, and certain foods should be avoided.

■ Ulcers

Ulcers are lesions that can occur on any body surface where necrotic tissue forms as a result of inflammation and is sloughed off, leaving a hole. Ulcers of the stomach and small intestine are termed **peptic ulcers.** They are due in part to the action of pepsin, a proteolytic enzyme secreted by the stomach. Figure 10–5 shows a peptic ulcer of the stomach. There are differences between ulcers of the stomach and those of the duodenum.

■ *Gastric Ulcer.* The patient with a **gastric ulcer** experiences nausea, vomiting, and abdominal pain that is relieved by antacids. At times bleeding from the upper part of the digestive tract occurs. A potential complication of any ulcer is hemorrhage.

Another danger in an ulcer patient is perforation. As the ulcer erodes deeper into the underlying tissue, the wall of the organ can actually rupture. The contents of the organ then spill out into the peritoneal cavity, setting up the conditions for a potentially fatal infection.

Obstruction of the gastrointestinal tract can result from an ulcer and the scar tissue surrounding it. This is most likely to occur in a narrow area of the stomach, such as the area of the pyloric sphincter. The pain of the ulcer can cause the sphincter to go into spasm, also resulting in obstruction.

In the case of a gastric ulcer, acid secretion by the stomach may be normal or even below normal. The ulceration is thought to be caused by

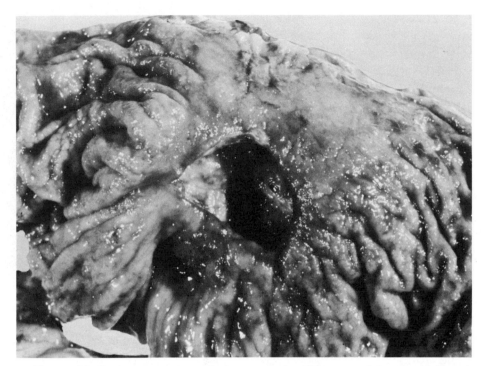

Figure 10-5. A peptic ulcer of the stomach. (*Courtesy of Dr. David R. Duffell.*)

intestinal juice, including bile, that is regurgitated through the pyloric sphincter. The gastric mucosa becomes irritated by this bile-containing secretion and the lesion develops.

To assure the proper diagnosis of the lesion, the methods described earlier for viewing and testing the inner surface of the stomach should be performed. An ulcer may be either malignant or benign; a biopsy and cell study will differentiate between the two.

■ Cancer of the Stomach

Pain is not an early sign of stomach cancer. Carcinoma of the stomach, which is more common in men than in women, may be very advanced before it is detected. It may even have spread to the liver and surrounding organs through the lymph and blood vessels. Figure 10–6 shows an infiltrating adenocarcinoma that has invaded the liver. Early symptoms are vague; loss of appetite, heartburn, and general stomach distress. Blood may be vomited or appear in the feces. Pernicious anemia generally accompanies cancer of the stomach. In both diseases, the gastric mucosa fails to secrete intrinsic factor. Gastric analysis by means of a stomach tube demonstrates

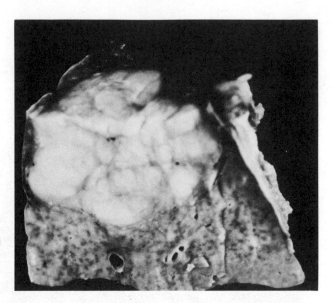

Figure 10-6. An infiltrating adenocarcinoma of the stomach invading the liver. (*Courtesy of Dr. David R. Duffell.*)

the absence of hydrochloric acid, or **achlorhydria.** Biopsy of any lesions seen through the gastroscope is an essential diagnostic procedure for carcinoma of the stomach.

The malignancy may be a large mass projecting into the lumen of the stomach or it may invade the stomach wall, causing it to thicken. These patterns of growth are illustrated in Figure 10–7A. As the tumor grows, the lumen is narrowed to the point of obstruction. The remainder of the

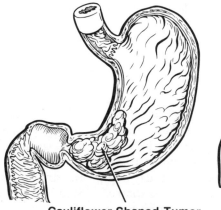 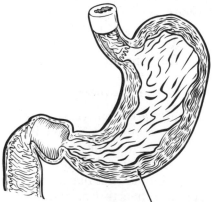

Cauliflower-Shaped Tumor Projecting into Lumen   **Malignant Invasion of Stomach Wall Causing it to Thicken**

Figure 10-7. A. Forms of gastric carcinoma.

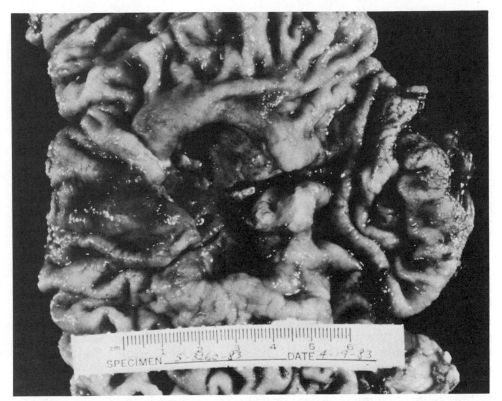

Figure 10-7. **B.** Photograph of a stomach cancer. (*Courtesy of Dr. David R. Duffell.*)

stomach becomes extremely dilated due to the blockage. Pain is experienced from the pressure on nerve endings. Infection frequently accompanies cancer, which causes additional pain. Figure 10–7B shows an actual photograph of a specimen of stomach cancer.

The etiology of this malignancy is not known. Current research is investigating the relationship between food preservatives and cancer. Studies correlating dietary habits and the incidence of stomach carcinoma are also being made. Good prognosis for this disease depends on early detection and treatment.

DISEASES OF THE INTESTINES

■ Duodenal Ulcer

The patient with **duodenal ulcers** usually has an excessive secretion of hydrochloric acid. This acid secretion of the stomach is carried into the duodenum, where the ulceration develops. The mucous membrane becomes necrotic; the acid eats away the dead tissue, leaving a hole.

Hydrochloric acid secretion is under nerve and hormonal control. An ulcer patient frequently has a nervous temperament, is high-strung, and prone to worry. Stressful situations affect the nerves that increase acid secretions.

Ulcer pain is caused by the action of hydrochloric acid on the raw surface of the lesion. Normally, the inner lining of the digestive tract is protected from the acid by a thick layer of mucus. The muscular contractions of peristalsis also intensify the pain.

Abdominal ulcer pain is relieved by antacids and temporarily by food, which acts as a protection from the acid. Bleeding from the ulcer is common and may appear as hematemesis, bloody vomitus, or as dark blood in the stools. Blood from the upper part of the digestive tract gives the stools a dark, tarry appearance, which is referred to as **melena.**

Ulcers can usually be healed by medication, antacids, and proper diet, the avoidance of irritants, gas producers, and fried food. If the ulcer is stress- or tension-related, certain changes in the patient's life might be advantageous. Even a change in the patient's psychological approach to the stressful situation can be beneficial.

If the ulcer is untreated, serious consequences can result. Severe hemorrhage, which may even lead to shock, is a complication of ulcers. It is possible for a large artery at the base of the ulcer to rupture as the erosion of the lesion goes deeper into underlying tissues. If an ulcer perforates, that is, breaks through the intestinal or gastric wall, there is sudden and intense abdominal pain. Surgery is required immediately. **Peritonitis,** inflammation of the lining of the abdominal cavity, usually results when the digestive contents enter the cavity, as this material contains numerous bacteria. The spread of peritonitis throughout the entire abdominal cavity is sometimes impeded by adhesions. The fibrous tissue of the adhesions can serve a purpose in localizing the inflammation.

Obstruction in the digestive tract is another complication of ulcers. It develops from the swelling of the inflamed area and fibrous scar tissue that forms around the ulcer. The complications of peptic ulcers are summarized in Figure 10–8.

■ Regional Enteritis (Crohn's Disease)

Regional enteritis is an inflammatory disease of the intestine. It affects most frequently young adults, particularly females. The intestinal walls become thick and rigid. As the wall thickens with the formation of fibrous tissue, the lumen is narrowed and a chronic obstruction can develop.

The cause of regional enteritis is not known. There seems to be a psychogenic element involved; stress or emotional upsets are frequently related to the onset of relapse of the disease.

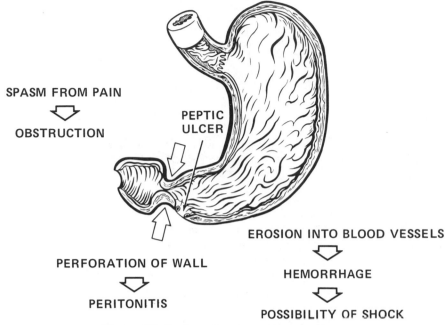

SPASM FROM PAIN

⇩

OBSTRUCTION

PEPTIC ULCER

EROSION INTO BLOOD VESSELS

⇩

HEMORRHAGE

⇩

POSSIBILITY OF SHOCK

PERFORATION OF WALL

⇩

PERITONITIS

Figure 10-8. Complications of peptic ulcers.

The pain of regional enteritis resembles that of appendicitis; it is in the lower right quadrant of the abdomen. A tender mass may be felt in this area. There is frequently an alternation between diarrhea and constipation. Melena, dark stools containing blood pigments, is common. The severe diarrhea can cause an electrolyte imbalance because of the large amount of water and salt lost in the stools.

Anorexia, nausea, and vomiting lead to a loss of weight. Periods of exacerbation and remission are common. In severe cases, hemorrhage or perforation is a threat.

Regional enteritis is usually treated with medication such as cortico-steroids. Surgery is not performed unless complications demand it.

■ Appendicitis

Appendicitis is an acute inflammation of the appendix usually caused by infection or obstruction. The wormlike shape of the appendix and its location on the cecum make it a trap for fecal material, which contains bacteria, particularly *Escherichia coli*. Figure 10–9 illustrates this potential site of infection.

The pain of appendicitis is not always typical. It often begins in the middle of the abdomen and shifts to the lower right quadrant. Nausea, vomiting, and fever are often symptoms. Leukocytosis is indicative of the

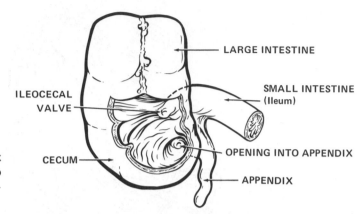

Figure 10-9. Appendix attached to cecum, into which the small intestine empties.

inflammation. Perforated ulcer, kidney stones, pancreatitis, and other diseases have similar symptoms, making diagnosis difficult.

The inflamed appendix becomes swollen, red, and covered with an inflammatory exudate. Because the swelling interferes with circulation, it is possible for **gangrene** to develop. The appendix then becomes green and black.

The wall of the appendix can become thin and rupture. Fecal material then spills out into the peritoneal cavity, causing peritonitis. Before antibiotic treatment, peritonitis was almost always fatal. Rupture of the appendix tends to give relief from the pain, which is very misleading. Surgery should be performed before rupture occurs.

■ Malabsorption Syndrome

A person unable to absorb fat or some other substance from the small intestine is said to have **malabsorption** syndrome. Defective mucosal cells can account for this abnormality. Because fat cannot be absorbed from the intestine it passes into the feces. The result is unformed, fatty, pale stools that have a terrible stench. The fat content causes the stools to float.

Many other diseases cause secondary malabsorption syndrome. A diseased pancreas or blocked pancreatic duct deprives the small intestine of lipases. In the absence of the enzymes, fat is not digested and cannot be absorbed.

Inadequate bile secretion, due to liver disease or a blocked bile duct, will also prevent lipid digestion and cause secondary malabsorption. One of the complications of the malabsorption syndrome is a bleeding tendency. Vitamin K, a fat-soluble vitamin that is essential to the blood clotting mechanism, cannot be absorbed.

Treatment for malabsorption syndrome depends on its cause. Diet is carefully controlled. Supplements are administered, such as the fat-soluble vitamins A, D, E, and K, which are not being absorbed.

■ Diverticulosis

A diverticulum is a little pouch or sac that forms in the intestine as the mucosal lining pushes through the underlying muscle layer. If there are many of these pouches, and their number tends to increase with age, the condition is called **diverticulosis.** There are usually no symptoms, but the diverticula can be seen on x-rays.

■ Diverticulitis

Diverticulitis is an inflammation of the diverticula. The inflammation occurs when the sacs become impacted with fecal material and bacteria. The patient experiences low cramplike pain, usually on the left side of the abdomen. As inflammation spreads, the lumen of the colon is narrowed and an obstruction can develop. Abscesses frequently form. Antibiotic therapy, together with a controlled diet, is usually effective. Figure 10–10 shows an example of diverticulitis.

■ Chronic Ulcerative Colitis

Chronic ulcerative colitis is a serious inflammation of the colon, the origin of which is unknown. A **psychogenic factor** may be involved, as the condition is often aggravated by stress. Persons of high-strung, neurotic temperament are most prone to the disease. Hypersensitivity to certain foods may play a part in the course of the disease. Chronic ulcerative colitis may be an

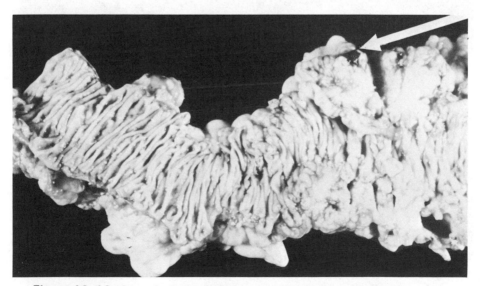

Figure 10–10. Diverticulosis with diverticulitis. Arrow indicates the thickened inflamed wall. (*Courtesy of Dr. David R. Duffell.*)

autoimmune disease in which the person's antibodies destroy the body's own tissue. Periods of remission and exacerbation are characteristic of ulcerative colitis.

There is extensive ulceration of the colon and rectum. Diarrhea with pus, blood, and mucus in the stools is the typical symptom. Cramplike pain is experienced in the lower abdomen. Anemia often accompanies ulcerative colitis because of the chronic blood loss through the rectum.

The colon of a chronic ulcerative colitis patient has a characteristic appearance on x-ray examination. The normal pouchlike markings of the colon, the haustra, are lacking. The colon appears straight and rigid, and is referred to as a "pipe-stem" colon (Figure 10–11A).

There is a high risk of a colon malignancy developing as a complication of long-standing ulcerative colitis. The incidence of this is high. Figure 10–11B shows a large polyp, which may become malignant.

Treatment of any chronic disease is difficult. The symptoms of chronic ulcerative colitis may be alleviated if certain stressful conditions are removed. Foods found to aggravate the disease should be avoided. Because the patient is usually of a very nervous temperament, mild sedation may be helpful. Corticosteroids are sometimes administered.

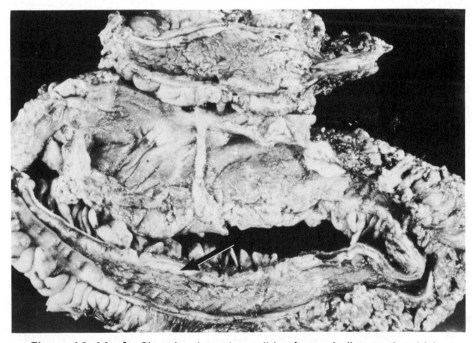

Figure 10–11. A. Chronic ulcerative colitis. Arrow indicates the thickened rigid wall referred to as a "pipe-stem" colon. (*Courtesy of Dr. David R. Duffell.*)

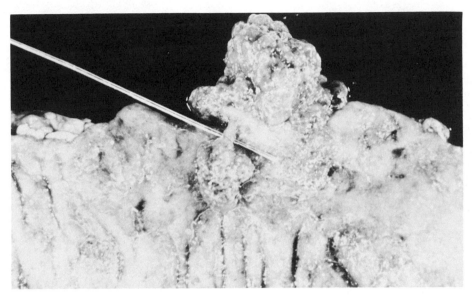

Figure 10-11. B. Large polyp (seen over probe) in chronic ulcerative colitis. (*Courtesy of Dr. David R. Duffell.*)

If the patient does not respond to these treatments, surgery may be necessary, occasionally requiring a colostomy. A **colostomy** is an artificial opening in the abdominal wall with a segment of the large intestine attached. Evacuation of the feces is through this opening. A colostomy may be temporary or permanent depending on the nature of the colon surgery.

■ Carcinoma of the Colon and Rectum

Carcinoma of the colon and rectum is a leading cause of death from cancer in the United States, yet it can be more easily diagnosed than many other cancers. The mass is often felt by rectal examination or seen with the protoscope or colonoscope, endoscopes used for the rectum and colon. If detected early, it responds well to surgical treatment.

The symptoms vary according to the site of the malignancy. A change in bowel habits—diarrhea or constipation—is symptomatic. As the tumor grows there may be abdominal discomfort and pressure. Blood often appears in the stools. Continuous blood loss from the malignant tumor causes anemia.

The mass can partially or completely obstruct the **lumen** of the colon. As the tumor invades underlying tissue, the cancer cells spread through the lymph vessels and veins.

As in all cancers, early detection and treatment are essential to prevent its spread. Most malignancies of the large intestine are in the rectum or the sigmoid colon (see Figure 10-9). This makes their detection and removal easier than malignant tumors in other areas of the digestive tract. A colostomy may be necessary.

There are two diseases that predispose to cancer of the colon: longstanding ulcerative colitis, which has been described, and familial polyposis of the colon. Familial polyposis is a hereditary disease in which numerous polyps develop in the intestinal tract. The polyps give no symptoms until a malignancy develops, but this is the usual outcome. An example of familial polyposis is seen in Figure 10–12.

■ Intestinal Obstructions

An obstruction can occur anywhere along the intestinal tract, and the contents within the tract are unable to move forward. **Obstructions** are classed as **organic** when there is some material blockage, or as **paralytic,** in which case there is a decrease in peristalsis preventing the propulsion of intestinal contents.

Tumors and hernias, both hiatal and inguinal, can cause organic obstructions. The intestine may be twisted on itself, a condition known as **volvulus** that may be unwound surgically. The intestine may be kinked, allowing nothing to pass. Adhesions, the linking together of two surfaces normally separate, can distort the tract. Abdominal adhesions sometimes follow

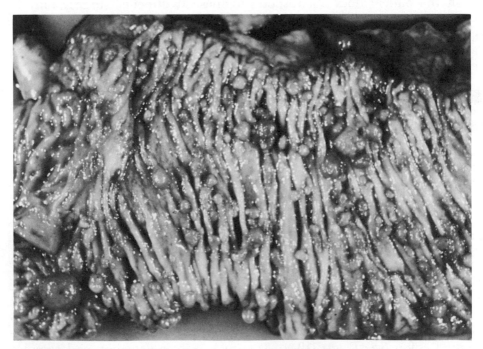

Figure 10–12. Familial polyposis. Note number of polyps. (*Courtesy of Dr. David R. Duffell.*)

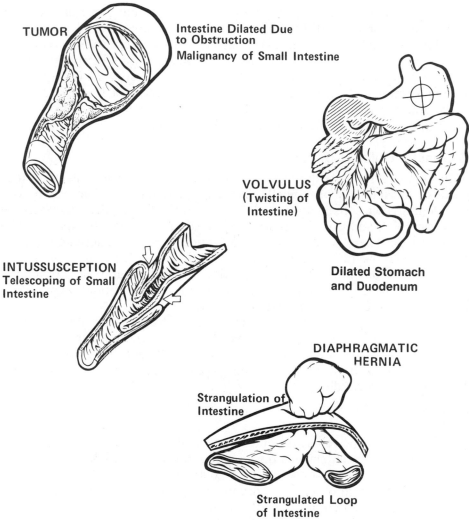

Figure 10-13. Organic obstructions of the intestinal tract.

surgery, when fibrous connective tissue grows around the incision. Adhesions also develop as a result of inflammation. Another type of organic obstruction is **intussusception,** in which a segment of intestine telescopes into the part forward to it. This occurs more often in children than in adults. Figure 10–13 shows various types of organic obstructions.

A paralytic obstruction can result from peritonitis. If a loop of small intestine is surrounded by pus from the infection, the smooth muscle of the intestinal wall cannot contract. Sphincters can go into spasm and fail to open as a result of intense pain.

If an acute organic obstruction develops, the patient experiences severe pain. The abdomen is distended and vomiting occurs. There is complete constipation; not even gas (**flatus**) is passed. This is a very serious condition, and the patient must be watched closely. Sometimes the obstruction can be relieved by means of a suction tube, but frequently surgery is required. If the obstruction is a strangulated hernia, a protrusion of intestine through the abdominal wall, surgery is required. The blood supply is cut off to the strangulated segment, and it can become gangrenous.

■ Spastic Colon (Colitis)

Many of the symptoms described for diseases of the lower intestinal tract are also characteristic of a **spastic colon,** or irritable bowel. These symptoms include diarrhea, constipation, and abdominal pain. The difference between a spastic colon and the diseases already discussed is that the spastic colon has no lesion. There is no tumor or ulceration. It is a functional disorder of motility, the movement, of the colon.

Certain foods and beverages, particularly coffee and alcohol, can irritate the bowel. The patient with a spastic colon should avoid these irritating foods. Laxatives should also be avoided.

Emotional stress has an adverse effect on the digestive system. Digestion is very much affected by the nerves of the autonomic nervous system. For the patient with a spastic colon, emotional stress and upset are even more disruptive. If stressful situations can be alleviated, the colon will function more normally.

■ Dysentery

People often use the terms dysentery and diarrhea interchangeably, which is not accurate. Dysentery is a disease; diarrhea is a symptom. **Dysentery** is an acute inflammation of the colon, a colitis. It can be caused by bacteria, parasitic worms, and other microorganisms. Its major symptom is diarrhea in which the stools contain pus, blood, and mucus. Severe abdominal pain accompanies the diarrhea. Dysentery is principally a disease of the tropics, where sanitation is poor. Infective organisms enter the body through uncooked food and contaminated water. Organisms invade the wall of the colon and cause numerous ulcerations, which account for the pus and blood in the stools. Antibiotics can be effective depending on the causative organism.

GENERAL DISORDERS OF THE DIGESTIVE TRACT

The symptoms describing the diseases of the digestive system are common phenomena. Vomiting, diarrhea, and constipation are some of these symptoms. The physiologic basis of each symptom will be described briefly.

■ Vomiting

Vomiting is a protective mechanism, a means of ridding the digestive tract of an irritant or of alleviating overdistention. Sensory nerve fibers are stimulated by the irritant, and the message is conveyed to the vomiting center in the medulla of the brain. Motor impulses then stimulate the diaphragm and abdominal muscles. Contraction of these muscles squeezes the stomach. Normal peristalsis is reversed so movement of the stomach contents is upward. The sphincter at the base of the esophagus is opened, and the gastric contents are **regurgitated.**

A feeling of nausea often precedes vomiting. The cause of the nausea may be nerve factors other than a gastric or intestinal irritant. Motion sickness produces this effect. A very unpleasant smell or a sickening sight can cause nausea with possible subsequent vomiting.

■ Diarrhea

Diarrhea results when the fluid contents of the small intestine are rushed through the large intestine, causing watery stools. It was stated earlier that the main function of the large intestine is to reabsorb water and minerals. In an attack of diarrhea there is no time for this reabsorption. The smooth muscle in the walls of the intestine is so stimulated that peristalsis is intensified.

Nervous states can cause this increased motility of the large intestine, as most people have experienced. An infection such as food poisoning can bring about the same effect. If any area of the mucosal lining is infected, the glands pour out copious amounts of their mucous secretions. This helps to flush out the invading organisms and infection.

■ Constipation

The cause of constipation is the reverse of diarrhea. Feces remain in the colon too long, with excessive reabsorption of water; they then become hard and dry. Poor habits of elimination are a major cause of constipation. Defecation should be allowed to occur when the defecation reflexes are strong, usually in the morning after breakfast. A proper diet is also important, one that contains adequate amounts of fiber. Fiber is obtained from fresh fruits, vegetables, and cereals. Various disorders of the digestive system cause constipation. Any obstruction of the lumen or interference with motility will result in this condition.

DISEASES INDICATED BY STOOL CHARACTERISTICS

In addition to the diagnostic procedures described for gastrointestinal disorders, examination of the stools is also important. Symptoms of several of the diseases discussed include blood in the stools. But blood appears differently, depending upon the site of bleeding.

Streaks of red blood can indicate bleeding hemorrhoids. Discussed in a previous chapter, hemorrhoids are varicose veins of the rectum or anus. If the blood in the stools is bright red, the bleeding is from the distal end of the colon, the rectum. This symptom can indicate cancer of the rectum.

Dark blood may appear in the stools giving them a dark, tarry appearance; the condition of melena. This blood was altered as it passed through the digestive tract, so it is from the stomach or duodenum. A bleeding ulcer or cancer of the stomach may be indicated by melena. It should be mentioned here that certain medications, those containing iron for instance, can also give this tarry appearance to the stools.

Blood may not be apparent to the naked eye, but a chemical test is required to show its presence. This is referred to as **occult blood.** It can indicate bleeding ulcers or a malignancy in the digestive tract.

If the stools are large and pale, appear greasy, and float on water, they contain fat. This is a symptom of the malabsorption syndrome. It may also indicate a diseased liver, gallbladder, or pancreas. Diseases of these organs will be discussed in the next chapter.

SUMMARY

The anatomy and physiology of the digestive system was reviewed to understand the diseases of each organ. The importance of such diagnostic procedures as barium x-rays, endoscopy, and microscopic cell study was stressed.

Certain diseases are characteristic of a particular organ, such as varicose veins of the esophagus, esophageal varices. Others occur in certain areas of the gastrointestinal tract; ulcers, for example, which develop in both the stomach and duodenum. Inflammation and cancer develop in all parts of the digestive system.

Some disorders result from anatomic abnormalities: A hiatal hernia, twisting of the intestine on itself (volvulus), and a kink in the intestine due to adhesions are of this type.

A psychogenic element, stress or emotional upset, is a factor in regional enteritis and chronic ulcerative colitis. Nervous states also aggravate duodenal ulcers and a spastic colon.

Any number of disorders—tumors, hernias, and gallstones—can cause an obstruction of the digestive tract. The motility of peristalsis can be inhibited by severe inflammation, as in the case of peritonitis. Motility can be increased in the colon, so that diarrhea results.

STUDY QUESTIONS

1. Name four procedures used to diagnose diseases of the digestive system.
2. What are the symptoms of carcinoma of the esophagus?
3. Explain the cause of esophageal varices.
4. What are the complications of an incompetent (a) cardiac sphincter and (b) pyloric sphincter?
5. Name three major diseases of the stomach.
6. How is chronic atrophic gastritis related to stomach cancer?
7. Name three possible complications of an ulcer.
8. What is the principal cause of a duodenal ulcer?
9. What do regional enteritis and chronic ulcerative colitis have in common? How do they differ?
10. What are the possible complications of appendicitis?
11. Explain the difference between diverticulosis and diverticulitis.
12. What is the most characteristic symptom of malabsorption syndrome?
13. Distinguish between an organic obstruction and a paralytic obstruction. Give examples of each.
14. How can a spastic colon be treated?
15. What is significant about the way blood appears in the stools?

CHAPTER 11

Diseases of the Liver, Gallbladder, and Pancreas

Diseases of the digestive tract were explained in the previous chapter, and references were made to the accessory organs of digestion. This chapter will treat these accessory organs—the liver, gallbladder, and pancreas—as they themselves are affected by disease.

FUNCTIONS OF THE LIVER

The liver is the largest glandular organ of the body, and it is unique in several ways. It has great powers of regeneration; it can replace damaged or diseased cells. The liver has countless functions essential to life, and even a small part of this organ can carry out these functions. The liver has a dual blood supply: It receives oxygenated blood from the hepatic artery and blood rich in nutrients from the portal vein. Figure 11-1 shows the arrangement of blood vessels associated with the liver.

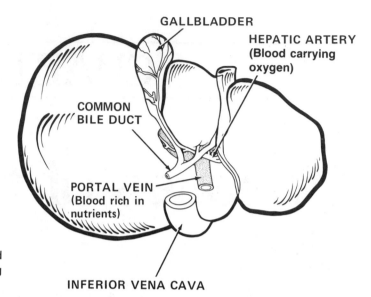

GALLBLADDER

HEPATIC ARTERY
(Blood carrying
oxygen)

COMMON
BILE DUCT

PORTAL VEIN
(Blood rich in
nutrients)

INFERIOR VENA CAVA

Figure 11-1. Liver viewed from below showing dual blood supply.

The blood reaching the liver through the portal vein comes from the stomach, intestines, spleen, and pancreas. Blood from the small intestines carries absorbed nutrients such as simple sugars and amino acids. One of the functions of the liver is to store any of these substances that are in excess. The liver plays an important role in maintaining the proper level of glucose in the blood. It acts as a buffer, taking up excess glucose and storing it as **glycogen.** When the level of circulating glucose falls below normal, the liver releases glucose. Iron and vitamins are also stored by the liver.

Another function of the liver is to synthesize various proteins. These proteins include enzymes necessary for various cellular activities. One means of evaluating liver function is to determine the level of these enzymes in the blood. The liver also synthesizes blood proteins. Albumin is the blood protein that has a water-holding power within the blood vessels. If the albumin level is too low, plasma seeps out of the blood vessels and into the tissue spaces, causing edema. The development of this condition in certain kidney diseases, in which albumin is lost in the urine, was explained in Chapter 9. Other essential blood proteins synthesized by the liver are those required for blood clotting, fibrinogen and prothrombin. If the liver is seriously diseased or injured and is unable to make these proteins, a bleeding tendency will result.

The liver can detoxify various substances, i.e., make poisonous substances harmless. Ammonia, which results from amino acid metabolism, is converted to urea by the liver. The urea then enters the bloodstream and is excreted by the kidneys. Certain drugs and chemicals are also **detoxified** by the liver. Specialized cells called **Kupffer's cells** line the blood spaces within the liver. These cells engulf and digest bacteria and other foreign substances thus cleansing the blood.

Bile, necessary for fat digestion, is secreted by the liver. As mentioned in the previous chapter, bile is an emulsifier, acting on fat in such a way that the lipid enzymes can digest it. The end product of lipid digestion can then be absorbed by the walls of the small intestine. In the absence of bile, the fat-soluble vitamins A, D, E, and K cannot be absorbed. Various functions of the liver are shown in Figure 11–2.

Bile consists of water, bile salts, cholesterol, and bilirubin, which is a colored substance resulting from the breakdown of hemoglobin. It is bilirubin that gives bile its characteristic color of yellow or orange.

Bile is secreted continuously by the liver and channeled into the hepatic duct. The body is very conservative. The bile is sent into the small intestine only as needed, when there is fat to be digested. Until it is needed, bile is stored in the gallbladder, a small saclike structure on the undersurface of the liver. The gallbladder releases the bile into the cystic duct when it receives neural and hormonal signals to do so. Bile is concentrated in the gallbladder, with water and salts being absorbed out of it. Figure 11–3 shows the relationship between the liver and gallbladder, as well as the duct system. The common bile duct empties into the duodenum.

DISEASES OF THE LIVER

If the liver is injured by a virus or a chemical agent such as alcohol, the cells become necrotic. If the injury is slight, the dead cells are removed and replaced with new ones. If the damage is extensive, however, fibrous connective tissue replaces normal cells. When this occurs, the functioning of the liver is impaired.

■ Jaundice

One symptom frequently associated with liver disease is jaundice. **Jaundice** is a yellow or orange discoloration of the skin and tissues. The whites of the eyes frequently show this pigmentation. It is caused by a build up of bilirubin, the pigment normally secreted in the bile and removed from the body in the feces, in the blood.

Causes of Jaundice. The liver may be normal and secreting bile as usual, but an obstruction may cause the bile to back up. The obstruction might be a tumor or a gallstone in the duct system. Since the bile cannot move forward, it leaks into the blood, with bilirubin coloring the plasma. When the blood reaches the kidneys, the bile filters into the glomeruli and appears in the urine, giving it a dark color. Since the bile is unable to reach the

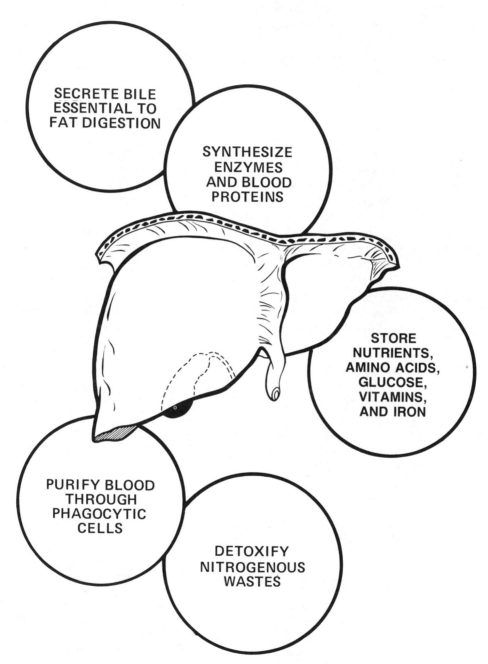

Figure 11-2. Functions of the liver.

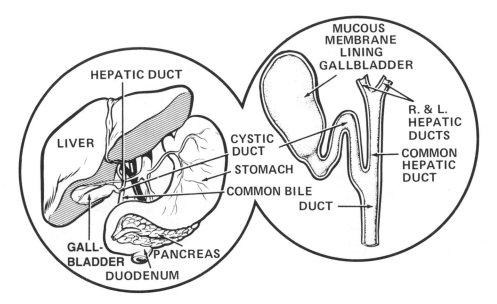

Figure 11-3. Bile duct system of liver and gallbladder.

duodenum, because of the obstruction, the stools are light in color. They are usually described as clay-colored.

Complications can result from this blockage to bile flow. Any condition of stasis, a stagnation, can lead to infection. Lack of bile interferes with fat digestion and absorption. This means that the fat-soluble vitamins are not being absorbed. In the absence of vitamin K, bleeding tendencies will develop. The obstruction can also cause liver damage.

Jaundice can also occur if the liver is diseased. If the cells are unable to function normally in secreting bile, bilirubin escapes into the blood. This condition will be discussed in more detail under hepatitis and cirrhosis.

Hemolytic jaundice has an entirely different cause, or etiology. This symptom accompanies the hemolytic anemias explained in Chapter 6. The condition may be congenital or acquired. In these anemias, the red blood cells hemolyze, and an excess of bilirubin results from the breakdown of released hemoglobin. Abnormal discoloration follows. Figure 11–4 illustrates the causes of jaundice and the complications of inadequate bile secretion.

■ Viral Hepatitis

Hepatitis, or inflammation of the liver, is caused by a number of factors. Certain viruses have been identified as causing two particular forms of hepatitis. They are hepatitis virus type A and hepatitis virus type B.

Hepatitis virus type A, formerly called infectious hepatitis, is the less serious form. It can develop as an isolated case or in an epidemic. Con-

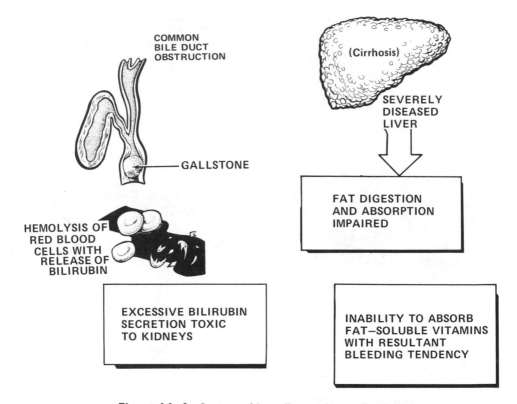

Figure 11-4. Causes of jaundice and complications.

taminated water or food is the usual source of the infection, which spreads under conditions of poor sanitation. The virus is excreted in the stools and urine, infecting soil and water.

The incubation period, the time from exposure to the development of symptoms, is from 2 to 6 weeks. The symptoms include anorexia, nausea, and mild fever. The urine becomes dark in color, and jaundice appears in some cases. On examination, the liver may be found to be enlarged and tender.

Hepatitis virus type A is usually mild in children; it is sometimes more severe in adults. Prognosis is usually good, with no permanent liver damage resulting.

Hepatitis virus type B, formerly called serum hepatitis, is a more serious disease. It can lead to chronic hepatitis or cirrhosis of the liver. Hepatitis virus type B is usually transmitted by blood or serum transfusions in which the donated blood contains the virus. It is also transmitted through the use of contaminated needles or syringes used by drug addicts.

The symptoms are similar to those of hepatitis virus type A but develop more slowly. The incubation period is long, lasting from 2 to 6 months. The severity of the disease varies greatly. A person's physical condition at the onset of the disease makes a difference in the seriousness of the infection. A person with poor nutritional status, for example, will be more adversely affected by hepatitis.

Occasionally a **fulminating** case of hepatitis virus type B develops, and it is fatal. This form has a sudden onset and progresses rapidly. The patient becomes delirious, then becomes comatose, and dies.

Let us relate the functions of the liver previously described to the failure of these functions, causing death. In the fulminating case, the liver becomes necrotic, so the cells stop functioning. They no longer produce the blood proteins necessary for blood clotting, so hemorrhage results. The liver cells are not able to detoxify poisonous substances. As these molecules accumulate in the blood they affect the brain. This causes delirum and coma. Bilirubin is no longer secreted in the bile. Instead, it is carried to the kidneys in large amounts.

There is now a specific blood test for hepatitis type B. A particular antigen, called the **Australia antigen,** is always present in an infected person's blood. Discovery of this antigen should reduce the incidence of hepatitis infection stemming from blood transfusions. A potential donor's blood can be tested for the specific antigen and rejected if the antigen is discovered. Blood and plasma in banks can also be carefully screened for the presence of the antigen.

Hospital personnel should be well informed of the hazards that can lead to acquiring hepatitis. Great precautions must be taken by nurses, laboratory technicians, dialysis workers, and blood bank personnel to prevent becoming infected.

A vaccine called **Hepatavax B** is now available that provides immunity for viral type B hepatitis. High-risk health care professionals are strongly urged to get vaccinated. **Immunoglobulin** injections provide temporary protection against hepatitis virus type A for people exposed to it. Once a person has had either type of hepatitis, he or she is immune to that particular type for life.

■ Cirrhosis of the Liver

Cirrhosis of the liver is a very serious disease. There are several types of cirrhosis but the symptoms for each are similar. Most people associate cirrhosis of the liver with chronic alcoholism, which is the leading cause. Severe chronic hepatitis can develop into cirrhosis. A chronic inflammation of the bile ducts can also have the same effect. Certain drugs and toxins can cause necrosis of the liver cells, which is the first step in the development of cirrhosis.

Cirrhosis is chronic destruction of liver cells and tissues with a nodular, bumpy, regeneration. In the normal liver there is a highly organized ar-

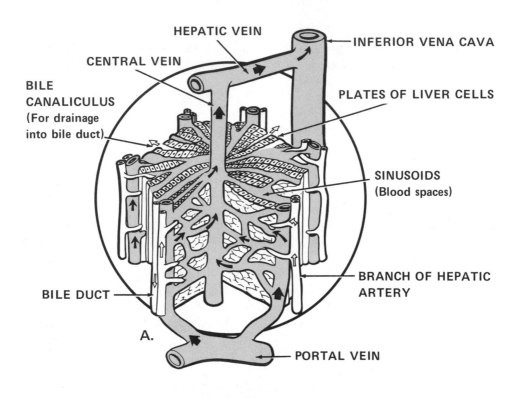

HEPATIC VEIN

INFERIOR VENA CAVA

CENTRAL VEIN

BILE
CANALICULUS
(For drainage
into bile duct)

PLATES OF LIVER CELLS

SINUSOIDS
(Blood spaces)

BILE DUCT

BRANCH OF HEPATIC
ARTERY

A.

PORTAL VEIN

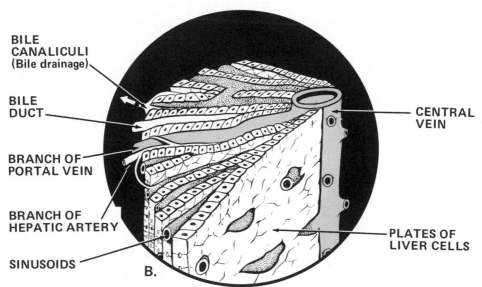

BILE
CANALICULI
(Bile drainage)

BILE
DUCT

BRANCH OF
PORTAL VEIN

BRANCH OF
HEPATIC ARTERY

SINUSOIDS

CENTRAL
VEIN

PLATES OF
LIVER CELLS

B.

Figure 11-5. Arrangement of liver cells, bile ducts, and blood vessels in a liver lobule.

rangement of cells, blood vessels, and bile ducts. A cirrhotic liver loses this organization and as a result the liver cannot function. Figure 11–5 illustrates the normal arrangement of liver cells, bile ducts, and blood vessels.

As the liver cells are damaged by excessive alcohol, drugs, or viral infection, they die. Fibrous connective tissue and scar tissue replace them. This tissue has none of the liver cell functions. At first the liver is generally enlarged due to regeneration but then becomes smaller as the fibrous connective tissue contracts. The surface acquires a nodular appearance. This liver, sometimes referred to as a "hobnailed" liver, is pictured in Figure 11–6.

Alcoholic cirrhosis, the most common type of cirrhosis, is the one that will be described in detail. This disease is also called portal, Laennec's, or fatty nutritional cirrhosis. An accumulation of fat often develops within the liver. Cirrhosis is more common in males than in females. The exact effect of excessive alcohol on the liver is not known, but it may be related to the malnutrition that frequently accompanies chronic alcoholism, or the alcohol itself may be toxic. The interior of a cirrhotic liver is shown in Figure 11–7. Rather than name the symptoms of cirrhosis as a dull list to be memorized, each symptom will be related to the malfunctioning liver to be more meaningful.

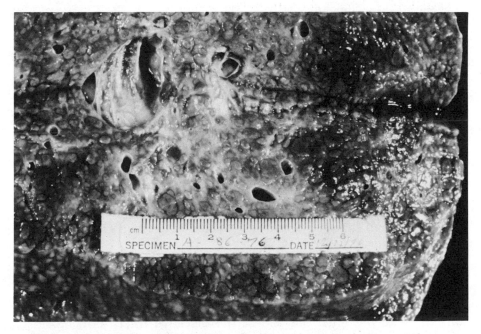

Figure 11-6. Typical "hobnailed" appearance of a liver affected by cirrhosis. (*Courtesy of Dr. David R. Duffell.*)

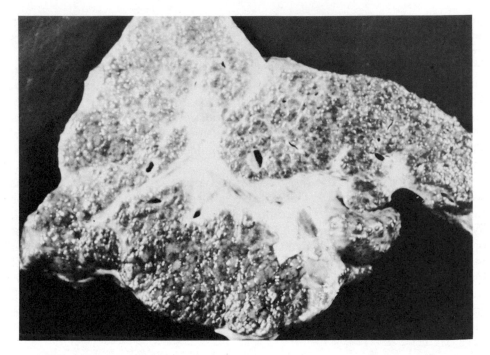

Figure 11-7. Interior of a cirrhotic liver. (*Courtesy of Dr. David R. Duffell.*)

The important portal vein passes through the liver and empties into the vena cava, returning blood to the heart. This vein becomes obstructed because of the disorganization, destruction, and nodular regeneration of the liver tissue. The blood backs up, affecting the organs drained by the portal vein: the stomach, intestines, spleen, and pancreas. Frequently the spleen becomes greatly enlarged, a condition known as **splenomegaly.**

Unable to flow through the portal vein, blood seeks alternative routes to bypass the liver, forming a **collateral circulation.** These large dilated veins become prominent on the abdominal wall in the area of the navel.

Pressure builds within the veins of the esophagus as a result of blockage of the portal vein. Esophageal varices, described in Chapter 8, develop. These varices tend to rupture, causing severe hemorrhages that can lead to shock and even death.

Hemorrhage can also occur in the stomach and intestines. Hematemesis, vomiting of blood, is often the first symptom of cirrhosis. The bleeding occurs because damaged liver cells fail to secrete the blood proteins essential to the blood-clotting mechanism. Alcohol, which causes the liver damage, is an irritant to the inner surface of the digestive tract. As a result, the stomach lining becomes inflamed. Another disease, acute hemorrhagic gastritis, often accompanies cirrhosis.

A characteristic symptom of cirrhosis is distention of the abdomen due to the accumulation of fluid in the peritoneal cavity. This fluid is called **ascites** and develops as a result of liver failure. The pressure within the obstructed veins forces plasma into the abdominal cavity, as illustrated in Figure 11–8. This fluid often has to be drained.

It is one function of the liver cells to produce an important blood protein, albumin. When an albumin deficiency (**hypoalbuminemia)** develops, fluid leaks out of the blood vessels and causes edema. Since the necrotic cells of the cirrhotic patient fail to produce albumin ascitic fluid develops, as does edema, particularly in the ankles and legs.

Jaundice usually results from obstruction of the bile ducts. The blockage of these ducts, like that of the blood vessels, follows the disorganization of the liver. Bile accumulates in the blood, giving the characteristic yellow

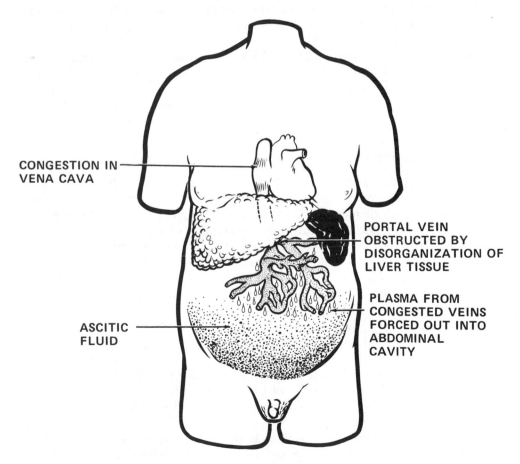

Figure 11–8. Accumulation of ascitic fluid.

coloration. Since bile is not secreted into the duodenum, stools are clay-colored. The excess of bile, carried by the blood to the kidneys, gives a dark color to urine.

A group of symptoms are related to the fact that the diseased liver cannot perform its usual biochemical activities. Normally, the liver inactivates small amounts of female sex hormones secreted by the adrenal glands in both males and females. Estrogens then have no effect on the male. The cirrhotic liver does not inactivate estrogens. They accumulate and have a feminizing effect on males. The breasts enlarge, a condition known as **gynecomastia.** The palms of the hand are red due to the estrogen level. Hair on the chest is lost, and a female-type distribution of hair develops. Atrophy of the testicles can also occur.

The necrotic liver cells are unable to carry out their normal function of detoxification, so blood is not cleansed by Kupffer's cells. As a result, ammonia and other poisonous substances accumulate in the blood and affect the brain. Various neural disorders follow. The patient becomes confused and disoriented, even to the point of stupor. A characteristic tremor or shaking develops. This shaking, together with halucinations, is referred to as delirium tremens, or DTs. Somnolence, or abnormal sleepiness, may lead to **hepatic coma.** This is a possible cause of death in cirrhosis. The typical signs and symptoms of cirrhosis are shown in Figure 11–9.

■ Carcinoma of the Liver

Hepatocarcinoma, cancer of the liver, is sometimes a complication of cirrhosis. This is a primary malignancy of the liver. Cancer often detected in the liver is a result of metastasis from other organs such as the breast, the colon, or the pancreas. These tumors are secondary carcinomas.

As mentioned in the chapter on neoplasia (Chapter 3), cancer spreads by way of the blood vessels and lymphatics. Because of the arrangement of these vessels through the liver, it is a frequent site of metastases. Cancer also spreads by invading surrounding tissue. A malignancy of the gallbladder or pancreas can grow into the liver.

The symptoms of hepatocarcinoma vary according to the site of the tumor. If the tumor is obstructing the portal vein, ascites develops in the abdominal cavity, as it does in cirrhosis. If the fluid is found to contain blood, a malignancy is indicated. A tumor blocking the bile duct will cause jaundice, as a result of the escape of bile into the blood. General symptoms may include loss of weight, an abdominal mass, and pain in the upper right quadrant of the abdomen.

Prognosis for cancer of the liver is poor. Usually the malignancy has developed elsewhere and has spread to the liver. Techniques such as the liver scan and needle biopsy are used in diagnosing the condition.

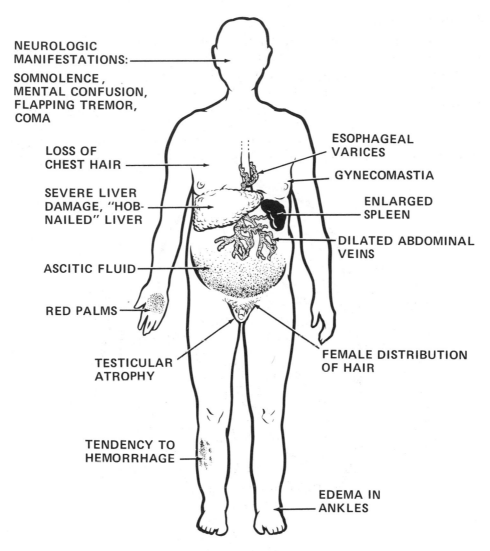

NEUROLOGIC
MANIFESTATIONS:

SOMNOLENCE,
MENTAL CONFUSION,
FLAPPING TREMOR,
COMA

LOSS OF
CHEST HAIR

SEVERE LIVER
DAMAGE, "HOB-
NAILED" LIVER

ASCITIC FLUID

RED PALMS

TESTICULAR
ATROPHY

TENDENCY TO
HEMORRHAGE

ESOPHAGEAL
VARICES

GYNECOMASTIA

ENLARGED
SPLEEN

DILATED ABDOMINAL
VEINS

FEMALE DISTRIBUTION
OF HAIR

EDEMA IN
ANKLES

Figure 11-9. Signs and symptoms of advanced cirrhosis.

DISEASES OF THE GALLBLADDER

The function of the gallbladder is to store and concentrate bile. The bile is sent to the duodenum when fat is present. This little muscular saclike structure does a lot of work. Like any organ it can become diseased or prevented from working by an obstruction.

■ Cholecystitis

Cholecystitis is an inflammation of the gallbladder. Note how meaningful the word is. The root word *chole* always refers to bile. A cyst is a sac. The gallbladder is a sac containing bile. The suffix, *itis,* indicates inflammation.

Cholecystitis is usually caused by an obstruction, a gallstone, or tumor. Because of the blockage, bile cannot leave the gallbladder. The bile becomes more concentrated and irritates the walls of the gallbladder. The typical inflammatory response occurs, and the gallbladder becomes extremely swollen. Figure 11–10 illustrates various forms of bile obstruction. Pain is

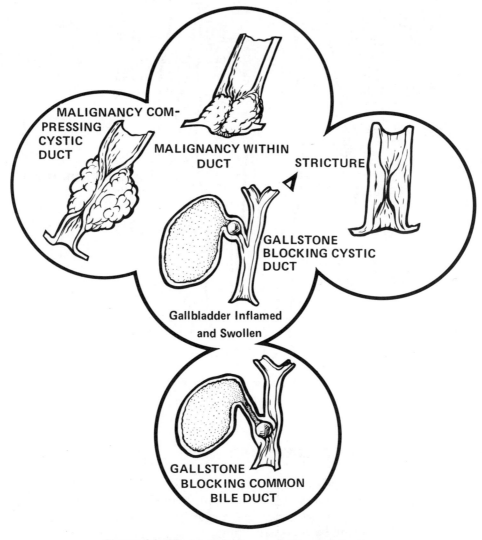

Figure 11-10. Various forms of bile obstruction.

experienced under the right rib cage and radiates to the right shoulder. At this point the gallbladder can usually be felt (palpated). The patient experiences chills and fever. Nausea and vomiting are also common symptoms.

Serious complications can result from cholecystitis. Lack of blood flow due to the obstruction brought about by the swelling can cause an infarction. With the death of the tissues, gangrene can set in. The acutely inflamed gallbladder, like an inflamed appendix, may rupture, causing peritonitis. A complication of chronic cholecystitis is that bile accumulates in the bile ducts of the liver. This causes necrosis and fibrosis of the liver cells lining the ducts. This is another form of cirrhosis, **biliary** (bile) **cirrhosis.** Possible complications of bile duct obstruction are summarized in Figure 11–11.

A patient with chronic cholecystitis experiences distress after eating fatty foods. The presence of fat in the duodenum stimulates the gallbladder to contract and release bile. The contraction of the inflamed gallbladder causes pain. Nausea and indigestion, accompanied by belching, follow eating a heavy meal.

Prolonged inflammation causes the gallbladder to lose its ability to concentrate bile. The walls of the gallbladder may thicken, making it impossible for the gallbladder to contract properly.

■ Gallstones (Cholelithiasis)

Gallstones, also called **biliary calculi,** may be present in the gallbladder and give no symptoms. There may be one gallstone present or several hundred, which can be large or small. Small stones, referred to as gravel, are the ones that enter the cystic duct and cause an obstruction. Excruciating pain follows. The formation or presence of gallstones is called **cholelithiasis;** the word element *lith(o)* refers to a stone.

Gallstones form when substances that are normally soluble precipitate out of solution. The stones consist principally of cholesterol, bilirubin, and calcium when in excess. Certain factors tend to stimulate gallstone formation such as obesity and pregnancy (because of an increased cholesterol level). The incidence of gallstones is higher in women.

The danger of gallstones is obstruction of the bile ducts, which causes inflammation. The converse is also true; inflammation of the gallbladder

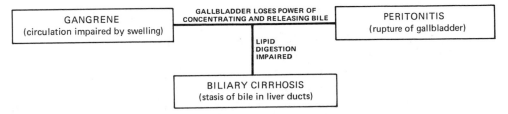

Figure 11–11. Complications of bile duct obstruction.

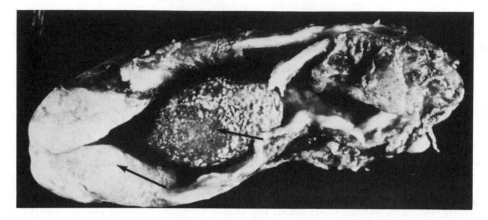

Figure 11-12. Gallbladder with chronic cholecystitis. Center arrow illustrates the thickened inflamed wall. Left arrow points to the gallstone. (*Courtesy of Dr. David R. Duffell.*)

causes gallstone formation. Figure 11–12 shows a gallbladder with chronic cholecystitis and cholelithiasis. Stones can sometimes be dissolved by medication, depending on their chemical composition.

Diagnosis of Gallbladder Disease

X-rays, used in combination with **radiopaque dyes,** will usually show the presence of gallstones, tumors, or a malfunctioning gallbladder. These x-rays of the gallbladder are called **cholecystograms** and those of the bile duct system, **choleangiograms.** These dyes may be given orally or intravenously. If the gallbladder does not become opaque with the dye, it is not filling and concentrating its contents properly. Any area in the duct system that does not become opaque indicates an obstruction.

STRUCTURE AND FUNCTION OF THE PANCREAS

The pancreas is a unique organ, having glands of both internal and external secretion. The glands of internal secretion are located in patches of tissue called the islands of Langerhans. They make up the endocrine part of the pancreas. These glands secrete two important hormones, insulin and glucagon, which regulate the level of circulating blood glucose. **Endocrine glands** have no ducts but secrete their hormones directly into the blood and lymph. Diseases of this part of the pancreas will be studied with those of other endocrine glands. Hormones of one endocrine gland effect another. Figure 11–13 shows the structure of the pancreas.

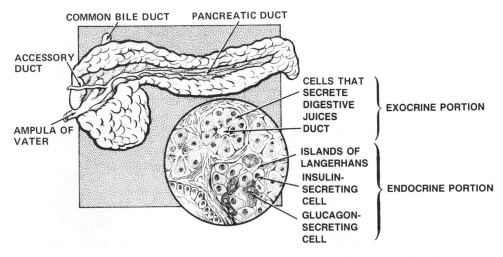

Figure 11-13. The pancreas—an endocrine and exocrine gland.

The glands of external secretion comprise the exocrine part of the pancreas. These glands secrete the digestive enzymes and juices that are carried to the duodenum by the pancreatic duct. The pancreatic duct and the common bile duct generally enter the duodenum at a common point, the ampulla of Vater.

The pancreas is a fish-shaped organ extending across the abdomen behind the stomach. The head fits into the curve of the duodenum, and it is here the pancreatic duct empties. Figure 11-14 shows the relationship between the pancreas and other digestive organs.

The pancreas is one of the most important organs of digestion. It secretes enzymes specific for carbohydrate, protein, and fat digestion. Amylase breaks down carbohydrates, **trypsin** and **chymotrypsin** digest protein, and lipase breaks down lipid or fat. The proteolytic enzymes are in an inactive state until they reach the duodenum.

Diseases of the pancreas severely interfere with the digestive process. The great number of digestive enzymes contained within the pancreas make it a threat to itself, as will be explained in a particular disease condition.

DISEASES OF THE PANCREAS

■ Pancreatitis

Acute **pancreatitis** is a serious inflammation of the pancreas that can result in death. For some reason, the protein- and lipid-digesting enzymes become activated within the pancreas and begin to digest the organ itself. Severe

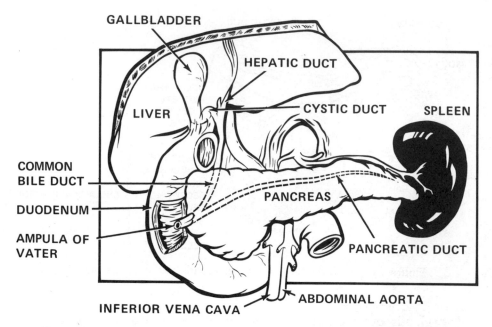

Figure 11-14. Relationship between pancreas and other digestive organs.

necrosis and edema of the pancreas result. The digestion can extend into blood vessels, which, of course, causes bleeding. If hemorrhaging occurs, the patient may go into shock. When the condition becomes this severe, it is called acute hemorrhagic pancreatitis. This is shown in Figure 11-15.

Severe, steady abdominal pain of sudden onset is the first symptom. The intense pain radiates to the back. It can resemble the sharp pain of a perforated ulcer. The patient feels some relief by drawing up the knees or assuming a sitting position. There may also be nausea and vomiting. Jaundice sometimes develops if the swelling of inflammation blocks the common bile duct.

Several factors can cause pancreatitis, but the most common one is excessive alcohol consumption. Inflammation of pancreatic ducts due to the presence of gallstones is another possible cause. Many cases of pancreatitis cannot be attributed to either of these causes. The etiology is said to be idiopathic, its cause is unknown. Pancreatitis is more common in women than in men and usually occurs after age 40.

If a large area of the pancreas is affected, both endocrine and exocrine functions of the gland become inadequate. Digestion is severely impaired. In the absence of lipid enzymes from the pancreas, fat cannot be digested. Stools are then greasy and have a terrible stench. Secondary malabsorption syndrome develops, as fat that is not digested cannot be absorbed.

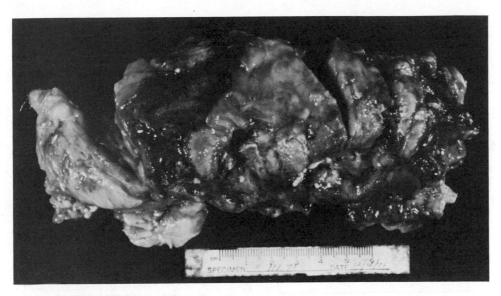

Figure 11-15. Acute hemorrhagic pancreatitis. (*Courtesy of Dr. David R. Duffell.*)

The most significant diagnostic procedures for pancreatitis are blood tests and urinalysis. High levels of pancreatic enzymes, particularly **amylase,** confirm the diagnosis of pancreatitis.

■ Cancer of the Pancreas

Cancer of the pancreas, an **adenocarcinoma** because the pancreas is a gland, has a high mortality rate. It occurs more frequently in males than in females. If the malignancy is in the head of the pancreas, it can block the common bile duct. This will give earlier symptoms than cancer in the body or tail, which can be very advanced before it is discovered.

Obstruction of the bile duct causes jaundice, as explained previously. Digestion is impaired if the pancreatic enzymes and bile cannot enter the duodenum. This causes malabsorption of fat and clay-colored stools. The patient cannot eat properly and loses weight. Great pain is experienced as the tumor grows. The cancer usually metastasizes to the surrounding organs: the duodenum, stomach, and liver. Prognosis for cancer of the pancreas is poor and death occurs in a relatively short time.

■ Cystic Fibrosis

Cystic fibrosis is a disease not only of the pancreas, but one that affects all the **exocrine glands** of the body, the glands of external secretion. Exocrine glands secrete mucus, perspiration, and digestive enzymes. It is called fibro-

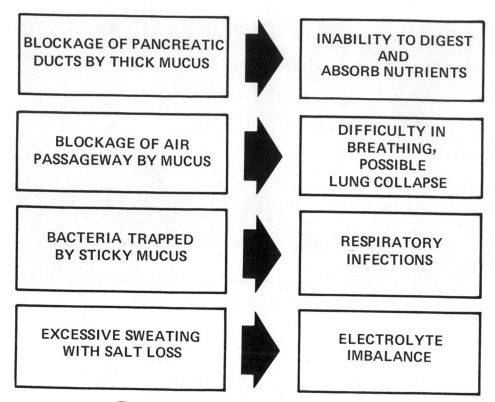

Figure 11-16. Complications of cystic fibrosis.

cystic disease of the pancreas because this organ is so highly secretory. Cystic fibrosis is a hereditary disease affecting young children. It is transmitted through a recessive gene carried by each parent (see Chapter 4). Before the disease was understood, the mortality rate of afflicted children was extremely high.

The abnormality in cystic fibrosis is excessively viscous mucus secretion of the glands. This mucus blocks the ducts of the pancreas, preventing the release of digestive enzymes. The absence of these enzymes impairs digestion. The child cannot benefit from the food eaten and becomes underweight. Lack of fat digestion results in large, bulky, foul-smelling stools. In the pancreas the glands become dilated and are converted into cysts that contain the thick mucus. Fibrous tissue then develops. This is how cystic fibrosis gets its name.

The most serious manifestation of cystic fibrosis is in the respiratory system. The trachea and bronchi secrete this thick mucus. As it accumulates the air passageway is blocked. This can lead to lung collapse. Most deaths occur as a result of respiratory failure.

Symptoms of cystic fibrosis are wheezing, persistent cough, and thick sputum. The child experiences difficulty in breathing because of the blocked airways. The child is particularly susceptible to respiratory infections due to the abnormal mucosal lining of the respiratory tract. Normally, bacteria are carried away by mucosal secretions, but in cystic fibrosis the bacteria adhere to the sticky mucus. The unmoved secretions serve as a breeding ground for bacteria. **Bronchiectasis** is a common complication of cystic fibrosis. Lung collapse can result from the inability to inflate them. Most deaths occur as a result of respiratory failure.

Not only are the mucous-secreting glands affected, but also the sweat glands. The child perspires excessively and loses large amounts of salt. Susceptibility to heat exhaustion is a result. This abnormal excretion of salt is the basis for the "sweat test" that confirms cystic fibrosis. Complications of cystic fibrosis are summarized in Figure 11–16.

Now that the disease is better understood the lives of many more children are being saved. Antibiotic treatment reduces the incidence of respiratory tract infection, and respiratory therapy can relieve congestion in the respiratory tract. Supplements for the lacking pancreatic enzymes can be given with food.

SUMMARY

The normal functions of the liver were reviewed, so that symptoms of liver disease would be meaningful. Liver cells become necrotic when injured, but the liver is able to regenerate new cells if the injury is slight. If the liver damage is extensive and liver cells are replaced by fibrous scar tissue, liver function fails.

Jaundice is frequently associated with liver disease because of abnormal bile production or release. Bile deficiency impairs digestion of fat and absorption of fat-soluble vitamins. In the absence of vitamin K, bleeding tendencies develop.

Hepatitis and cirrhosis are the serious liver diseases that were considered. Chronic hepatitis can lead to cirrhosis, but the most common cause of cirrhosis is alcoholism.

Cholecystitis, inflammation of the gallbladder, can cause gallstone formation, which in turn can cause inflammation. The most serious complication of gallstones is obstruction of the bile duct.

Inflammation of the pancreas, pancreatitis, is a serious disease in which enzymes intended for the digestive tract digest the pancreas itself. Carcinoma of the pancreas is a malignancy with a very poor prognosis.

Cystic fibrosis affects more than the pancreas. It is a disease condition of all the exocrine glands of the body. The most serious ramifications are in the respiratory system.

STUDY QUESTIONS

1. Name three causes of jaundice.
2. Why does a bleeding tendency often accompany liver disease? Give two reasons.
3. Compare and contrast hepatitis virus type A and hepatitis virus type B as to: (a) cause, (b) symptoms, (c) incubation period, and (d) prognosis.
4. What has reduced the incidence of hepatitis infection stemming from blood transfusions?
5. How are high-risk health professionals protected against virus type B hepatitis?
6. What are the complications of portal vein obstruction in cirrhosis of the liver?
7. Why does acute hemorrhagic gastritis frequently accompany cirrhosis?
8. Explain the feminizing effect on males afflicted with cirrhosis.
9. Why do neural disorders result from severe hepatitis and cirrhosis?
10. Explain the relationship between gallstones and cholecystitis.
11. What are the symptoms of cholecystitis?
12. Name three factors that predispose to gallstone formation.
13. What are the symptoms of pancreatitis?
14. Why is carcinoma of the pancreas detected more easily if the malignancy is in the head of the pancreas?
15. How does cystic fibrosis manifest itself?
16. What is the greatest danger in cystic fibrosis?

CHAPTER 12

Diseases of the Respiratory System

The need for an adequate blood supply to all the cells and tissues of the body has been stressed in every chapter. Why is the requirement for blood so critical? The blood supplies nutrients and minerals to the cells and removes waste products of cellular metabolism. But cellular metabolism is dependent on oxygen. The respiratory system provides a fresh oxygen supply to the circulatory system, so the two work hand in hand. A significant determination of pulmonary function is by blood gas analysis of the levels of oxygen and carbon dioxide.

STRUCTURE AND FUNCTION OF THE RESPIRATORY SYSTEM

The respiratory system consists of a tubular air passageway from the external environment to the lungs. Smooth muscle comprises the walls of these tubes, a significant factor in asthma. Air enters the nasal cavity, passes through the pharynx, or throat, to the trachea, the windpipe. The entrance to the trachea is the larynx, the voice box. The trachea branches out to the bronchi, one of each going to each lung. The bronchi continue to branch into smaller and smaller tubules called bronchioles. The structure resembles an inverted tree and is often called the "bronchial tree." The bronchioles terminate in the lungs as small air sacs called the alveoli. Figure 12–1 illustrates the air passageway.

The alveoli are very thin-walled sacs surrounded by blood capillaries where the exchange of gases occurs. Oxygen that is inspired, or inhaled, diffuses from the alveoli into the blood capillaries. The hemoglobin molecules

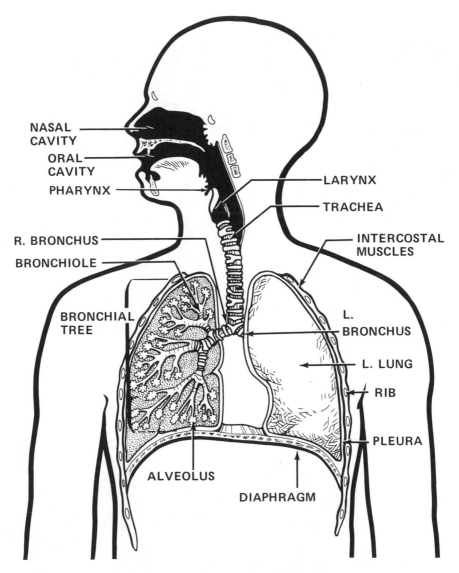

Figure 12-1. Air passageway to lungs.

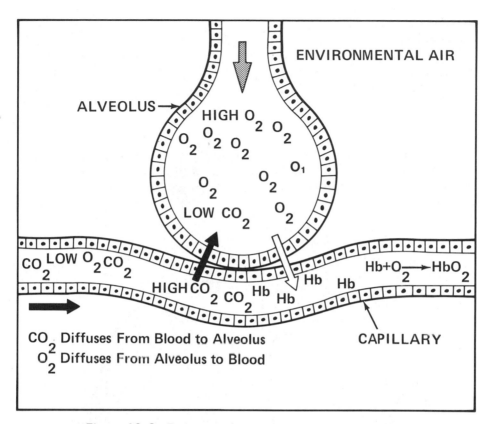

Figure 12-2. Exchange of gases between lungs and blood.

of the red blood cells become saturated with oxygen. Carbon dioxide, a waste product of cellular metabolism, diffuses from the blood capillaries into the alveoli to be expired, or exhaled. This exchange of gases is illustrated in Figure 12-2. In obstructive respiratory disease, this exchange of gases is impaired.

Why does air move in and out of the lungs? The movement occurs constantly without your thinking about it. You can only hold your breath so long and are then forced to breathe. Respiration is controlled by a center in the medulla of the brain. The respiratory center is regulated by the level of carbon dioxide in the blood: The more carbon dioxide, the greater the need for oxygen. This center stimulates the muscles of inspiration—the diaphragm and the muscles between the ribs called intercostals (*costa* means rib).

When the muscles of inspiration contract, the volume of the chest cavity increases. The pressure within the lungs decreases and air rushes in. The same muscles relax, the volume of the chest cavity decreases, and air is pushed out. There are also special muscles of expiration, the abdominal and internal intercostal muscles, but they are only needed in difficult breathing. These muscles are used in emphysema for example.

The lungs are encased by a double membrane consisting of two layers of pleura. One layer of this membrane covers the lungs, and the other lines the inner chest wall or thoracic cavity. There is only a potential space, the **pleural cavity,** between them, containing a small amount of fluid. This fluid lubricates the surfaces, preventing friction as the lungs expand and contract. The fluid also reduces surface tension, which helps to keep the lungs expanded. The air tight space between the lungs and the chest wall has a pressure slightly less than the pressure within the lungs. This difference in pressure acts as a vacuum and prevents the lungs from collapsing, as shown in Figure 12–3.

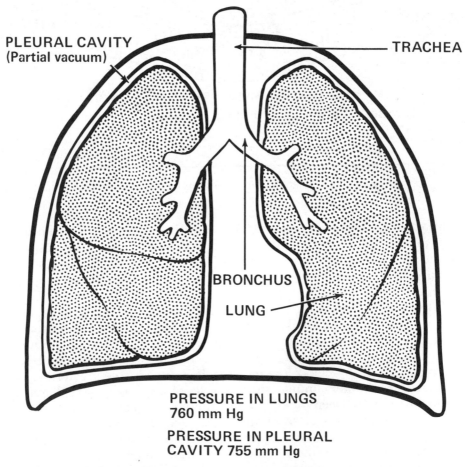

PLEURAL CAVITY
(Partial vacuum)

TRACHEA

BRONCHUS

LUNG

PRESSURE IN LUNGS
760 mm Hg

PRESSURE IN PLEURAL
CAVITY 755 mm Hg

Figure 12-3. Air pressure difference between lungs and pleural cavity.

The lungs have a double blood supply. Unoxygenated blood is carried from the right ventricle of the heart through the pulmonary artery. Oxygenated blood is carried through the bronchial arteries to the lungs. Blood, rich in oxygen, returns to the left side of the heart to be distributed to the entire body. (See Chapter 7 for a review of heart–lung blood flow.)

The entire respiratory tract is lined with a mucous membrane, the **respiratory epithelium.** Numerous hairlike projections **(cilia)** are contained within this mucosa. When air is inspired, it is moistened and warmed as it passes to the lungs. The cilia exert a sweeping action, preventing dust and foreign particles from reaching the lungs. The breakdown of this mucous membrane paves the way for infection.

The lungs are in direct communication with the external environment because of the open air passageway. Bacteria and viruses, entering with inspired air, can set up various sites of infection along the respiratory tract. Diseases of the nose and throat are called **upper respiratory diseases.** Those of the trachea, bronchi, and lungs are **lower respiratory diseases.**

UPPER RESPIRATORY DISEASES

■ The Common Cold

The common cold is a disease that is within everyone's experience. The symptoms would not even have to be written. What causes the stuffed-up head, runny nose, watery eyes, and fever? Countless strains of a tiny virus are capable of causing this misery. The common cold is highly contagious. Unlike many other diseases, having had a cold provides no immunity. Another strain of virus is always ready to attack.

A cold is an acute inflammation of the mucous membrane lining the upper respiratory tract. The initial stuffed-up feeling is due to the swelling of the mucous membrane, which narrows the air passageway. Then the mucous glands begin their copious secretion.

Many people believe that you catch a cold by such ways, for example, as getting soaked in the rain, sleeping in a draft, or getting chilled. This is not true. It is a virus that causes a cold; however, these factors can lower your resistance, making you less able to fight off the viral attack.

There is no known cure for the common cold. The symptoms can be treated by using aspirin for the fever and antihistamines for relieving the congestion. Drinking fluids may help, but generally the disease has to run its course.

Very often with a viral disease, bacteria come in as secondary invaders. These are usually streptococci, staphylococci, or pneumococci. Bacterial infection frequently develops with the cold and may spread to the sinuses, the spaces within the skull bones, or down the trachea. Many bacteria are pyogenic, and this accounts for the change in consistency of nasal secretion from watery to thick and yellow.

■ Hay Fever

Hay fever is an allergic disease. Although it is not inherited, it does tend to run in families. A person does inherit a predisposition to become sensitive to certain foreign proteins called **antigens.** The most common offenders are the pollens of ragweed and grasses.

Chapter 2 discussed allergies in general. The allergic person has an abundance of antibodies called **reagins** or **immunoglobulins,** specifically **IgE.** These antibodies attach to the **mast cells** of the mucous membrane lining the nose and to the inner surface of the eyelids. When pollen, the antigen, contacts the antibodies, a complex is formed. This complex breaks down certain cells, causing the release of **histamine.** Histamine dilates small blood vessels that increase blood flow into the area. Histamine also makes the walls of blood vessels leaky. Fluid oozes out of the blood vessels into the surrounding tissue, causing edema. This accounts for the feeling of congestion in the nasal passages. Figure 2–7 is a diagrammatic representation of the allergic reaction.

The irritation of the mucosal cells stimulates an excessive secretion of mucus, causing the runny nose and watery eyes. Because the release of histamine causes these unpleasant effects, a substance which counteracts its action, an **antihistamine,** may give relief. Antihistamines do have side effects, such as drowsiness, dizziness, or muscular weakness. Antihistamines have a drying effect on the mucous membranes, and the mouth and throat tend to become dry. Because patients who use antihistamines can become drowsy, they are warned about driving or operating heavy machinery.

Many hay fever sufferers take allergy injections to **desensitize** them to pollen or other allergens. By administering small doses of antigen and gradually increasing the dosage, the patient produces antibodies against it. It is hoped that these antibodies can inactivate the pollen before it interacts with the reagins attached to the nasal mucosa.

■ Tonsillitis

The same bacteria that cause strep throat, the streptococci, can cause tonsillitis, or inflammation of the tonsils. The tonsils are patches of **lymph tissue** at the entrance to the throat (Figure 12–4). Lymph tissue is very important, serving a protective function against disease. Lymph tissue, such as the tonsils, filters out bacteria. It then destroys them through the action of **phagocytic cells.** Antibodies produced to fight foreign antigens are also produced by lymph tissue.

At times, too many strep organisms are trapped by the tonsils, and they themselves become infected. The tonsils become very enlarged and red. The

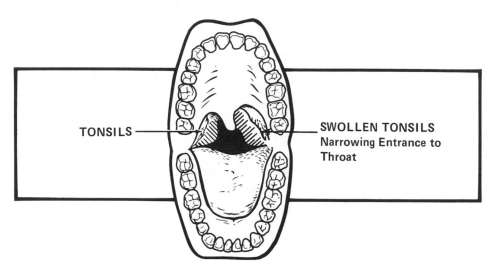

TONSILS

SWOLLEN TONSILS
Narrowing Entrance to
Throat

Figure 12-4. Tonsils—normal and enlarged.

opening to the throat narrows due to the swelling, and swallowing is difficult. The throat is very sore, and a high fever develops due to the strep toxins. The surface of the tonsils may become covered with pus. A blood count shows an elevated number of leukocytes, or leukocytosis, due to the infection.

Antibiotics are effective in counteracting the strep invasion. If the tonsillitis recurs frequently, it may be recommended that the tonsils be removed. This procedure used to be done routinely in children. Now that the protective function of tonsils is better understood, they are not removed unnecessarily.

A danger of strep infections, strep throat, or tonsillitis, is the onset of other diseases resulting from them. In Chapter 7, Diseases of the Heart, it was explained that strep infections are the basis of rheumatic fever. The kidney disease glomerulonephritis also develops as the result of a strep infection.

■ Influenza

Influenza is a viral infection of the upper respiratory system. Everyone is familiar with the symptoms of the flu because it is so common. The onset of the disease is sudden. The patient experiences chills and a fever, a cough, sore throat, and runny nose. Chest pains, muscular aching, and gastrointestinal disorders may also be symptoms. Many different strains of viruses causing influenza are known.

Epidemics of Asian, Hong Kong, Russian, and swine flu have occurred in the United States within recent years. Unfortunately, immunity for one strain does not protect against another.

There is a broad range in the severity of flu cases. It can be very mild, or it can lead to pneumonia and be life-threatening. Influenza is particularly serious in the elderly and chronically ill. The virus can destroy the respiratory epithelium, a strong line of defense against bacterial invasion. With the loss of the protective epithelium, bacterial infection can invade any part of the respiratory tract. Pneumococci, streptococci, and staphylococci are all capable of causing pneumonia.

There is no medication that cures influenza. Sometimes antibiotics are prescribed to ward off secondary bacterial infection. Bedrest, fluids, and aspirin to reduce fever are the usual treatments. Flu vaccines are only beneficial before onset of the disease. These shots do not give immunity for all strains of the flu virus.

LOWER RESPIRATORY DISEASES

■ Chronic Obstructive Pulmonary Disease (COPD)

Chronic obstructive pulmonary disease (COPD), or chronic obstructive lung disease (COLD), includes a number of conditions in which the exchange of respiratory gases is ineffective. It includes, primarily, chronic bronchitis, emphysema, and asthma. The respiratory control center of COPD patients is often affected.

These patients lose the normal respiratory response to elevated levels of carbon dioxide. When this occurs, the only stimulus for respiration is low oxygen tension. In this case, oxygen therapy can be fatal, as the effective stimulus on the respiratory control center to breathe is removed.

■ *Bronchitis.* Bronchitis, inflammation of the **bronchi,** may be acute or chronic. The mucous membrane lining the bronchi becomes swollen and red, the typical inflammatory response. Irritants such as industrial fumes, automobile exhaust, viruses, or bacteria can cause acute bronchitis. If a pyogenic organism, a pus-forming bacteria such as streptococci, is the causative agent, pus can fill the lumen of the bronchi. The trachea as well as the bronchi may become inflamed, and the condition then is called **tracheobronchitis.**

Acute bronchitis is most serious in small children, the chronically ill, and the elderly. The tiny **bronchioles** of children can become easily obstructed. An obstructed bronchus is illustrated in Figure 12–5. The elderly or chronically ill are likely to have a secondary infection develop, such as pneumonia. Acute bronchitis often follows an upper respiratory infection. The patient experiences chest pains, **dyspnea,** a cough, fever, and sometimes chills. The

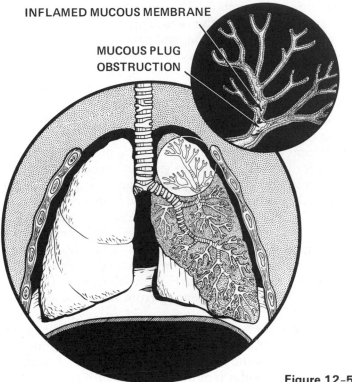

INFLAMED MUCOUS MEMBRANE

MUCOUS PLUG
OBSTRUCTION

Figure 12-5. Obstructed bronchus.

sputum coughed up may contain pus. Depending on the organism causing
the bronchitis, antibiotics may be administered. Viruses do not respond to
antibiotics. Vapors, sprays, and cough medicines may give relief.

Chronic bronchitis is indicated by repeated attacks of acute bronchitis,
coughing, with sputum production, lasting for several months for 2 consecu-
tive years. The symptoms are the same as in acute bronchitis, but they
persist. Chronic bronchitis may be a complication of another respiratory
infection. Chronic bronchitis can result form long-term exposure to air
pollutants or cigarette smoking. It is more common in men than women.

In chronic bronchitis there is an excessive secretion of **mucus** from the
mucous glands of the bronchial **mucosa.** The mucous glands hypertrophy,
and the mucosa itself is thickened and inflamed. The interference in the air
passageway due to the swelling and mucus reduces the patient's oxygen
level. **Hypoxia,** an insufficient oxygenation of the tissues, results. Poor
drainage of the mucus sets the stage for bacterial infection. Parts of the
respiratory tract can become necrotic, and fibrous scarring follows. Chronic
bronchitis is aggravated by other respiratory diseases such as the flu or a
cold.

There is no cure for chronic bronchitis. The symptoms can be treated with antibiotics and moist vapors to ease the breathing. A cigarette smoker should quit smoking. Pneumonia, emphysema, and bronchiectasis, diseases yet to be described, are frequent complications.

■ *Bronchial Asthma.*   A very common disease that can have serious consequences is bronchial asthma. Not only is the patient restricted in activities and likely to miss school or work, but the family also experiences a tension and anxiety when attacks are frequent or severe.

Bronchial asthma is not inherited, but there is a hereditary factor involved. A predisposition for hypersensitivity to various **allergens** is inborn. Common allergens are house dust, molds, pollens, animal dander, and various foods. Certain fabrics and cosmetics can also be highly allergenic.

What actually happens in an asthma attack that causes the characteristic wheezing and difficulty in breathing? It is a blockage of the airways, the bronchi. The smooth muscle in the walls of the bronchi suddenly contracts, narrowing the lumen of the tubes. The spasm is a sustained contraction of the musculature, making breathing, particularly expiration, very difficult. Figure 12–6 shows the narrowed bronchi resulting from muscular contraction.

The mucous membrane becomes swollen with fluid, also narrowing the lumen. Excessive secretion of mucus adds to the obstruction. Stale air becomes trapped, which decreases the amount of fresh air that can enter the lungs. The **wheezing** sound results from air passing through the narrowed tubes. The sound can be heard clearly by placing your ear on the patient's chest.

But another question must be asked. What causes the muscular spasm and abnormal reaction of the mucous membrane? This question brings us back to the concept of allergies or hypersensitivity developed in Chapter 2. Some asthmatic people have an excess of an allergic antibody, an immunoglobulin called reagin, or IgE. These reagenic antibodies have an affinity for, are attracted to, the smooth muscle and mucous membrane of the bronchi. They attach themselves, and when corresponding antigens such as dust, pollen, or mold are introduced, complexes are formed. These antigen–antibody combinations cause certain cells—called **mast cells**—to release histamine. Histamine stimulates the mucous secretion and muscular contraction.

Psychogenic factors are frequently associated with an asthma attack. A tense situation or an emotional experience can trigger one. Other nonallergic causes are overexertion, infection, or inflammation of the bronchi, bronchitis. Exposure of the bronchial mucosa to irritants such as cigarette smoke, aerosol sprays, or perfume may also bring about an attack.

There is no cure for asthma, but attacks may become less severe with age. It is important to identify the offending antigens and avoid contact with

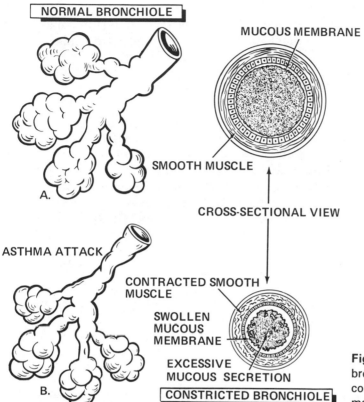

NORMAL BRONCHIOLE

MUCOUS MEMBRANE

SMOOTH MUSCLE

A.

CROSS-SECTIONAL VIEW

ASTHMA ATTACK

CONTRACTED SMOOTH MUSCLE

SWOLLEN MUCOUS MEMBRANE

EXCESSIVE MUCOUS SECRETION

B.

CONSTRICTED BRONCHIOLE

Figure 12-6. Normal bronchiole **(A)** and one constricted **(B)** in asthma attack.

them as much as possible. Skin tests, in which minute quantities of allergen are introduced into a scratch, can show various sensitivities. Development of a red hivelike lesion at the site of injection indicates an allergy.

Medication and allergy shots can reduce the incidence or severity of asthma attacks. To counteract an ongoing attack, substances that dilate the bronchi are effective. Ephedrine sprays and **epinephrine (adrenalin)** injections are often effective. Cortisonelike drugs are sometimes used, but these always carry a threat of side effects. All medications used in the treatment of asthma must be carefully controlled and under close supervision of the physician. Antihistamines, although somewhat effective for hay fever, should not be used for asthma.

The most severe form of an asthma attack is called **status asthmaticus,** in which the patient fails to respond to the usual treatment. A procedure as drastic as a **tracheotomy**—opening of the trachea surgically—may be required. Status asthmaticus may end in respiratory failure and death if not treated.

Great strides in asthma research have been made by the National Asthma Center at Denver. A reader with a particular interest in coping with this disease may wish to contact them for more detailed information. The following are suggestions offered by the National Asthma Center for reducing the frequency or severity of asthma attacks. These are listed in the Center's publication entitled *Asthma.*

Eliminate house dust as much as possible. Dust catchers such as wool carpeting, heavy draperies, and stuffed furniture should not be used in an asthmatic's bedroom. Dacron, rather than foam rubber pillows, should be used, as the latter can harbor mold spores. Pillows and animals stuffed with feathers or hair should be avoided. Animals should not be kept in the house and cigarette smoking should be avoided, at least in the presence of the asthmatic. Low humidity is desirable to reduce the growth of molds. When common allergens are high outside, the patient should stay in the house with windows closed. The patient should also avoid allergenic substances in food.

■ Bronchiectasis

Many respiratory diseases result from an already-existing disease. **Bronchiectasis** is an example of this. The word element *ectasis* means **dilation** or distention. In bronchiectasis, the smaller bronchi and bronchioles become chronically dilated as seen in Figure 12–7. If you envision this as a ballooning of these walls, you can understand how they are weakened.

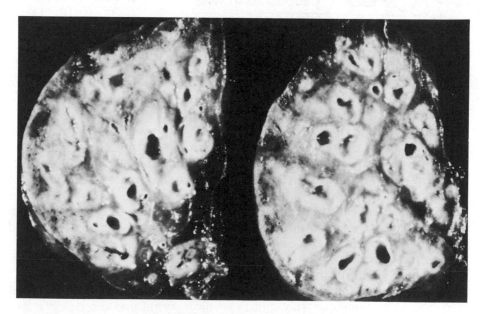

Figure 12-7. Bronchiectasis. Light areas are the thickened walls of the dilated bronchi. (*Courtesy of Dr. David R. Duffell.*)

This dilation of the bronchi results from obstruction or infection in the respiratory tract. Obstructions tend to cause infection, as was previously explained. Bronchitis can lead to bronchiectasis because of the mucous plugs that develop. Bronchiectasis is sometimes a complication of influenza, pneumonia, or a chronic sinus infection. Children can develop bronchiectasis after measles or whooping cough.

As the bronchi dilate, pockets are formed where infectious material collects. **Abscesses** develop, which cause pus to be coughed up in the sputum. The weakened walls of the bronchi become necrotic and are destroyed. With the destruction of the smooth muscle in the walls, the ability to cough up mucus is reduced. Stages of bronchiectasis development are shown in Figure 12–8.

The necrotic tissue causes foul-smelling, pus-containing material to be brought up. The patient's breath also has a very bad odor. This infection

STEPS IN DEVELOPMENT OF BRONCHIECTASIS

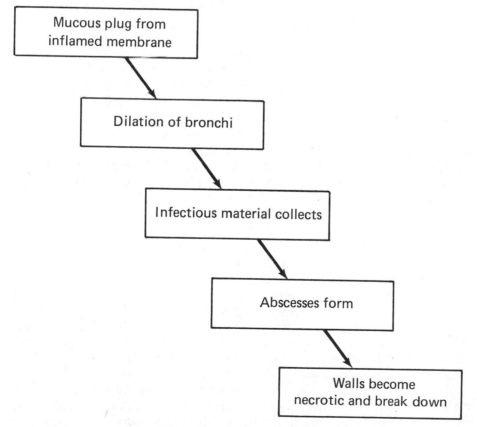

Figure 12–8. Bronchiectasis.

may spread to the **pleural membrane** on the lung, causing pleurisy. If the infection invades the pleural cavity, empyema results.

Bronchiectasis can be arrested in the early stages but not after the tissue destruction is advanced. Penicillin or other antibiotics prevent secondary bacterial infection. Conditions that promote general good health—fresh air, good diet, and rest—are important.

■ Emphysema

Emphysema is a crippling and **debilitating** disease. It is neither a contagious nor an infectious disease, but one of chronic lung obstruction and destruction. The cause of emphysema is not known, but it is most frequently associated with heavy cigarette smoking. Air pollution and long-term exposure to irritants of the respiratory tract also seem to be factors of its etiology. Emphysema is a frequent complication of chronic bronchitis.

The word *emphysema* means inflation. The lungs become filled with stale air high in carbon dioxide. This air cannot be adequately exhaled to allow oxygen to enter. The patient experiences a suffocating feeling and great distress from the inability to breathe. Severe pain accompanies the difficult breathing.

The emphysema patient shows an increased rate of breathing and a greater than normal expansion of the chest. The chest wall becomes permanently expanded, producing a characteristic "barrel chest." A stethescope placed on the chest detects abnormal respiratory sounds called rales.

Let us go back one step and see what causes this inflation of the lungs with trapped air. The irritants mentioned—smoke, fumes, and pollutants—have their first effect on the cilia of the respiratory mucosa. When their sweeping, cleansing action fails, the mucosa becomes inflamed from the accumulation of foreign particles. In response, the mucosa secretes an excess of mucus that clogs the air passageways. Inadequate oxygen and excess carbon dioxide in the **alveoli,** the tiny air sacs of the lung, cause their thin walls to break down. Deterioration of the walls between alveoli results in a fusion of these tiny air sacs into larger spaces called **bullae.** Fewer alveoli are left to function. Elasticity of the lungs is lost with alveolar deterioration. An emphysematous lung is shown in Figure 12–9.

Emphysema patients are sometimes classified as "pink puffers" or "blue bloaters." The "pink puffers" maintain relatively normal blood gas volumes. They experience progressive dyspnea but no **cyanosis.** It seems that "pink puffers" are able to hyperventilate and they show an increase in lung capacity. The "blue bloaters," by contrast, show marked cyanosis. They have repeated episodes of right-sided heart failure and hypoxemia.

The loss of elasticity plus the narrowed airways explain the difficulty in exhaling the stale air. As the lungs become less efficient in moving air in and out, a strain is placed on the heart, as the circulatory and respiratory

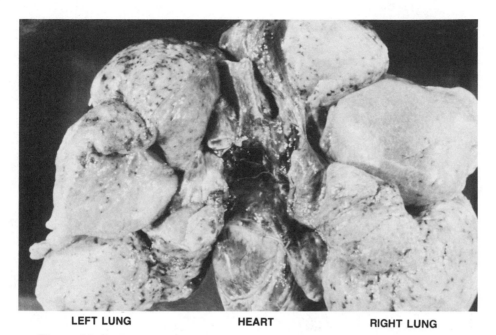

LEFT LUNG   **HEART**   **RIGHT LUNG**

Figure 12-9. Emphysematous lungs viewed posteriorly. (*Courtesy of Dr. David R. Duffell.*)

systems work together. The heart tries to pump more blood to meet the body's oxygen needs. This overworking of the heart causes it to enlarge.

Emphysema can last for many years, during which time the damage to the lungs is irreversible. As in any serious disease, complications often develop. With the breakdown of alveolar walls, the surrounding blood capillaries are damaged. This interference with circulation in the lungs can lead to an obstruction of the pulmonary artery.

The large air sacs formed by the fusion of the alveoli, tend to rupture. This allows air into the pleural cavity, the space between the lungs and the chest wall. Air in this space causes the lung to collapse. A ruptured bulla is shown in Figure 12-10.

Early detection of emphysema can slow its further development. Symptoms such as a chronic cough (often called smokers cough), shortness of breath, and abnormally rapid breathing indicate a respiratory disease. A physician should be consulted. The respiratory rate is increased in emphysema as the body attempts to get more oxygen. The patient tires easily and feels great distress after the slightest exertion, due to the lack of oxygen.

The most significant diagnostic test for emphysema is an evaluation of the patient's lung capacity. A simple instrument, a **spirometer,** measures the ability to move air in and out of the lungs. X-rays do not show emphysema

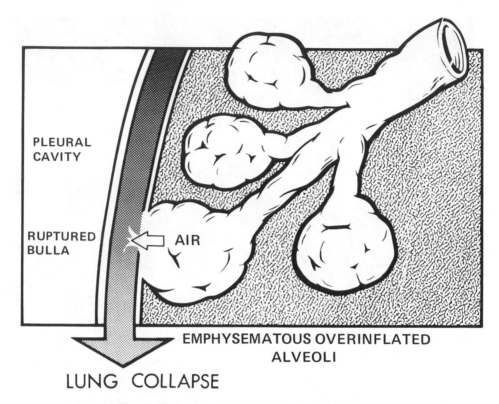

PLEURAL
CAVITY

RUPTURED
BULLA

AIR

EMPHYSEMATOUS OVERINFLATED
ALVEOLI

LUNG COLLAPSE

Figure 12-10. Ruptured bulla in emphysema.

in the early stages. Treatment involves stopping the source of the irritation if possible. A smoker will be told to stop smoking and to avoid polluted air, air filled with smoke, fumes, and irritating dust.

The patient should observe ozone warnings and limit outdoor activity when the ozone level is high.

Medications can be administered to clear mucus from the lungs. This prevents infection due to stagnation. Some medications give relief from the feeling of not being able to breathe. Physical therapy is sometimes helpful in teaching the patients to use all possible muscles of respiration in the abdomen and chest wall.

■ Pneumothorax

The lungs are surrounded by an airtight space. This is the pleural cavity between the two layers of pleural membrane. An air pressure in the cavity less than that within the lungs keeps the lungs expanded (see Figure 12–3). If air or gas enters this pleural cavity on either side, the lung will collapse. Admission of air or gas into the pleural cavity is known as a **pneumothorax.**

A pneumothorax can occur in one of two ways. A weakened area of the lung can rupture, letting air into the space. Rupture of a bulla formed in emphysema is a common cause of a pneumothorax. Sometimes ruptures occur spontaneously in young adults. Air can also be admitted into the pleural cavity from outside the body. A chest wound, a stabbing, gunshot, or fractured rib can cause a pneumothorax. The increased air in the pleural cavity puts pressure on the lung and causes it to collapse. The patient experiences sudden, severe chest pain. Breathing becomes difficult and the pulse is rapid and weak.

Treatment depends on the cause of the pneumothorax. If it occurred spontaneously from within it will probably heal itself and the lung will reinflate. In the meantime, the patient must be rested. Drawing out the air from the pleural space, **pleurocentesis,** is sometimes required.

A pneumothorax can be used as a surgical procedure to rest a lung. A measured amount of air is admitted into the pleural cavity. This is sometimes done in the treatment of tuberculosis to give a tuberculous lesion time to heal. Collapse of a lung by this method may follow lung surgery to temporarily immobilize it.

■ Atelectasis

In the discussion of emphysema it was noted that bulging, weakened walls of the alveoli can rupture, admitting air into the pleural cavity. Entrance of air into the pleural cavity is the condition of pneumothorax. The increased pressure in the pleural cavity causes the lung to collapse. Collapse of the lung is called **atelectasis.**

Atelectasis can occur in one of two ways. A lung can collapse when it is compressed. The compression can be due to increased air pressure as in a pneumothorax. Increased fluid secreted by the pleural membranes also compresses the lungs. An accumulation of pus in the pleural cavity resulting from a ruptured lung abscess or malignant tumor can also cause atelectasis.

A lung will also collapse if the air passageway is obstructed. Air is unable to enter and inflate the lung. Severe chronic bronchitis can cause obstruction of a bronchi, because of the excessive secretion of mucus. This occurs if the mucus cannot be coughed up. A malignant tumor growing into the lumen of a bronchi also blocks the airway. Atelectasis can result from any of these events. Figures 12–11A and 12–11B show lung collapse due to compression and obstruction.

■ Pneumonia

There are many different kinds of pneumonia caused by both bacteria and viruses. Pneumonia is an acute inflammation of the lung. It can affect one lung or both. If both lungs are affected, it is called double pneumonia. Primary pneumonia is usually caused by pneumococci, streptococci, or

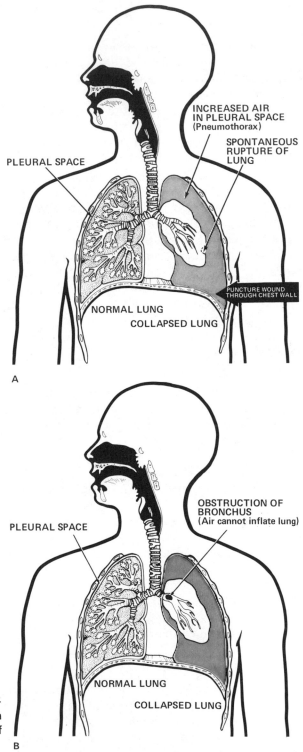

INCREASED AIR
IN PLEURAL SPACE
(Pneumothorax)

SPONTANEOUS
RUPTURE OF
LUNG

PLEURAL SPACE

PUNCTURE WOUND
THROUGH CHEST WALL

NORMAL LUNG

COLLAPSED LUNG

A

OBSTRUCTION OF
BRONCHUS
(Air cannot inflate lung)

PLEURAL SPACE

NORMAL LUNG

COLLAPSED LUNG

B

Figure 12-11. Causes of atelectasis due to **(A)** compression of lung and **(B)** obstruction of air passageway.

staphylococci. Pneumonia can develop as a secondary disease after influenza, bronchiectasis, bronchitis, or congestive heart failure. One of the difficulties in treating pneumonia is recognizing the causative agent. This is necessary to prescribe the most effective antibiotics. More than one kind of pneumonia may be present at the same time, which makes treatment more difficult.

Lobar pneumonia is generally acquired by pneumococci. The bacteria may come from a person with the disease or from one who carries the organisms in his or her throat.

A person with low resistance is more likely to develop pneumonia. It often develops after surgery or immobilization resulting from a severe fracture. Chronic alcoholism is also a predisposing factor to pneumonia.

Lobar pneumonia has a sudden onset. The patient experiences a severe chill possibly accompanied by shaking. A fever develops and both heart rate and respiration rate are increased. Chest pains on breathing may be very severe.

The inflammatory response that produces **inflammatory exudate** was described in Chapter 2. In lobar pneumonia a great amount of exudate containing plasma, leukocytes, and fibrin seeps out of the capillaries into the air spaces, the alveoli. Fibrin, a plasma protein essential to blood clotting, becomes stringy when activated. This causes the exudate to solidify. The affected part of the lung becomes solid or **consolidated.** Capillaries can break down, causing the release of red blood cells into the exudate. The exudate takes the place of air in the alveoli. The inflammation spreads rapidly through the lung tissue and may affect an entire lobe. That is the reason for the name lobar pneumonia. It may affect the entire lung.

The severe pain is due to the pleurisy that generally accompanies lobar pneumonia. The pleural membranes, normally very smooth, become covered with exudate. This exudate is described as shaggy because of the consistency produced by the fibrin. A creaking sound is heard with the stethoscope as the two pleural membranes rub on each other.

Lobar pneumonia can be very severe at the onset, but it is relatively short lived, lasting about a week. Antibiotics are effective treatment. The crisis is passed when sweating occurs and the temperature drops. The causative organisms are killed and the exudate softens. Much of the exudate is removed by coughing it up in the sputum. Phagocytic white blood cells digest some of it. The return of the lung to a normal condition is called **resolution.** There is usually no permanent lung damage after lobar pneumonia and the lung returns to normal. As there is no destruction of lung tissue, abscesses do not form.

The symptoms of lobar pneumonia can be related to their causes. The patient's face is flushed due to the fever. Fever develops in response to toxins, the poisonous substances produced by the pneumococci. Fever is considered to be a protective body mechanism, as the elevated temperature kills some microorganisms. Cellular activity, or metabolism, is increased. More antibodies against the invaders are produced with this increase in activity. The respiratory rate is increased, but breathing is shallow. The poor uptake of oxygen by the consolidated lungs stimulates the rapid breathing. Breathing is painful because of the pleurisy that accompanies lobar pneumonia.

Coughing is a reflex, protective mechanism to rid the respiratory tract of an irritant. The sputum that is coughed up is sticky due to the fibrin in the exudate. The sputum may contain red blood cells, as well as white blood cells and the pneumococci.

Bronchopneumonia (bronchial pneumonia) is primarily an inflammation of the bronchioles, a bronchitis. The infection then spreads into the alveoli at the termination of the bronchioles. The consolidation that develops is spotty. The entire lobe or lung is not consolidated as it is in lobar pneumonia. One or both lungs may be affected.

Bronchopneumonia is more common than lobar. The symptoms are less severe, and it develops more slowly, running a longer course than lobar pneumonia. There is a tendency for bronchopneumonia to recur, and the recurrences can be more serious. Abscesses tend to develop, and the lungs can be scarred with fibrosis.

Predisposing causes to bronchopneumonia are chronic bronchitis and bronchiectasis. It occurs most frequently in children and in the aged. In children, bronchopneumonia sometimes follows measles or whooping cough. In the aged and cancer patients, bronchopneumonia can be the cause of death. Predisposing causes of bronchopneumonia are summarized in Figure 12–12.

The same organisms that cause lobar pneumonia cause bronchopneumonia; staphylococci, streptococci, and pneumococci. The infection is spread by coughing. Sometimes antibiotic-resistant staphylococci develop in hospitals and cause serious infections. The weakened patients are very susceptible to pneumonia from this source.

Primary atypical pneumonia is caused by a variety of viruses. Viral pneumonia is the most common pneumonia. It often develops as a complication of a viral disease such as measles or influenza. Primary atypical pneumonia is an acute inflammation of the upper respiratory tract involving the lungs to a lesser degree.

Influenzal pneumonia is a very serious inflammatory disease of the respiratory system. When you hear of great flu epidemics that killed millions of people, it was this disease that was responsible.

The influenza develops when a virus is inhaled and sets up an infection in the nose and throat. The infection spreads into the sinuses and down the trachea and bronchi. The patient becomes very weak, and resistance to bacterial invasion is lessened. Bacteria then attack the susceptible lungs with the development of pneumonia.

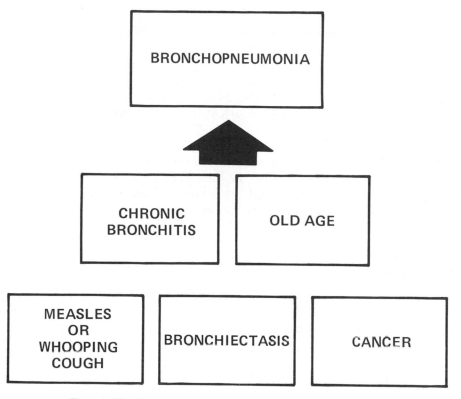

Figure 12-12. Predisposing causes of bronchopneumonia.

Both lungs are always involved. The exudate is not thick as it is in lobar pneumonia, so the lungs are not consolidated. Instead, the exudate is watery and contains blood. The bleeding is from ruptured capillaries, and abscesses form throughout the lung. These often rupture into the pleural cavity, spreading the pus and causing empyema, a disease yet to be described.

The patient is totally debilitated, has no strength, and experiences dyspnea. The fluid in the alveoli prevents the normal exchange of carbon dioxide for oxygen. The patient becomes cyanotic due to the absence of oxygenated hemoglobin. A cough persists from the irritation within the respiratory tract, while the sputum is watery and contains blood. For a patient with lowered resistance, the disease can be fatal. Figure 12-13 summarizes the condition of alveoli in the diseased states described.

■ Pleurisy

Reference has been made to **pleurisy,** inflammation of the pleural membranes, as a complication of various lung diseases. Pleurisy may result from infection, pneumonia, or tuberculosis. It may follow an injury or tumor formation. Pleurisy is extremely painful; a sharp, stabbing pain accompanies each inspiration. It is treated with antibiotics, heat applications, and bed rest.

There are two kinds of pleurisy: dry pleurisy, the more painful form, and pleurisy with effusion. Dry pleurisy is a complication of lobar pneumonia. Each layer of pleura is congested, swollen, and covered with a shaggy exudate. Friction results as the pleura rub on each other. They may stick together, forming adhesions.

Pleurisy with effusion results from an excessive amount of exudate in the pleural cavity. It can interfere with breathing by compressing the lung. Enough fluid may collect to cause the lung to collapse. This type of pleurisy is associated with lung cancer and tuberculosis. Pleural fluid can be drawn out with a needle for diagnostic purposes. Figure 12–14 illustrates the two kinds of pleurisy.

■ Empyema

If the exudate in the pleural cavity contains pus, the condition is known as **empyema.** (The word element, *py*, refers to pus). Empyema has become rare since the development of antibiotics. Pus can enter the pleural cavity from

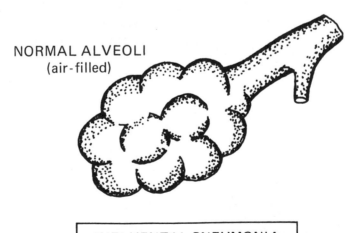

LOBAR PNEUMONIA
(consolidated exudate)

EMPHYSEMA
(overinflated with stale air)

NORMAL ALVEOLI
(air-filled)

INFLUENZAL PNEUMONIA
(watery, hemorrhagic exudate)

Figure 12-13. Comparison of alveoli in diseased states.

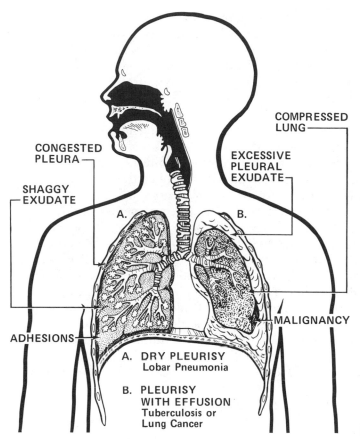

CONGESTED PLEURA

SHAGGY EXUDATE

A.

COMPRESSED LUNG

EXCESSIVE PLEURAL EXUDATE

B.

MALIGNANCY

ADHESIONS

A. **DRY PLEURISY**
   Lobar Pneumonia

B. **PLEURISY WITH EFFUSION**
   Tuberculosis or Lung Cancer

Figure 12-14. Pleurisy.

a ruptured lung abscess or from an ulcerated malignant tumor that grows into the pleural space. Empyema also results from the spread of infection into the pleural cavity in bronchiectasis. Atelectasis, or collapse of the lung, can follow the filling of the pleural cavity with pus.

■ Tuberculosis

The incidence of tuberculosis has been greatly reduced in recent years in the United States, but it is still a serious disease that affects many people. It is primarily a disease of the lungs, but it can spread to other organs such as the kidney, brain, or bone.

Tuberculosis is contracted by the inhalation of infectious material and is spread by coughs and sneezes. The organism that causes tuberculosis, *Mycobacterium tuberculosis*, has a protective waxy coat, enabling it to live outside the body for a long time. Infected droplets of sputum dry up and the microorganisms remain as dust. They are killed only by direct sunlight.

Several reasons account for the decrease in the number of tuberculosis cases. Better living conditions, less crowding, and more available fresh air are among them. Chest x-rays are required for admission to hospitals, for certain jobs, and are often part of complete physical examinations. If tuberculosis is detected in the early stages, it is easier to treat. Tuberculous patients are taught good hygiene in the management of their infectious sputum.

The symptoms are fever (particularly in the afternoon), night sweats, weight loss, and weakness. A productive cough accompanies the more advanced stages. The outcome of tuberculosis depends on the dosage of the bacilli received and the resistance of the patient. A healthy person fights off the disease, often not even aware of the infection. In the early stages, tuberculosis can be **asymptomatic,** that is, produce no symptoms. A person living in crowded conditions, poorly nourished, overworked, or suffering from chronic alcoholism is susceptible to serious tubercular infection.

The first infection with tuberculosis is called a primary infection. The lung lesion is a small spot, called a Ghon lesion, that drains to a nearby lymph node. The **tubercle bacilli** are surrounded by blood cells, macrophages, lymphocytes, and multinucleated giant cells. Antibodies are produced against the tubercle bacillus and its toxin. The disease can be overcome at this stage. A small scar of fibrous tissue, which limits the spread of the infection, may result. With the production of antibodies, the cells become hypersensitive to the tubercle bacillus, or allergic, so that a reinfection takes a different course.

It is this hypersensitivity to the organism that is the basis for the tuberculin test. Injection of the tuberculin protein into the skin triggers an immune response if the antibodies are present. Development of a red, raised area within 48 to 72 hours at the site of injection indicates sensitivity to the organism or previous exposure.

A secondary lesion occurs when there is reactivation of organisms from previously dormant tubercles. The tuberculosis bacillus can lie dormant for many years before a secondary lesion occurs. The reactivation may occur because of a decrease in the body's immune defense.

Most often the tuberculous lesion will heal with only a fibrous scar remaining. The scar may contain calcium deposits, which can be seen on x-ray. A minimum of lung tissue is actually destroyed.

The standard lesion of chronic tuberculosis is called a **tubercle.** It consists of a clump of bacilli surrounded by inflammatory cells. Within the tubercle, cells are killed by the bacilli—so the core becomes necrotic. It resembles a cheesy mass that is referred to as **caseous** material. Formation of this cheesy mass is called **caseation.**

The mass becomes liquefied and is coughed up in the sputum, leaving a cavity in the lung. Formation of cavities is the way lung tissue is destroyed in advanced tuberculosis. Numerous tubercles form and fuse, and caseation occurs. The result is the formation of large cavities. Blood vessels spanning a cavity can rupture, with a hemorrhage following. Blood is then coughed up which is known as **hemoptysis.** This advanced form of the disease is called chronic fibrocaseous tuberculosis. The name refers to the fibrous scarring and caseation or destruction. Pleurisy is always a complication of chronic tuberculosis.

You have probably heard the term "galloping consumption" used to describe a killing disease. This lethal course of the disease is acute tuberculous pneumonia. The resistance of the patient is totally overwhelmed by the infecting organisms, and no defense is made against them. Frequently, because of the low resistance, secondary bacterial invaders enter, causing the severe pneumonia. If the tuberculosis spreads by means of the bloodstream, setting up minute tubercles in other organs, the condition is called acute miliary tuberculosis. Numerous bacilli enter the bloodstream, as blood vessels are destroyed by the disease.

Antituberculous drugs control the progression of the disease in many people. Surgery is sometimes performed to remove the diseased parts of the lung.

■ Bronchogenic Carcinoma

Cancer of the lung, **bronchogenic carcinoma,** arises from the bronchial tree. It can be observed with the **bronchoscope,** a lighted tube that can be placed down the trachea. A biopsy can be made using this instrument. Although bronchogenic cancer is easily diagnosed in this way, it is a most lethal form of cancer. The prognosis is poor.

Lung cancer is more common in men than in women. Although the cause is not known, it is linked to smoking and the inhalation of carcinogens, cancer-causing agents. This can be an occupational hazard among workers who are constantly exposed to air pollution, exhaust gases, and industrial fumes.

The great danger in bronchogenic carcinoma is blockage of the airway by the malignant tumor as it grows into the lumen of the bronchus. The affected part of the lung collapses for lack of air. A malignant lung tumor is shown in Figure 12–15.

Blockage of any secretions leads to infection. Abscesses form in the obstructed bronchus, and walls become weakened and dilated, resulting in bronchiectasis. Bronchopneumonia is likely to develop and may be the cause of death.

The symptoms of lung cancer are a persistent cough and hemoptysis. The blood in the sputum results from the erosion of blood vessels by the growing malignancy. Anorexia, weight loss, and weakness accompany the disease. The poor oxygenation of the blood explains the generalized weak-

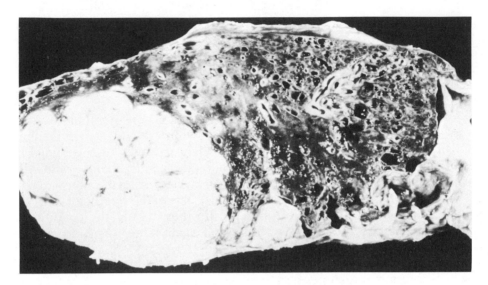

Figure 12-15. Carcinoma of the lung (large white area). (*Courtesy of Dr. David R. Duffell.*)

ness. The patient experiences difficulty in breathing due to the obstructed airway.

Diagnosis of lung cancer is made from a biopsy of the tumor, detecting cancer cells in the sputum, or washings from the bronchoscopy examination. Treatment may be surgery, radiation, or chemotherapy, depending on the particular tumor. In addition to primary carcinoma of the lungs, the lungs are a frequent site of metastases from other organs.

■ Hyaline Membrane Disease

Hyaline membrane disease is a condition, usually fatal, in which the lungs of a premature newborn infant collapse. A hyalinelike membrane forms, lining the alveoli of the immature lungs and thus interfering with air exchange. The normal amount of surfactant, a substance necessary to reduce surface tension, is not produced, causing the lungs to collapse.

■ Hiccoughs

Most everyone has experienced the annoyance of hiccoughs. What causes this phenomenon? Hiccoughs result from a spasm of the muscles of inspiration, particularly the diaphragm. Air is inhaled and the air passageway then closes abruptly, producing the characteristic sound. Hiccoughs can occur in normal people after eating or drinking. They can usually be stopped by holding the breath, drinking water, or rebreathing from a paper bag.

Hiccoughs can accompany certain diseases and are then more difficult to stop. Persistent hiccoughs are sometimes treated with medication. If this fails, one of the nerves that stimulates the diaphragm—one of the phrenic nerves—can be blocked with local anesthesia.

SUMMARY

Reviewing the respiratory structure and function laid the foundation for understanding diseases of the system. The interaction of the respiratory and circulatory systems in providing the entire body with oxygen was explained.

Diseases of the upper respiratory system can be caused by both viruses and bacteria. Many viral infections, such as the common cold and influenza, are followed by bacterial infections. Pyogenic bacteria—streptococci, staphylococci, and pneumococci—cause the formation of pus. This is added to the excessive mucous secretion resulting from inflammation of the mucous membranes.

In allergic diseases—hay fever and asthma—the cause is hypersensitivity to foreign proteins. The allergy sufferer has abnormal antibodies, or reagins, also called immunoglobulins or IgE, that sensitize parts of the respiratory tract. The sensitization is in the nasal passages with hay fever and in the bronchi with asthma.

Certain respiratory diseases are related as a result of obstruction in the airways. Blockage of secretions sets the stage for bacterial infections. Chronic bronchitis can lead to pneumonia, bronchiectasis, and emphysema. Influenza and pneumonia can also cause bronchiectasis.

Pneumonia is caused by both viruses and bacteria. The elderly and chronically ill are very susceptible to pneumonia, which may even prove fatal. Predisposing causes of bronchopneumonia are chronic bronchitis and bronchiectasis. Again, the relationship between one respiratory disease and another is seen.

The severity of tuberculosis depends on the dosage of tubercle bacilli received and the resistance of the patient. The incidence of tuberculosis has greatly decreased with better living conditions, greater caution in the presence of infectious sputum, and earlier detection of the disease.

Lung cancer, although easily diagnosed, has a poor prognosis. The greatest danger is that the malignancy will obstruct the air passageway and the affected part of the lung will collapse.

STUDY QUESTIONS

1. Explain the cause of the common cold's symptoms.
2. Why is not everyone allergic to ragweed?

3. Why is acute bronchitis most serious in small children, the aged, and chronically ill?
4. Explain the hypoxia that can develop in chronic bronchitis.
5. What is the cause of the muscular constriction of the bronchi in bronchial asthma?
6. What is the theory behind allergy shots?
7. Explain the development of bronchiectasis.
8. Why is the sputum foul-smelling in bronchiectasis?
9. How does emphysema develop?
10. Explain the difficult breathing in emphysema.
11. Name two ways in which a pneumothorax develops.
12. Describe two ways in which atelectasis can occur.
13. Differentiate between lobar pneumonia and bronchopneumonia as to (a) onset of symptoms, (b) length of course, (c) consolidation of lung, and (d) condition of lungs after each type.
14. Explain the causes of symptoms in influenzal pneumonia.
15. Describe the two kinds of pleurisy and the major problem of each.
16. How are pneumothorax and empyema related to atelectasis?
17. Explain the process of cavity formation in chronic fibrocaseous tuberculosis.
18. How is bronchogenic carcinoma diagnosed?
19. What are some possible complications of lung cancer?
20. Name several precautions that should be taken in dealing with tuberculous patients.
21. Describe the impairment in chronic obstructive pulmonary disease.
22. Why is hyaline membrane disease usually fatal?
23. What causes hiccoughs?

CHAPTER 13

Diseases of the Endocrine System

The functions of the endocrine system cover a broad range of action. Endocrine activity affects the entire body: growth and development, metabolism, sexual activity, and even mental ability and emotions. The endocrine system is a means of communication between one body part and another.

All the glands of internal secretions are included in this system. These glands secrete directly into the bloodstream or lymph and possess no ducts. The pituitary gland, the thyroid, the adrenals, and the parathyroids are all part of the endocrine system. A certain area of the pancreas is endocrine in function, as are the sex glands. The sex glands—the ovaries and testes—will be studied with the Reproductive System in Chapter 14. Figure 13-1 shows the endocrine glands.

The secretions of endocrine glands are **hormones**—the chemical messengers that circulate in the blood. Some of these hormones affect the whole body, whereas others act only on a distant organ, a target organ. Hormones may be steroids, small proteins, or modified amino acids.

Most glandular activity is controlled by the pituitary, which is sometimes called the master gland. The pituitary itself is controlled by an area of the brain called the hypothalamus.

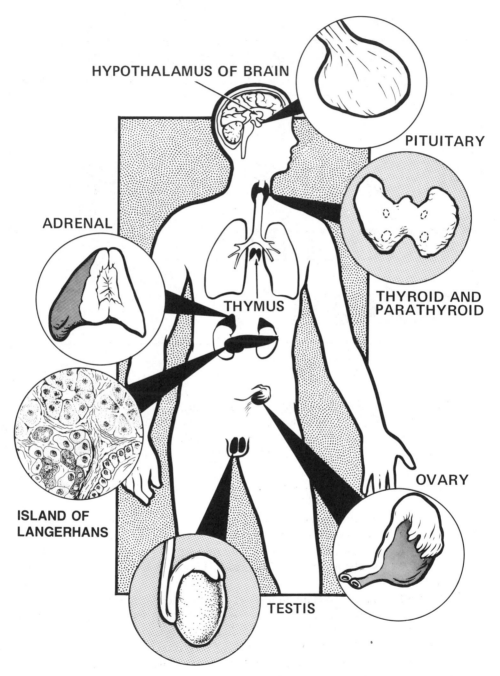

Figure 13-1. The endocrine glands.

The body is conservative and secretes hormones only as needed. For example, insulin is secreted when the blood sugar level rises. Another hormone, glucagon, works antagonistically to **insulin** and is released when the blood sugar level falls below normal. Hormones are potent chemicals, so their circulating levels must be carefully controlled. When the level of a hormone is adequate, its further release is stopped. This type of control is called a **negative feedback mechanism.** Its importance will become clearer as specific diseases of the endocrine system are considered.

Overactivity or underactivity of a gland is the malfunction that most commonly causes endocrine diseases. If a gland secretes an excessive amount of its hormone, it is hyperactive. This condition is sometimes caused by a hypertrophied gland or by a glandular tumor.

A gland that fails to secrete its hormone or secretes an inadequate amount of it is hypoactive. The gland may be diseased, tumorous, or it may have been adversely affected by trauma, surgery, or radiation. A gland that has decreased in size and consequently is secreting inadequately is said to be atrophied. Each endocrine gland will be discussed with an emphasis on normal function and importance. The diseases caused by hypoactivity and hyperactivity of each gland will then be explained.

STRUCTURE AND FUNCTION OF THE PITUITARY GLAND

The wonder of the pituitary gland is its tiny size and yet its tremendous functions. It is only the size of a pea suspended from the base of the brain by a small stalk. The pituitary gland fits into a bony depression in one of the skull bones that carefully protects it from injury. The pituitary gland is illustrated in Figure 13–2.

Another name for the pituitary gland is the **hypophysis.** The hypophysis has two parts to it, each of which acts as a separate gland. Each part is stimulated differently to secrete, and each secretes entirely different hormones.

The anterior and larger portion of the hypophysis is the **adenohypophysis.** *Adeno* means gland, and this part is truly glandular. It is in direct communication with the hypothalamus of the brain. Portal blood vessels extending through the stalk connect the two. The hypothalamus is an extremely important coordinating center for the brain. It directs which hormones the anterior pituitary gland should secrete at a particular time. It does this by sending substances called **releasing factors** to the anterior pituitary through the connecting blood vessels. The pituitary then secretes the proper hormone.

The posterior pituitary, or posterior hypophysis, works differently. It receives hormones secreted by the hypothalamus and stores them for

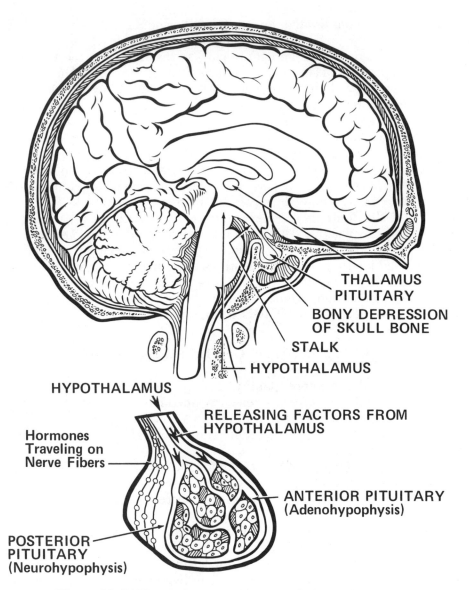

Figure 13-2. The pituitary gland and its relation to the brain.

subsequent release. These hormones travel over nerve fibers from the hypothalamus to the posterior hypophysis. Because of the neural connection with the hypothalamus, this posterior portion of the pituitary gland is called the **neurohypophysis.**

What can this little pea-sized structure control that makes it the master gland? The anterior pituitary, the adenohypophysis, secretes six hormones called tropic hormones. The word element *tropic* means going toward. That is what these six hormones do. They go toward a particular target organ.

Hormones of the Anterior Pituitary Gland

Growth hormone (GH; also called **somatotropin**) affects all parts of the body by promoting growth and development of the tissues. Before puberty, it stimulates the growth of long bones, increasing the child's height. Soft tissues—organs such as the liver, heart, and kidneys—also increase in size and develop under the influence of growth hormone. After adolescence, growth hormone is secreted in lesser amounts but continues to function in promoting tissue replacement and repair.

The thyroid gland regulates metabolism, the rate at which the body produces and uses energy. Secretion of thyroid hormone is controlled by the anterior pituitary. The pituitary hormone that stimulates the thyroid gland is thyroid stimulating hormone (TSH; also called **thyrotropin**). In the absence of TSH, the thyroid gland stops functioning.

The adrenal glands, essential to life, are also regulated by the anterior pituitary. The adrenal glands have an inner part, the medulla, and an outer portion, the cortex. It is the cortex that is controlled by the anterior pituitary. The tropic hormone affecting the adrenal cortex is adrenocorticotropic hormone **(ACTH).**

The anterior pituitary regulates sexual development and function by means of a group of hormones known as the **gonadotropins.** These are not sex hormones, but they affect the sex organs, the gonads. They are follicle stimulating hormone (FSH), luteinizing hormone (LH), and prolactin (LTH). These gonadotropic hormones regulate the menstrual cycle and secretion of male and female hormones. The relationship between the anterior pituitary and its target organs is seen in Figure 13-3.

DISEASES OF THE ANTERIOR PITUITARY GLAND

■ Hyperpituitarism

The most noticeable result of **hyperpituitarism** is the effect of excessive growth hormone. The condition produces a giant if the hypersecretion of growth hormone occurs before puberty. Normally at puberty the ends of the long bones seal with the shafts and no further height is attained. Excessive growth hormone retards this normal closure of the bones. Sexual development is usually decreased and mental development may be normal or retarded. Gigantism is usually the result of a tumor, an **adenoma,** of the anterior pituitary. Removal of the tumor or radiation treatment to reduce its size decreases the secretion of growth hormone. Gigantism is illustrated in Figure 13-4.

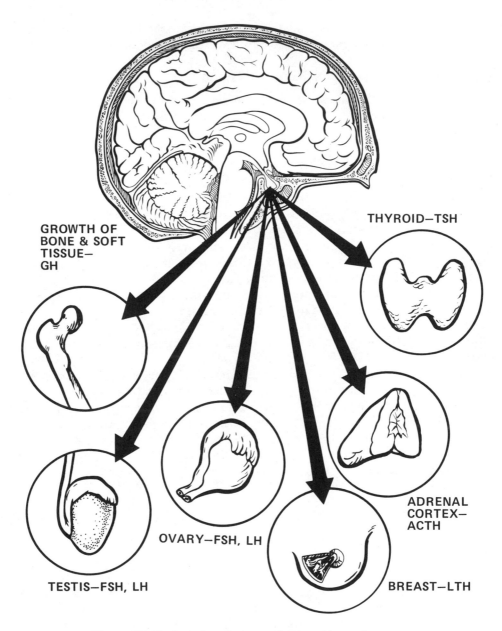

GROWTH OF BONE & SOFT TISSUE— GH

THYROID—TSH

TESTIS—FSH, LH

OVARY—FSH, LH

BREAST—LTH

ADRENAL CORTEX— ACTH

Figure 13-3. Anterior pituitary gland and its target organs.

If the excessive production of growth hormone occurs after puberty, when full stature is attained, the result is different. This is the condition of **acromegaly;** the word element *megaly* means enlargement. The long bones can no longer grow, but the bones of the hands, feet, and face enlarge. There is also excessive growth of soft tissues. The features of the face

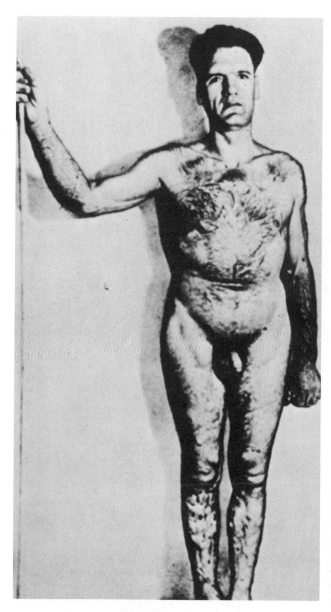

Figure 13-4. A 36-year-old pituitary giant approximately 6'9" tall. The head is large, and enlargement of the hands and feet is progressive. (*From Kosowicz. Atlas of Endocrine Diseases, 1978. Courtesy of The Charles Press.*)

become coarsened; the nose and lips enlarge, and the lower jaw protrudes, producing an overbite that interferes with chewing. The skin and tongue thicken, the latter causing slurred speech. A curvature of the spine often develops, giving the patient a bent appearance. The curvature is due to an overgrowth of the vertebrae. This hyperactivity of the pituitary gland is generally due to a tumor. A patient with acromegaly is illustrated in Figure 13-5.

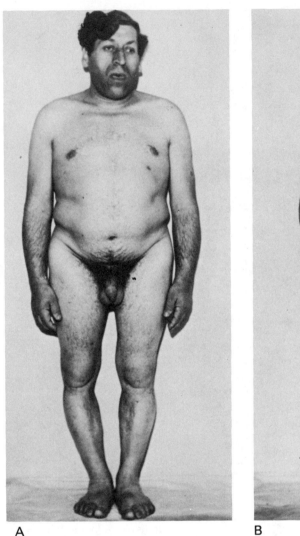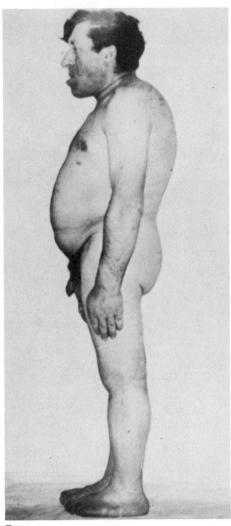

A   B

Figure 13-5. A. A 43-year-old patient with acromegaly. Note heavy,
stocky build; broad chest; large head; and heavy hands and feet. B.
Curvature of the spine causes the arms to appear excessively large.
Thickening of the fingers interferes with manual dexterity. (*From Kosowicz.
Atlas of Endocrine Diseases, 1978. Courtesy of The Charles Press.*)

■ Hypopituitarism

Hypopituitarism can result from damage to the anterior lobe of the pituitary
gland or from an inadequate secretion of hormones. A fracture at the base
of the skull, a tumor, or ischemia (lack of blood flow) can cause pituitary
destruction. Lack of blood flow causes an infarction, and the tissue becomes
necrotic. Hypopituitarism can be mild or severe. If the entire anterior lobe

of the pituitary is destroyed, the condition is called **panhypopituitarism,** *pan* meaning all. No pituitary hormones are secreted.

The abnormalities that result from the absence of tropic hormones are numerous. The thyroid gland, for example, is dependent on thyroid stimulating hormone from the pituitary for its functioning. Without that tropic hormone, the thyroid atrophies and the functions of the thyroid cease. Mental dullness and lethargy, a condition of drowsiness, develop.

Lack of ACTH causes the adrenal cortex to atrophy. Inadequate cortical hormones result in a salt imbalance and improper metabolism of nutrients. The adrenal cortical hormones are essential to life.

Absence of the gonadotropic hormones depresses sexual functions. The gonads atrophy without stimulation of the tropic hormones. If the lack of hormones exists before puberty, sexual development is impaired. In an adult woman menstruation ceases; an adult male will lack sex drive or have aspermia, that is, no formation or emission of sperm. Figure 13–6 illustrates the glandular failure caused by severe hypopituitarism.

Hypopituitarism caused by a tumor may show additional symptoms. Pressure of the tumor may cause pain, a headache, or a peculiar form of blindness. Figure 13–7 shows the closeness of the pituitary gland to the optic nerves. As the tumor enlarges, it interferes with these nerves.

The patient suffering from hypopituitarism must be treated with hormonal supplements. Administration of **thyroxine, cortisone,** growth hormone, and sex hormones can compensate for the dysfunctional glands. It is significant that all these failures result from hypoactivity of the anterior pituitary. For this reason the anterior pituitary is called the master gland.

A different form of hypopituitarism sometimes occurs in children. Inadequate growth hormone can cause a pituitary dwarf. This patient is mentally bright but small and underdeveloped sexually. All growth processes are retarded; teeth, for example, are late in erupting. A 28-year-old pituitary dwarf is shown in Figure 13–8. Growth hormones to prevent this condition are now being synthesized and tested.

Simmond's syndrome, a form of premature senility, is the result of chronic pituitary insufficiency, a case of panhypopituitarism. A child with this disease has the appearance of an old man or woman with pale, wrinkled skin and fine, soft hair. A 29-year-old man with pituitary insufficiency is shown in Figure 13–9.

Simmond's syndrome develops in an adult if the anterior pituitary becomes necrotic. This can follow a serious head injury or pituitary ischemia. Blood vessels to the pituitary occasionally collapse after a hemorrhage from a difficult delivery. A patient affected with this condition is seen in Figure 13–10. The breasts lack normal engorgement after a delivery, and pigmentation around the nipple is decreased. Simmond's syndrome may also be caused by an undifferentiated tumor of the pituitary that secretes no hormones.

Symptoms of this disease include weakness, dry, smooth skin with no

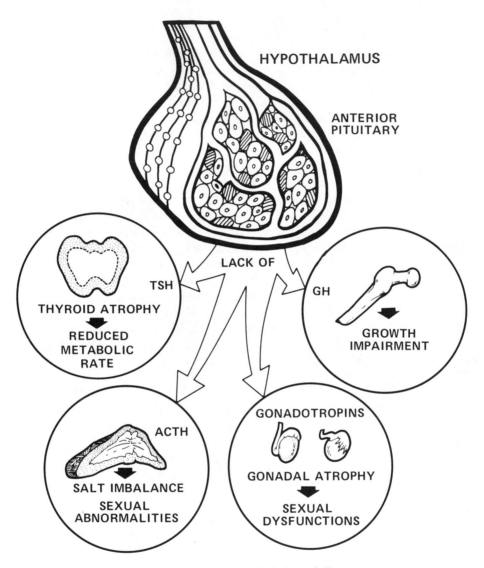

Figure 13-6. Effects of pituitary failure.

sweating, and a loss of pubic and axillary hair. Both blood pressure and the rate of metabolism are low. Menstruation ceases in a woman, and sex drive is decreased. Since Simmond's syndrome is a form of panhypopituitarism, the symptoms result from widespread glandular failure. The thyroid, adrenal cortex, and gonads cease to function because of inadequate stimulation by the anterior pituitary gland.

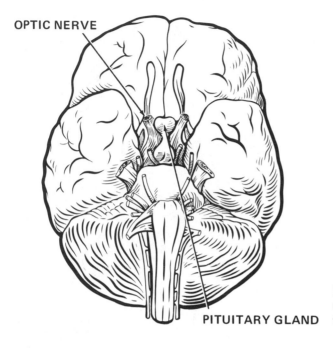

OPTIC NERVE

PITUITARY GLAND

Figure 13-7. Base of brain showing proximity of pituitary gland to optic nerves.

FUNCTION OF THE POSTERIOR PITUITARY GLAND

The posterior pituitary, or neurohypophysis, secretes two hormones: **oxytocin** and vasopressin, also called **antidiuretic hormone** (ADH). Oxytocin causes smooth muscle, particularly that of the uterus, to contract. It strengthens contractions during labor and helps to prevent hemorrhage after delivery. Antidiuretic hormone prevents excessive water loss through the kidneys and makes the collecting ducts permeable to water. Water is then reabsorbed back into the bloodstream by the kidney tubules.

DISEASE OF THE POSTERIOR PITUITARY GLAND

■ Diabetes Insipidus

In the absence of ADH, water is not reabsorbed and is lost in the urine. **Polyuria,** excessive urination, results. This is the condition of **diabetes insipidus,** a disease not related to **diabetes mellitus.** The posterior pituitary fails to secrete ADH, and a copious amount of dilute urine is therefore passed. This excessive water loss could quickly lead to dehydration. The body compensates, however, through an insatiable thirst, a condition known as **polydipsia.** Treatment of diabetes insipidus is the administration of ADH.

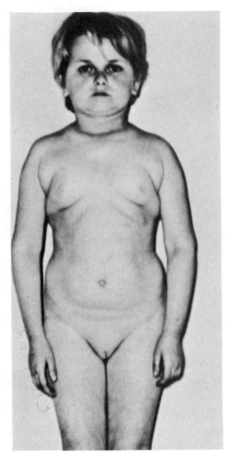

Figure 13-8. This 28-year-old pituitary dwarf is 45 inches tall, with the characteristic round face and fat deposits in breasts and abdomen. No sexual development is observed. (*From Kosowicz. Atlas of Endocrine Diseases, 1978. Courtesy of The Charles Press.*)

Figure 13–11A shows the normal action of ADH, and Figure 13–11B shows the effects of its absence.

STRUCTURE AND FUNCTION OF THE THYROID GLAND

The activity of the thyroid gland affects the whole body. It regulates the metabolic rate, the rate at which calories are used. The thyroid gland, through its hormone thyroxine, governs cellular oxygen consumption and, thus, energy and heat production. The more oxygen that is used, the more calories are metabolized ("burned up"). Thyroxine assures that enough body heat is produced to maintain normal temperature even in a cold environment.

Many people blame obesity on an underactive thyroid, a low rate of metabolism. Although there is a relationship between a person's body weight and metabolic rate, diet is still the critical factor in controlling obesity. A person with a low rate of metabolism requires fewer calories than someone who uses them at a faster rate.

Structure of the Thyroid Gland

The thyroid gland is located in the neck region, one lobe on either side of the trachea. A connecting strip, or isthmus, anterior to the trachea connects the two lobes. The thyroid gland lies just below the Adam's apple, the protrusion formed by part of the larynx. Figure 13–12 illustrates the thyroid gland. Internally, the thyroid gland consists of countless follicles, microscopic sacs. Within these protein-containing follicles, the thyroid hormones thyroxine and **triiodothyronine** are made. Thin-walled capillaries run between the follicles in a position ideal to receive the thyroid hormones.

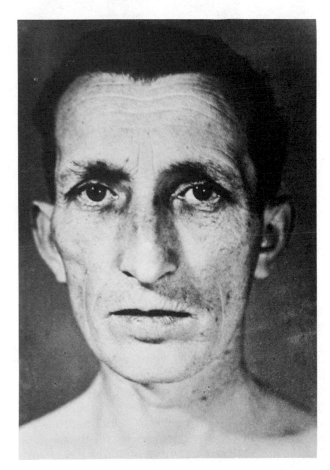

Figure 13-9. Face of a 29-year-old patient with a pituitary tumor and insufficient pituitary hormones. Note premature aging. The skin shows many fine wrinkles and lack of beard growth. (*From Kosowicz. Atlas of Endocrine Diseases, 1978. Courtesy of The Charles Press.*)

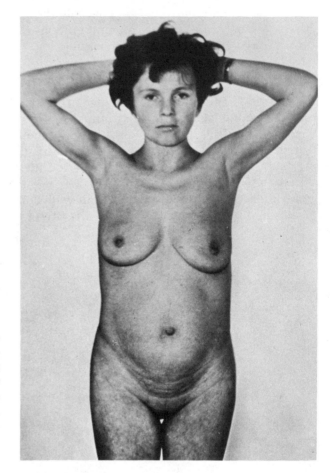

Figure 13-10. A 26-year-old patient with hypopituitarism after childbirth. Her skin is pale, and pubic and axillary hair has ceased to grow. Note lack of breast development. (*From Kosowicz. Atlas of Endocrine Diseases, 1978. Courtesy of The Charles Press.*)

Function of the Thyroid Gland

The thyroid gland synthesizes, stores, and releases thyroid hormones, which contain iodine. In fact, most of the iodide ions of the body are taken into the thyroid gland by a mechanism called the iodide trap. Iodine combines with an amino acid. Two of these groups join, and the thyroid hormones are formed.

The hormones are stored until needed and then released into the blood capillaries. In the blood the thyroid hormones combine with plasma proteins. Tests to determine the activity of the thyroid gland are based on this combination of triiodothyronine (T_3) and thyroxine (T_4) with plasma proteins. In the T_3 and T_4 tests, a sample of the patient's serum is incubated with radioactive thyroid hormones and resin. The resin absorbs the hormones that are not bound to the blood proteins. Radioactivity counts of the serum and resin are made and the percentage of thyroid hormones absorbed by the resin is calculated. A low percentage of absorption indicates a poorly functioning thyroid gland. A high percentage of absorption indicates hyperactivity. In the latter case, the patient's own thyroid hormones had saturated the plasma proteins, and the radioactive hormones were absorbed by the resin. This is a more accurate means of measuring thyroid activity than the test used for many years, the BMR, or basal metabolic rate. The term basal metabolic rate, however, is still used. It refers to a person's oxygen consumption while at rest.

Effects of Thyroid Hormones

Although there is more than one thyroid hormone, for clarity the thyroid hormones are referred to here as thyroxine, the one that is secreted in the largest quantity. Thyroxine stimulates cellular metabolism by increasing the rate of oxygen use with subsequent energy and heat production.

Keeping in mind that thyroxine stimulates the rate of cellular metabolism, the effect of an increased thyroxine level on heart activity becomes clear. Think of it this way: Faster cellular metabolism increases the cell's demand for oxygen. More oxygen must be circulated to the cells. Nutrients are

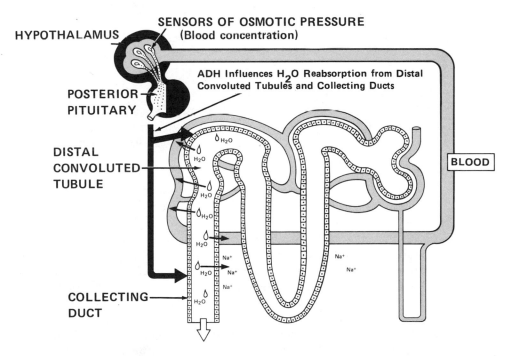

Figure 13-11. A. Normal action of antidiuretic hormone (ADH).

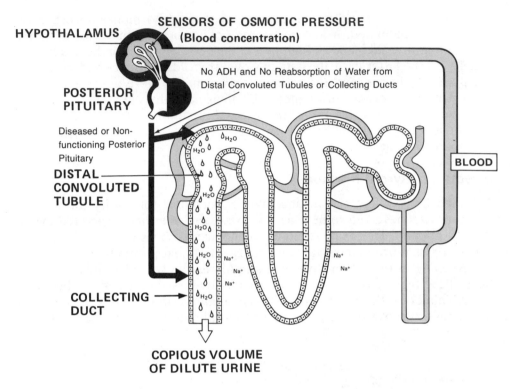

Figure 13-11. B. Effect of antidiuretic hormone (ADH) deficiency.

converted to energy in the presence of oxygen and the waste products of metabolism, including carbon dioxide, are formed. These must be carried away from the cells. The circulatory system can meet these needs by increasing blood flow to the cells. Increased blood flow is obtained by greater cardiac output, more heart activity.

What about the effect of increased cellular metabolism on respiration? The greater need for oxygen and a corresponding accumulation of carbon dioxide stimulate the respiratory center of the brain. Stimulation of the respiratory center results in a faster rate and greater depth of breathing.

How does thyroxine affect body temperature? Heat is produced through cellular metabolism, and thyroxine stimulates this process. In a cold environment, thyroxine secretion increases to assure adequate body heat. If excessive body heat is produced, it is dissipated in two ways. Blood vessels of the skin dilate, increasing blood flow at the body surface, and giving the body a flushed appearance. As the blood flows through the skin blood vessels, excess heat escapes. The body is also cooled by the perspiration mechanism. Body temperature is controlled by a regulatory center in the brain.

Thyroxine also has a stimulatory effect on the gastrointestinal system. It increases the secretion of digestive juices and the movement of material through the digestive tract. Absorption of carbohydrates from the intestine is also increased under the influence of thyroxine, assuring adequate fuel for cellular metabolism. The effects of thyroxine are illustrated in Figure 13–13.

An understanding of these effects of thyroxine will make the diseases of the thyroid gland meaningful. Basically, the results of inadequate or excessive thyroxine secretion will be considered. The symptoms of each disease will be related to the function of thyroxine.

Control of Circulating Thyroxine Level

The anterior pituitary gland stimulates the thyroid by releasing thyroid stimulating hormone, TSH. The thyroid in turn releases thyroxine, which circulates in the blood to all cells and tissues. When the level of circulating thyroxine is high, the anterior pituitary is inhibited and stops releasing TSH. This is an example of a negative feedback mechanism. An adequate level of thyroxine prevents further synthesis of the hormone. When the level of thyroxine falls, the anterior pituitary is released from the inhibition, and once again sends out TSH. This feedback mechanism is shown in Figure 13–14.

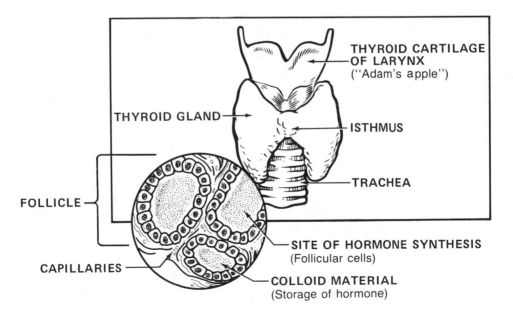

Figure 13-12. The thyroid gland.

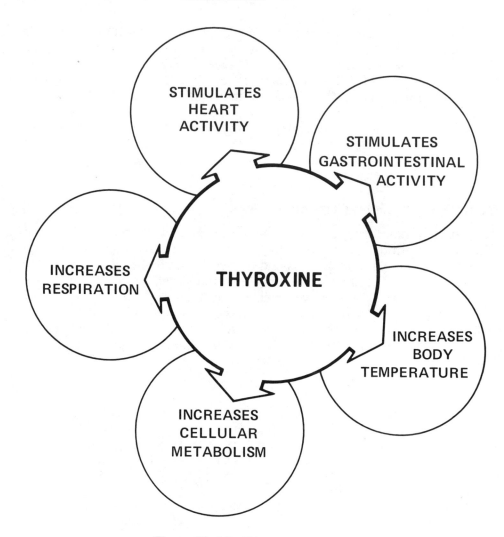

Figure 13-13. Effects of thyroxine.

At times this mechanism fails, constituting one basis for a thyroid disease. The thyroid gland may be perfectly healthy, but if the body's iodine supply is inadequate, the gland cannot produce thyroxine. It is possible for the thyroid gland to be overstimulated or understimulated by the anterior pituitary. The thyroid gland itself may be diseased, with a resultant hyperactivity or hypoactivity. These are some of the conditions that will be discussed.

DISEASES OF THE THYROID GLAND

■ Goiter

Goiter is an enlargement of the thyroid gland. The enlargement may be due to hypoactivity or hyperactivity of the thyroid. A goiter develops if the gland is unable to produce adequate thyroxine because of an iodine deficiency. The thyroid also enlarges if the gland is hyperactive.

The most common type of goiter is the **diffuse colloidal goiter,** or nontoxic goiter. The follicles of the thyroid gland normally contain colloid, a protein material. In this type of goiter an excessive amount of colloid is secreted into the follicles, increasing the size of the gland. A diffuse colloidal goiter is also called an endemic goiter because it is common in a particular geographic region.

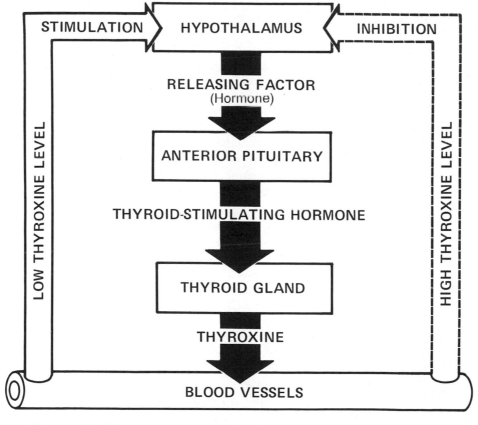

Figure 13-14. Control of thyroxine secretion (negative feedback mechanism).

The usual cause of an endemic goiter is insufficient iodine in the diet. Inland areas, such as the Great Lakes region, and mountainous regions, like the Alps, have a very low iodine content in the soil and water. As a result, the inhabitants are unable to synthesize thyroxine adequately.

Normally, when the proper level of thyroxine is circulating, the anterior pituitary stops secreting thyroid stimulating hormone. In the absence of thyroxine there is nothing to inhibit the anterior pituitary. As a result, the continuous secretion of thyroid stimulating hormone causes the thyroid gland to enlarge as a compensatory mechanism. The thyroid enlarges in an attempt to meet the demand of thyroid stimulating hormone.

An enlargement of the neck is generally the only symptom. Usually enough thyroxine is produced to prevent the symptoms of **hypothyroidism.** The condition responds well to treatment with iodines, so the use of iodized salt prevents endemic goiter formation. If the goiter is very advanced, surgery may be necessary. A very large goiter puts pressure on the esophagus, causing difficulty in swallowing, or presses on the trachea, causing a cough or choking sensation.

Other factors can cause a simple diffuse colloidal goiter, for example, a defect in the thyroxine-synthesizing mechanism. A young girl entering adolescence may develop this type of goiter because of an increased need for thyroxine at this time.

■ Hyperthyroidism

Another type of goiter is the **adenomatous** or **nodular goiter,** named from adenoma, a glandular tumor. These nodules are secretory and produce an excessive amount of thyroxine, a condition of **hyperthyroidism.** Various goiters are shown in Figure 13–15.

The effects of thyroxine have been discussed. An excessive amount of this hormone augments these effects. The hyperthyroid patient is very nervous and experiences tremors, a shakiness, particularly in the hands. The metabolic rate is high, causing sweating and a rapid pulse. A nodule or adenoma may put pressure on the trachea or esophagus. Surgery is sometimes necessary to remove part of the thyroid gland, but medication is often effective in preventing further enlargement.

Graves' disease is another type of goiter. In this case the entire gland hypertrophies, and there are no nodules. The patient suffers from severe hyperthyroidism. Graves' disease is far more common in women than in men and usually affects young women.

A patient with Graves' disease has a very characteristic appearance. The facial expression is strained and tense, and there is a stare in the eyes. The eyeballs protrude outward, a condition called **exophthalmos** (Figure 13–16). This is caused by edema in the tissue behind the eyes. The bulging of the eyes can be so severe that the eyelids do not close, and the swelling some-

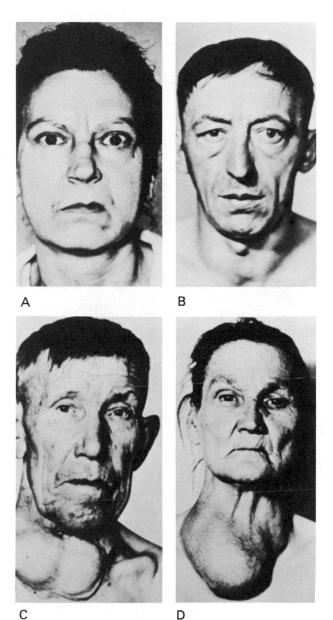

Figure 13-15. **A.** A nontoxic, nodular goiter. **B.** A 32-year-old man showing diffuse enlargement of the thyroid. **C.** An elderly man with a multinodular and cystic goiter. **D.** A diffuse, multinodular colloid goiter. (*From Kosowicz. Atlas of Endocrine Diseases, 1978. Courtesy of The Charles Press.*)

times damages the optic nerve. This symptom generally persists when the hyperthyroidism is corrected.

The patient has a tremendous appetite but loses weight to the point of appearing emaciated, as calories are burned up at a rapid rate. Thyroxine speeds the passage of food through the digestive tract. There is no time for

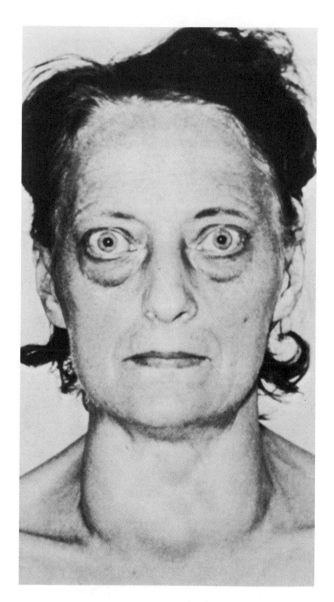

Figure 13-16. A Graves' disease patient with marked exophthalmos. The eyes have a fixed, staring expression. Note marked swelling of neck due to an enlarged thyroid. (*From Kosowicz. Atlas of Endocrine Diseases, 1978. Courtesy of The Charles Press.*)

the normal reabsorption of water from the large intestine, so diarrhea frequently accompanies the disease.

Tachycardia, rapid pulse rate, and palpitation are also among the symptoms. The patient is extremely nervous, excitable, and is always tired but cannot sleep because of the hyperactivity of the body. The high metabolic rate causes excessive heat production, which results in profuse perspiration.

The skin is always moist, and an insatiable thirst follows the loss of water. The symptoms of Graves' disease are shown in Figure 13–17.

The cause of Graves' disease is not understood although it may be related to the nervous system. A terrifying experience or shock can trigger its onset. Graves' disease may be an autoimmune condition in which antibodies to a thyroid antigen stimulate the hyperactivity.

Graves' disease can sometimes be treated with medication that inhibits the synthesis of thyroxine, but removal of the thyroid gland may be necessary. If the gland is removed, hormonal supplements must be given. Partial removal of the thyroid gland allows the remaining portion to secrete hormones.

■ Hypothyroidism

Myxedema is the condition of severe hypothyroidism, an inadequate level of thyroxine. The symptoms are just the opposite of those in Graves' disease. The patient's face is bloated, the tongue is thick, and the eyelids are puffy. The skin is dry and scaly, and there is little perspiration. The patient has no tolerance of a cold environment.

A person with myxedema experiences muscular weakness and **somnolence,** sleeping for 14 to 16 hours a day. The mental and physical processes are sluggish, the speech is slurred, and reflexes are slow. Heart rate is decreased, and the slowed circulation causes edema to develop. Lack

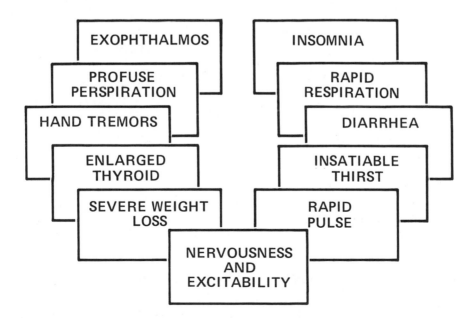

Figure 13–17. Symptoms of Graves' disease.

of thyroxine increases the amount of circulating lipids, which leads to the development of atherosclerosis (Chapter 8). The digestive system works sluggishly, so the patient suffers from constipation. Weight gain also accompanies the disease.

Myxedema affects women more than men, and usually women of middle age. It can result from radiation damage to the thyroid gland or after thyroid surgery if thyroxine is not administered. Myxedema can be a primary disease of the thyroid gland or secondary to pituitary disease. If the pituitary gland does not secrete thyroid stimulating hormones, the thyroid gland ceases to function. Patients with myxedema are shown in Figure 13–18. Myxedema is treated by administering thyroxine. The condition generally responds well to treatment and the symptoms disappear.

■ Cretinism

Cretinism is a congenital thyroid deficiency in which thyroxine is not synthesized. Thyroxine is essential to both physical and mental development. Lack of this hormone in an infant or young child causes mental retardation and an abnormal, dwarfed stature. Cretinism can result from an error in fetal development if the thyroid gland fails to form or is nonfunctional. Cretinism sometimes occurs in areas of endemic goiter where the mother suffers from an inadequate iodine supply.

The cretin is a dwarf with a stocky stature and a characteristically protruding abdomen. The sexual organs do not develop, and the face of the cretin is typically misshapen: a broad, sunken nose, small eyes set far apart, puffy eyelids, and a short forehead. A thick tongue protrudes from a wide-open mouth, and the face is expressionless. Figure 13–19 shows an example of a cretin.

The earlier this condition is diagnosed and treated with thyroxine, the more optimistic is the prognosis. Life-long hormonal therapy will be required. An untreated 14-year-old patient is shown in Figure 13–20.

Even less severe cases of hypothyroidism should be treated in infants. A baby may appear normal at first and only later give indication that the developmental processes are retarded. The baby may be slow in smiling, reaching, sitting, and standing. Valuable treatment time has been lost by then. The American Thyroid Association recommends that all newborn babies be given a simple blood test for hypothryoidism. Some hospitals have already adopted the practice. Figure 13–21 shows the effectiveness of thyroxine replacement therapy.

STRUCTURE AND FUNCTION OF THE ADRENAL GLANDS

The adrenal glands are located at the top of each kidney. Each of the glands consists of two distinct parts: an outer part, the cortex, and an inner section, the medulla. The cortex and the medulla secrete different hormones. The

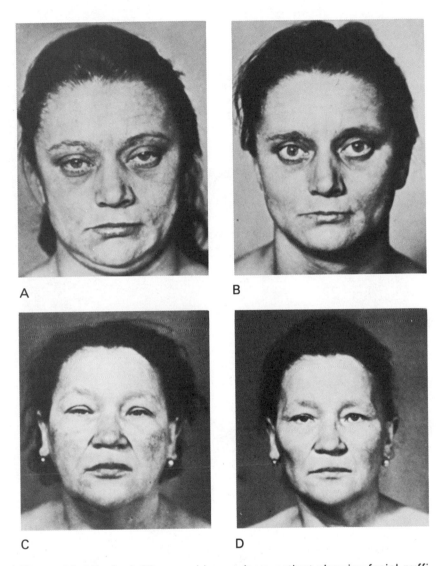

A

B

C

D

Figure 13–18. **A.** A 29-year-old myxedema patient showing facial puffiness, muscle weakness, and drooping eyelids, which give a sleepy appearance. **B.** The same patient after 2 months of thyroxine replacement. **C.** A 62-year-old patient with myxedema exhibiting marked edema of the face and a somnolent look. The hair is stiff and without luster. **D.** The same patient after 3 months of treatment with thyroxine. (*From Kosowicz. Atlas of Endocrine Diseases, 1978. Courtesy of The Charles Press.*)

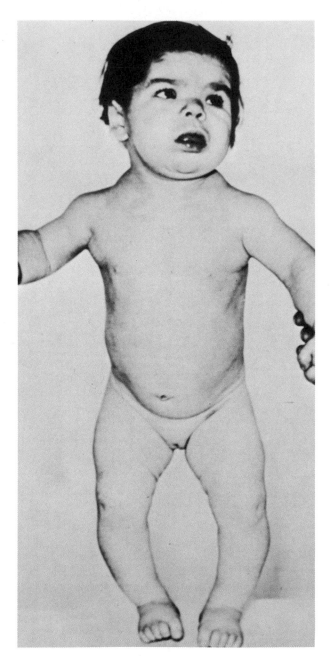

Figure 13-19. A 4-year-old child with congenital hypothyroidism. Note stunted growth (32 inches) and typical facial features: broad, flat nose; open mouth; and protruding tongue. The child cannot stand unsupported or speak. (*From Kosowicz. Atlas of Endocrine Diseases, 1978. Courtesy of The Charles Press.*)

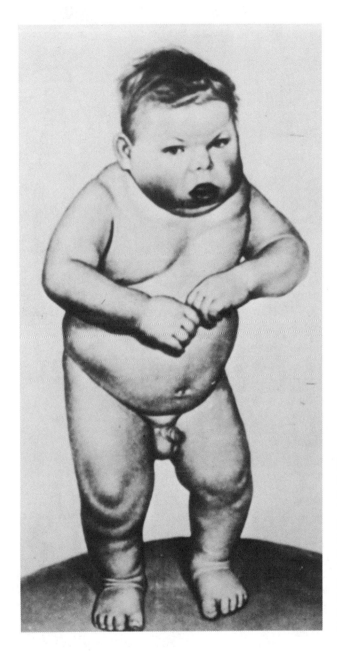

Figure 13-20. A 14-year-old untreated patient with severe, congenital hypothyroidism. The face is greatly swollen, the neck is obscured by fat, and the abdomen protrudes due to lack of muscle tone. The patient has difficulty in standing and walking. (*From Kosowicz. Atlas of Endocrine Diseases, 1978. Courtesy of The Charles Press.*)

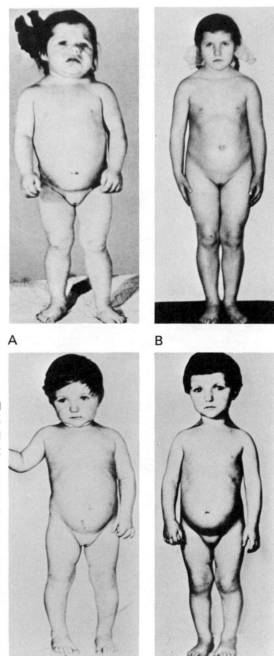

Figure 13–21. A. A 6-year-old child with congenital hypothyroidism, exhibiting marked mental and physical retardation. **B.** The same patient after 3 years of thyroxine therapy, which resulted in a spurt of growth and regression of pathological manifestations. Mental development is delayed. **C.** A 5-year-old patient with congenital hypothyroidism. Mental and physical development are delayed. **D.** The same patient after 3 months of thyroxine treatment. The child began to grow, lost weight, and became more alert. (*From Kosowicz. Atlas of Endocrine Diseases, 1978. Courtesy of The Charles Press.*)

adrenal cortex is stimulated by ACTH, adrenocorticotropic hormone, from the anterior pituitary gland. The adrenal glands are shown in Figure 13–22.

The adrenal cortex secretes many steroid hormones, which can be classified into three groups. One group, the mineralocorticoids, regulates salt balance. The principal hormone of this group is **aldosterone.** Aldosterone causes sodium retention and potassium secretion by the kidneys. Another group, the glucocorticoids, helps to regulate carbohydrate, lipid, and

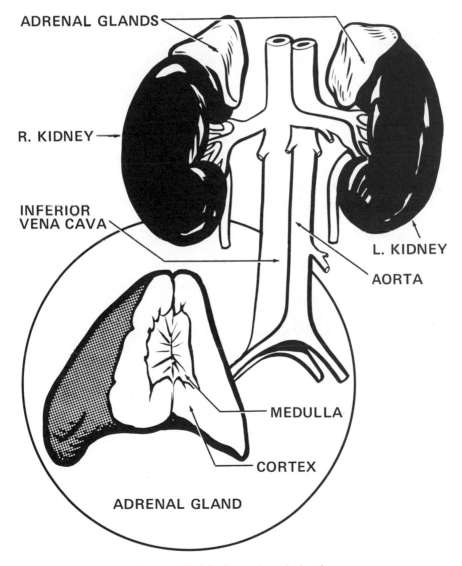

Figure 13-22. The adrenal glands.

protein metabolism. The principal hormone of this group is **cortisol** or hydrocortisone. The third group of hormones are sex hormones: **androgens,** the male hormones, and **estrogen,** the female hormone.

You may be familiar with one of the hormones of the adrenal cortex called cortisone. It is frequently used to treat nonbacterial inflammatory diseases such as rheumatoid arthritis, bursitis, and asthma. It can greatly relieve pain, but it must be understood that it relieves only the symptoms, not the cause of the disease.

There are many side effects to prolonged cortisone use. It can cause high blood pressure, peptic ulcers, and electrolyte imbalance that affects the heart. Cortisone reduces the body's inflammatory response and thus masks the symptoms of a bacterial or viral invasion. An infection therefore can be well established before the patient is aware of it. Cortisone causes a puffiness of the face, referred to as a "moon-face" appearance. This steroid hormone produces a drowsiness that is a danger when driving a car or using power equipment. Research is progressing to reduce the side effects of cortisone while maintaining its valuable actions.

The adrenal medulla secretes **epinephrine,** also called adrenalin. This hormone is secreted in stress situations when additional energy and strength are needed. Epinephrine raises the blood pressure, stimulates heart activity, and causes an increase in blood glucose. Epinephrine, through constriction of some blood vessels and dilation of others, shunts blood to active muscles where oxygen and nutrients are needed. The action of epinephrine is often called the "flight or fight" mechanism.

Hyperactivity of the adrenal glands is usually caused by hyperplasia (enlargement of the glands), a tumor, or administration of corticosteroids. Hyperactivity may also result from overstimulation by the anterior pituitary gland.

Hypoactivity of the adrenal cortex sometimes results from a destructive disease such as tuberculosis. Some steroid hormones can cause the adrenal glands to atrophy by interfering with the normal control mechanism for corticosteroid release.

DISEASES OF THE ADRENAL CORTEX

■ Hyperadrenalism

Overactivity of the adrenal cortex **(hyperadrenalism)** can take different forms depending on which group of hormones are secreted in excess. **Cushing's syndrome** develops from an excess of glucocorticoid hormones, the hormones that raise the blood sugar level. In excess they cause **hyperglycemia.** Elevation of blood glucose due to hypersecretion by the adrenal cortex is called **adrenal diabetes.** Glucocorticoids mobilize lipids increasing their level in the blood. A characteristic obesity develops that is confined to the trunk of the body. A fat pad forms behind the shoulders and is referred to as a buffalo hump, but the arms and legs remain normal. The face is round and described as moon-shaped.

The patient with Cushing's syndrome retains salt and water, resulting in hypertension. Atherosclerosis develops as a result of excess circulating lipid. Muscular weakness and fatigue accompany the disease, and the patient finds it difficult even to climb stairs. The skin is thin and tends to bruise easily. Red striae (stretch marks) develop on the abdomen, buttocks, and breasts as a result of a loss of elastic tissue and fat accumulation. Figure 13-23 shows a patient with Cushing's syndrome. Wounds heal poorly, and the patient is very susceptible to infection. Bones, particularly the vertebrae and ribs, are likely to fracture. These symptoms result from a decrease in

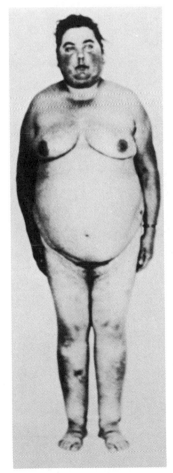 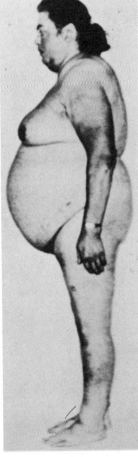

Figure 13-23. A. Cushing's syndrome patient showing round, red face; stocky neck; and marked obesity of the trunk with protruding abdomen. Note bruises on trunk and legs and also stretch marks. **B.** Note fat pads above the collarbone and on the back of the neck, which produce the "buffalo hump." (*From Kosowicz. Atlas of Endocrine Diseases, 1978. Courtesy of The Charles Press.*)

A   B

protein synthesis. Surgical removal of the enlarged glands or tumor can correct the condition. Hormonal therapy is then required to replace the hormones normally secreted by the adrenal cortex.

Conn's syndrome is another form of hyperadrenalism. In this disease aldosterone is secreted in excess. This causes retention of sodium and water, and abnormal loss of potassium in the urine. Hypertension develops as a result of the salt imbalance and water retention. Muscles become weak to the point of paralysis. The patient has an excessive thirst (polydipsia) due to the salt retention, and polyuria follows the great intake of water. Conn's syndrome is usually caused by a tumor that can be removed surgically, and the prognosis is usually good.

Adrenogenital syndrome is another form of hyperadrenalism, also called adrenal virilism. In this case androgens, male hormones, are secreted in excess. If this occurs in children, it stimulates premature sexual development. Sex organs of a male child greatly enlarge. In a girl, the clitoris enlarges, a male distribution of hair develops, and the voice deepens. This condition is seen in Figure 13–24A and B.

This excessive production of androgens is usually due to a block in the synthesis of cortisol from cortisone and other corticosteroids. Cortisone is

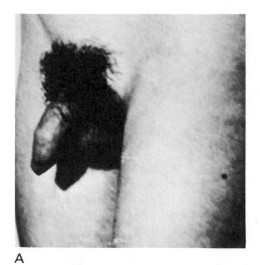
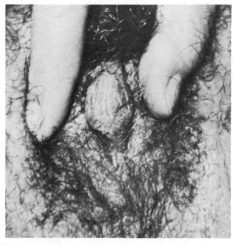

A   B

Figure 13–24. A. Genitalia of a 6-year-old boy with adrenogenital syndrome, showing precocious sexual development. The penis is enlarged but the testes remain small. **B.** Genitals of an 18-year-old woman with adrenogenital syndrome. The enlarged clitoris resembles a penis, and growth of pubic hair is excessive. (*From Kosowicz. Atlas of Endocrine Diseases, 1978. Courtesy of The Charles Press.*)

generally inactive until it is converted to cortisol. Cortisone is prepared synthetically from animal and plant tissue. Since steroids cannot be converted to cortisol, because of the blockage in the pathway, they are converted to androgens. Cortisol treatment can prevent this overproduction.

Excessive androgen secretion in a woman causes masculinization (adrenal virilism). Hair develops on the face, a condition called **hirsutism,** and the hairline recedes. The breasts diminish in size, the clitoris enlarges, and ovulation and menstruation cease. In an adult the cause is usually a tumor of the glands that secrete androgens. Adrenal virilism is shown in Figure 13–25.

■ Hypoadrenalism

Chronic **hypoadrenalism** is called **Addison's disease.** The indiscriminate use of steroid hormones can cause this disease in which the adrenal glands atrophy. An autoimmune mechanism may also result in destruction of the glands. Surprisingly, the adrenal cortex can still function adequately when up to 90 percent of it is destroyed. In Addison's disease the adrenal glands fail to secrete aldosterone, which renders the patient unable to retain salt and water. This causes dehydration and the blood level of potassium rises. Blood pressure is low due to the electrolyte imbalance. There is always a loss of weight, muscle weakness, and fatigue, and gastrointestinal disturbances are common.

A peculiar pigmentation—yellow to deep brown—develops. Normally pigmented areas such as the areola surrounding the nipples and parts of the genitals become even darker. Areas of the body subjected to friction, the palms and elbows, also darken and pigment develops in scars. This coloration is due to a pituitary hormone normally inhibited by cortisol, but cortisol is not secreted in Addison's disease. Steroid therapy can correct the salt imbalance, but it does not restore the adrenal glands.

STRUCTURE AND FUNCTION OF THE PARATHYROIDS

Structure of the Parathyroids

The parathyroids are four tiny glands located on the posterior side of the thyroid gland (see Figure 13–26). Before the function of the parathyroid glands was understood, they were sometimes removed with a thyroidectomy. The hormone secreted by the parathyroids is **parathormone.**

Function of the Parathyroids

The parathyroid glands are extremely important in regulating the level of circulating calcium and phosphate. Ninety-nine percent of the body's calcium is in bone, but the remaining 1 percent has many important functions.

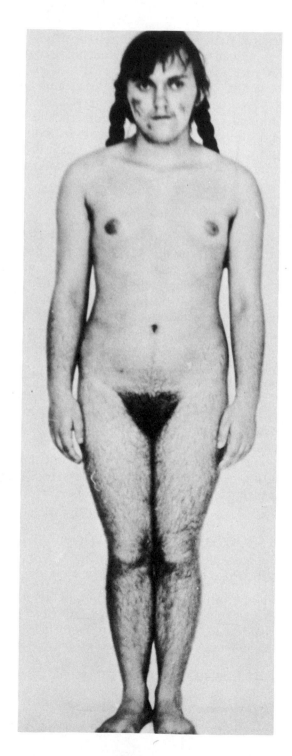

Figure 13-25. A 15-year-old girl with congenital adrenogenital syndrome. Note typical masculine build of broad shoulders and narrow hips. Breast development is poor, and excessive hair has developed on the face, abdomen, and legs. (*From Kosowicz. Atlas of Endocrine Diseases, 1978. Courtesy of The Charles Press.*)

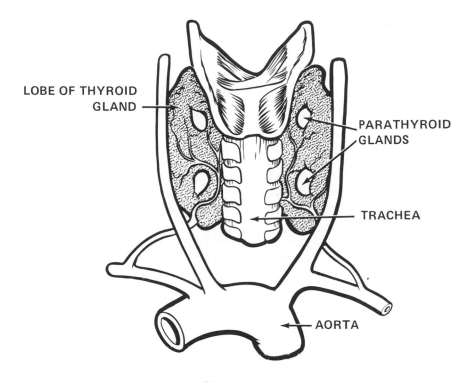

LOBE OF THYROID
GLAND

PARATHYROID
GLANDS

TRACHEA

AORTA

Figure 13-26. Parathyroid glands.

Calcium is essential to the blood-clotting mechanism. It increases the tone of heart muscle and plays a significant role in muscle contraction.

Bone is not inert. There is a constant exchange of calcium and phosphate between bone and the blood. Two kinds of cells are at work within bone: **osteoblasts** (bone-forming tissue) and **osteoclasts** (which resorb salts out of bone, dissolving it). These salts are then released into the blood. The balance between these two processes, osteoblastic and osteoclastic, is governed by the parathyroid hormone.

When the calcium level falls, parathormone is secreted. The hormone acts at three distinct sites to raise the level of calcium to normal. Parathormone increases the amount of calcium that is absorbed out of the digestive tract by interaction with ingested vitamin D. It prevents a loss of calcium through the kidneys and releases calcium from bones by stimulating osteoclastic activity. When the proper level of circulating calcium is restored, parathormone is no longer released. An excess or a deficiency of calcium can have disastrous results. These conditions are usually the result of hyperactivity or hypoactivity of the parathyroid glands.

DISEASES OF THE PARATHYROID GLAND

■ Hyperparathyroidism

An overactive parathyroid gland secretes too much parathormone **(hyperparathyroidism).** Excessive parathormone raises the level of circulating calcium above normal. This condition is called **hypercalcemia.** Much of the calcium comes from bone resorption mediated by parathormone. As the calcium level rises, the phosphate level falls.

What effect does this have on the bones? With the loss of calcium, the bones are weakened. They tend to bend, become deformed, and fracture spontaneously. Giant cell tumors and cysts of the bone sometimes develop. Excessive calcium causes formation of kidney stones because calcium forms insoluble compounds. Calcium deposited within the walls of the blood vessels makes them hard. It may also be found in the stomach and lungs. Effects of hyperparathyroidism are illustrated in Figure 13–27.

Hyperparathyroidism, with its concurrent excess of calcium, causes generalized symptoms. There may be pain in the bones that is sometimes confused with arthritis. The nervous system is depressed and muscles lose their tone and weaken. Heart muscle is affected and the pulse slows. Gastrointestinal disturbances, abdominal pain, vomiting, and constipation develop. These symptoms result from deposits of calcium in the mucosa of the gastrointestinal tract. Deposits of calcium sometimes form in the eye, causing irritation and excessive tearing. Hyperparathyroidism usually results from a tumor. If the tumor is removed, parathormone secretion returns to normal, and the level of circulating calcium is again properly controlled.

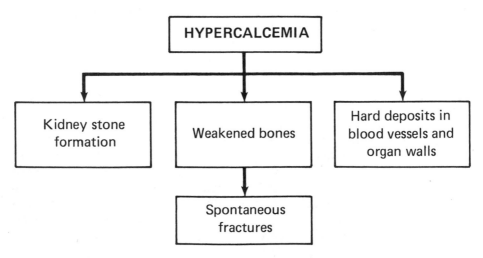

Figure 13-27. Complications of hyperparathyroidism—hypercalcemia.

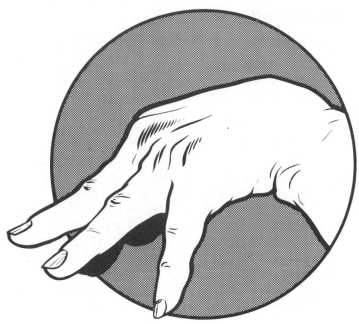

Figure 13-28. Tetany of the hand in hypoparathyroidism.

Hyperparathyroidism can develop from other conditions that reduce the level of circulating calcium. Any decrease in calcium stimulates the parathyroid glands to hypertrophy and to increase their rate of secretion. During pregnancy and lactation, the mother's supply of calcium is reduced. This reduction will stimulate the parathyroid glands to secrete parathormone.

◼ Hypoparathyroidism

The principal manifestation of **hypoparathyroidism** is **tetany,** a sustained muscular contraction. In hypoparathyroidism the muscles of the hands and feet contract in a characteristic fashion. The typical tetanic contraction of the hand is seen in Figure 13–28. Laryngeal muscles are very susceptible to these spasms, which can obstruct the respiratory tract, and death may follow.

The low level of calcium in the blood, **hypocalcemia,** makes the nervous system hyperexcitable. As the nerves discharge spontaneously, the skeletal muscles are overstimulated. Administration of calcium and vitamin D, which assists in the absorption of calcium from the gastrointestinal tract, will correct the condition.

ENDOCRINE FUNCTION OF THE PANCREAS

The structure of the pancreas and its role as an exocrine gland were described in Chapter 11. The pancreas has another critical function: the control of glucose level in the blood. This is accomplished through the secretion of two hormones, insulin and glucagon.

Insulin is secreted by certain cells of the pancreas called **beta cells,** located in patches of tissue named the islands of Langerhans. Glucagon is secreted by the **alpha cells** of the islets. This arrangement is illustrated in Figure 13–29. These hormones work antagonistically to each other. Insulin lowers the level of blood glucose and glucagon elevates it. The combined effect of these hormones maintains the normal level of blood glucose.

Insulin is secreted when the blood glucose level rises. Through a complex mechanism, not completely understood, insulin facilitates the entry of glucose into the cells where it is metabolized for energy. Glucose enters primarily skeletal muscle cells and fat cells. Glucose is metabolized, and energy is produced in the cells. As glucose enters cells, the level of blood glucose falls. The normal level of glucose in the blood is about 90 milligrams per 100 milliliters (90 mg/100 ml) of blood. This is also expressed as 90 mg percent.

When the level of blood glucose falls below normal, glucagon is released. Glucagon circulates to the liver and stimulates the release of glucose from

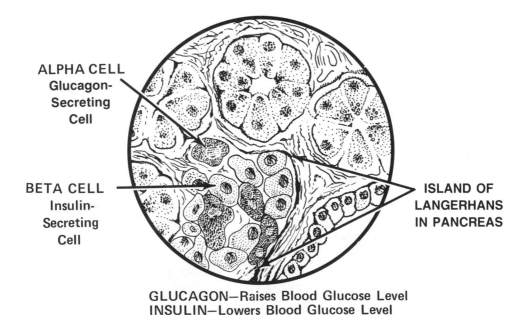

ALPHA CELL
Glucagon-
Secreting
Cell

BETA CELL
Insulin-
Secreting
Cell

ISLAND OF
LANGERHANS
IN PANCREAS

GLUCAGON—Raises Blood Glucose Level
INSULIN—Lowers Blood Glucose Level

Figure 13-29. Islands of Langerhans.

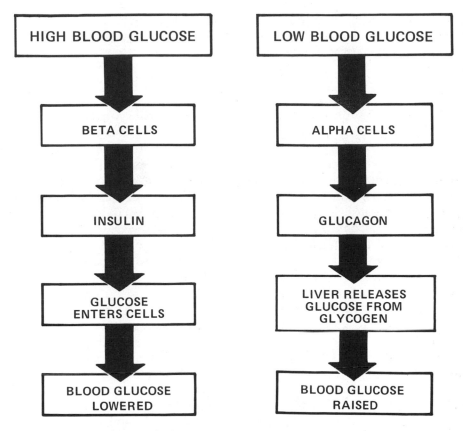

Figure 13-30. Control of blood glucose level.

its stored form, glycogen. This raises the level of blood glucose to normal. The control of glucose is illustrated in Figure 13–30.

■ Diabetes Mellitis (Hyperglycemia)

Diabetes mellitis is an endocrine disease in which the beta cells fail to secrete insulin or target cells fail to respond to insulin. In the absence of insulin, glucose cannot enter the cells. The glucose level in the blood increases greatly, resulting in **hyperglycemia.** A diabetic's sugar level can range from 300 to 1200 mg/100 ml of blood and even higher. The cells are deprived of their principal nutrient, glucose, for the production of energy.

Diabetes that develops in children is called juvenile-onset diabetes or **insulin-dependent diabetes mellitus (IDDM).** This is the more serious form, and the patient requires daily insulin injections. Diabetes that develops later in life, maturity-onset diabetes, or **non-insulin-dependent diabetes mellitus (NIDDM),** is less severe and can often be controlled by diet alone. It affects women more often than men, and usually women over 40. Maturity-onset diabetes frequently accompanies obesity. A prolonged, excessively high carbohydrate diet overstimulates the beta cells to secrete insulin. As a result, the beta cells "burn out" and stop functioning. Development of diabetes mellitus may have a genetic basis.

Symptoms of Diabetes Mellitus. One of the principal symptoms of diabetes mellitus is excessive urination, or polyuria. This is caused by the great amount of glucose that filters into the kidney tubule and the volume of water required to carry it away. The glucose acts as a diuretic. Normally, glucose that enters the kidney tubules is reabsorbed and does not appear in the urine. In diabetes, however, the amount of glucose that the kidney tubules can reabsorb, the tubular maximum, is surpassed. The excess glucose is excreted in the urine, a condition called **glycosuria.** Glycosuria is a major sign of diabetes mellitus.

The great loss of water with the glucose could result in dehydration, but the diabetic has an excessive thirst. By drinking large amounts of water, polydipsia, the diabetic compensates for the fluid loss. An unusual thirst is also one of the symptoms of diabetes.

Cells prefer to metabolize glucose. In its absence, cells metabolize fats first and proteins last. This is known as the "protein-sparing effect." Since glucose cannot enter the cells without the action of insulin, the diabetic metabolizes a large amount of fat. Fat metabolism produces a large number of fatty acids and **ketone bodies,** acetone and related substances. The presence of ketone bodies in the urine is another sign of diabetes mellitus.

The production of acids lowers the body's pH, and the condition of **acidosis** results. This is one of the most serious consequences of diabetes. The body tolerates only a very limited pH range of 7.35 to 7.45. If the pH drops below 6.9 to 7.0, the patient goes into a coma and will die if not treated.

Another sign of diabetes mellitus is weight loss, although the diabetic's appetite is good. The patient tires easily and lacks energy. In the absence of glucose to metabolize, the diabetic uses the body's tissue fat and protein, as well as that in the diet, which explains the loss of weight. There is an increased breakdown of tissue protein and a decrease in protein synthesis that results in poor wound healing. Susceptibility to infection also accompanies diabetes.

Complications of Diabetes Mellitus. Lipid is mobilized from fat tissue, and the level of blood lipid, particularly cholesterol, increases. Much of this lipid is deposited within the walls of the blood vessels causing atherosclerosis. This is one of the greatest dangers in long-term diabetes because blood vessels tend to become occluded. Blockage of a coronary artery causes a myocardial infarction, as explained in Chapter 7. Occlusion of a leg artery can result in gangrene. Atherosclerosis generally causes poor circulation. This is another reason for poor wound healing.

Another complication of diabetes is a vascular disorder of the retina that can result in blindness. The minute retinal blood vessels become sclerotic and rupture. The nervous system is affected by poor circulation, as manifested by pain, tingling sensations, loss of feeling, and paralysis. The kidneys are always affected by long-standing diabetes, and kidney failure is frequently the cause of death in the diabetic. The complications of diabetes are summarized in Figure 13–31.

Treatment of Diabetes Mellitus. The important factors in treating diabetes are diet, insulin, and exercise. The insulin dosage prescribed accompanies a carefully regulated diet that includes some carbohydrates. The diet cannot be altered without creating an insulin excess or deficiency. A person who exercises actively requires less insulin than one who does not. A diabetic's exercise pattern is a factor in prescribing insulin.

Regulation of the proper insulin dosage takes time. Certain factors—illness or emotional stress—can temporarily alter a patient's needs. There are different types of insulin (fast-, intermediate- and slow-acting), which are effective over various time periods. These are often prescribed in combination.

Insulin must be given by injection. It is a protein and would be digested in the gastrointestinal tract. There are oral compounds that can be used for mild diabetes, maturity-onset diabetes, but they are not insulin. These are oral hypoglycemic agents, which stimulate secretion of insulin from beta cells that still have some capacity.

Diabetic Coma and Insulin Shock. Diabetic coma develops when a severe diabetic fails to take enough insulin or deviates markedly from a prescribed diet. Acidosis and dehydration result, and death can follow if proper treatment is not given immediately. One symptom of diabetic coma is deep, labored breathing, which results from the effect of the acidosis on the respiratory center of the brain. The patient's breath has a fruity, acetone smell. The skin is flushed and dry, and the tongue is dry due to the dehydration. A diabetic coma may have a gradual onset, during which time the patient is drowsy and lethargic. If urine and blood samples are taken, a high level of sugar is found.

Treatment of the comatose patient requires a large dosage of insulin. Dehydration must be remedied by administration of fluids. Sodium chloride and sodium bicarbonate, which counteract the acidosis, are administered in the fluid. The patient's level of potassium must be checked; the entire electrolyte balance is affected by the dehydration.

Insulin shock, also called hypoglycemic shock, results from too much insulin, not enough food, or excessive exercise. The patient feels light-

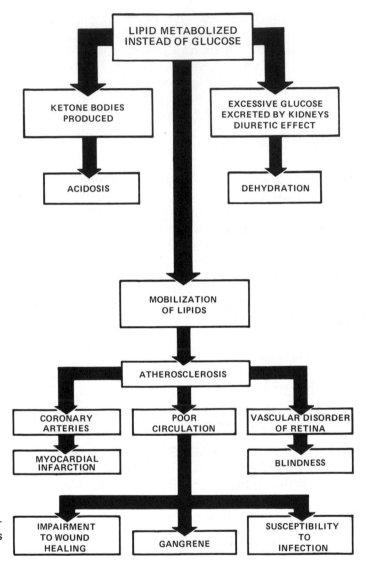

Figure 13-31. Complications of diabetes mellitus.

headed and faint, trembles, and begins to perspire. Taking sugar in some form, candy or orange juice for example, may be adequate treatment at this stage. If the glucose level is not raised, the condition becomes more serious. The patient's speech becomes thick and walking becomes unsteady. The low level of glucose affects the brain, causing these results. Double vision may be experienced, and loss of consciousness may follow.

If the patient becomes comatose, it is difficult for the untrained to determine if the cause is a diabetic coma or insulin shock. A significant difference is that the deep, rapid breathing and acetone breath characteristic of diabetic coma are not present in insulin shock. The patient in shock breathes shallowly. Intravenous injections of glucose must be given immediately for insulin shock. The administration of epinephrine also raises the blood sugar level. Figure 13–32 illustrates the differences between diabetic coma and insulin shock.

Tests for Diabetes Mellitus. A simple test can show the presence or absence of glucose in the urine. If glucose is found, a test of the blood after fasting is made to determine the glucose level. When diabetes is suspected, a glucose tolerance test is performed by having the patient, in a fasting state, drink a standard glucose solution. Blood and urine samples are then analyzed during the next 4 to 5 hours. No food is allowed during the test, but the patient is encouraged to drink water. Smoking and exercise are not permitted during the test period. No glucose should appear in the urine, and the blood level should not exceed 170 mg/100 ml of blood if insulin is being produced. Other glucose tolerance tests are also available.

Education of the Diabetic Patient. The American Diabetes Association, physicians, nurses, and dieticians have made a great effort to assist the diabetic patient in leading a normal life. The diabetic who understands the disease knows the importance of insulin dosage, diet, and exercise to lead an active life. A safety precaution advised by the American Diabetes Associa-

DIABETIC COMA	INSULIN SHOCK
Deep, labored breathing due to acidosis	Shallow breathing
Skin and tongue dry due to dehydration	Patient perspires
Fruity, acetone smell to breath	Odor of breath normal
Patient drowsy and lethargic before onset	Patient feels light-headed and faint before onset
Comatose	Comatose
Requires large dose of insulin	Requires glucose intravenously
Fluid and salts needed	

Figure 13-32. Differences between diabetic coma and insulin shock.

tion is that anyone who takes insulin carry an identification card explaining the emergency treatment required if an insulin reaction occurs.

■ Hypoglycemia

Hypoglycemia is an abnormally low level of glucose in the blood. Symptoms develop when the glucose level falls below 50 mg/100 ml as compared with the normal of 90 mg/100 ml. The symptoms of hypoglycemia have been described under hypoglycemic or insulin shock. They include faintness, sweating, nervousness, and mental confusion. A severe condition that is not treated results in coma and possibly convulsions and death. The patient, if conscious, should eat sugar in any form. If the patient is unconscious, glucose must be given by injection.

In addition to hypoglycemic shock in the diabetic resulting from too much insulin, insufficient food, or strenuous exercise, other factors can cause hypoglycemia. A tumor of the beta cells in the pancreas results in a hypersecretion of insulin that lowers blood glucose. A patient with Addison's disease, hypoactivity of the adrenal cortex, secretes an inadequate amount of glucocorticoids to raise the level of blood glucose.

Treatment of hypoglycemia depends on its cause. For the diabetic, precautionary measures can usually prevent its development: exact insulin dosage, careful observance of diet and times for meals, and exercise within the prescribed range. A tumor causing excessive insulin secretion should be removed. The patient with Addison's disease requires hormonal supplements.

SUMMARY

The endocrine system provides a means of chemical communication between body parts. The tiny anterior pituitary gland controls activities of the thyroid, adrenals, and sex glands. It also stimulates growth, development, and tissue repair. The pituitary is called the "master gland" for these reasons. Pituitary activity is governed by the hypothalamus of the brain.

Hyperpituitarism causes an excess of growth hormone. This condition, if present before puberty results in gigantism. In an adult, excessive production of growth hormone leads to abnormal enlargement of facial bones, bones of hands and feet, and soft tissue. This growth in an adult is called acromegaly.

Severe hypopituitarism impedes growth and development in a child, causing the child to be dwarfed in stature. Glands dependent on stimulation by the anterior pituitary—the thyroid, adrenals, and sex glands—cease functioning in hypopituitarism at any age. The posterior pituitary gland secretes vasopressin, also called antidiuretic hormone, and oxytocin. Hypoactivity of this gland causes diabetes insipidus.

The rate of metabolism is controlled by the thyroid gland. An enlargement of this gland is a goiter. Hyperthyroidism, an excess of thyroxine, accelerates heart and respiratory activity, increases metabolic rate, and raises body temperature. Graves' disease is an example of severe hyperthyroidism. A congenital lack of thyroxine results in cretinism, a condition of mental and physical retardation. Myxedema is a disease of severe hypothyroidism in an adult.

Hormones of the adrenal cortex are essential to life. Aldosterone regulates salt balance and cortisol affects the metabolism of nutrients. Accessory sex hormones are also produced by this gland. Hypoactivity of the adrenal cortex is called Addison's disease.

Hyperactivity of the adrenal cortex causes different diseases, depending on which hormones are in excess. Cushing's syndrome results from an excess of cortisol, and Conn's syndrome results from excessive aldosterone. Precocious puberty and adrenal virilism develop from too much androgen secretion.

The parathyroid hormone, parathormone, regulates the level of circulating calcium and phosphate. Hyperactivity of the parathyroids causes hypercalcemia. The high level of calcium is primarily from bone resorption that weakens the bones. Hypoparathyroidism reduces the level of calcium in the blood. This causes the nervous system to become hyperexcitable, skeletal muscles are overstimulated, and tetany results. Hormones of the pancreas, insulin and glucagon, control blood sugar level. Lack of insulin causes an increase in blood glucose, the condition of diabetes mellitus.

Hypoglycemia, abnormally low blood glucose, results from insulin excess. This condition can develop in the diabetic from an overdosage of insulin. A tumor of the insulin-producing cells of the pancreas can also cause hypoglycemia. The absence of glucocorticoids in an Addison's disease patient results in low blood glucose.

STUDY QUESTIONS

1. Explain the relationship between gigantism and acromegaly.
2. What are the effects of hypopituitarism on other glands?
3. Describe Simmond's syndrome. What are its possible causes?
4. Contrast diabetes insipidus and diabetes mellitus.
5. Explain the T_3 and T_4 tests to determine thyroid activity.
6. Name five effects of thyroxine.
7. Explain the negative feedback mechanism in secretion of thyroxine.

8. How is a goiter related to hypothyroidism and hyperthyroidism?
9. What are the symptoms of Graves' disease?
10. Describe the characteristic appearance of a cretin.
11. What causes myxedema? What are the symptoms?
12. What is the treatment of Cushing's disease?
13. Explain adrenal virilism.
14. What is the basis of Addison's disease?
15. Describe the effects of hyperparathyroidism.
16. Name four signs of diabetes mellitus.
17. Explain the possible complications of diabetes mellitus.
18. Describe the differences between diabetic coma and insulin shock as to cause, signs, and treatment.
19. What are the tests for diabetes mellitus?
20. Name three possible causes of hypoglycemia.

CHAPTER 14

Diseases of the Reproductive Systems and Sexually Transmitted Diseases

New life is created through the reproductive system. The female body produces ova, nurtures the developing fetus in the uterus, and nourishes the baby at the breast. The male body produces sperm and transmits it to the female. The fertilization that ensues combines characteristics of each parent, and an embryo begins to develop.

ANATOMY OF THE FEMALE REPRODUCTIVE SYSTEM

The female reproductive system consists of the vagina, the uterus, the fallopian tubes, and the ovaries. The vagina is a tubular structure extending backward and upward to the cervix, the lowest part of the uterus. The expanded, upper portion of the uterus tapers down to form the narrow cervix, giving the organ a pear-shaped appearance. The uterine wall is very strong, comprised of smooth muscle and lined with a mucosal membrane, the endometrium. It is responsive to hormonal changes. Figure 14–1 shows the female reproductive system.

The fallopian tubes extend laterally from each side of the uterus supported by the broad ligament. The outer ends of the tube are open to receive a released ovum. Fringelike projections at the outer ends, the fimbriae, propel the ova into the tube.

The ovaries, small oval-shaped glands, are anchored near the open end of the fallopian tubes by ligaments. The ovaries contain hundreds of thousands of ova, which are present at birth. Each ovum is surrounded by a single layer of cells comprising a primary follicle. The relationship between the ovaries and the fallopian tubes is shown in Figure 14–2.

The external genitalia, the **vulva,** consists of the mons pubis, the major and minor lips, the clitoris, and the vaginal opening. The urinary meatus is between the clitoris and the vaginal opening. The mons pubis, a pad of fat tissue over the pubic symphysis, becomes covered with hair at puberty. Extending back from the mons pubis to the anus are two pairs of folds, the

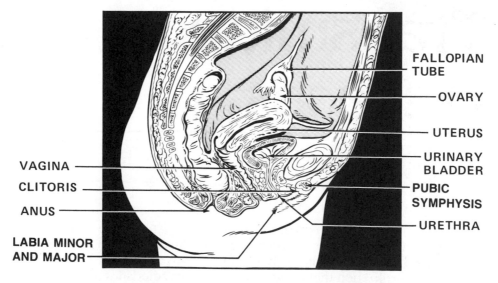

Figure 14-1. Sagittal view of female reproductive organs.

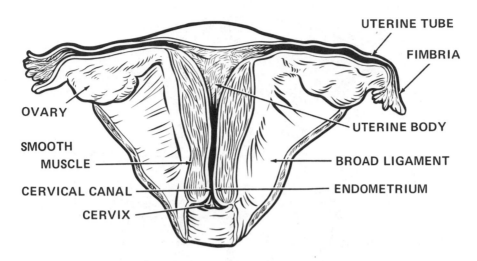

Figure 14-2. Relationship of ovaries to fallopian tubes.

major and minor lips. The clitoris, a tuft of erectile tissue, similar to that of the penis, is located at the anterior junction of the minor lips. A membranous fold, the **hymen,** partly or completely closes the vaginal opening. Occasionally this membrane is imperforate or abnormally closed and requires a minor surgical procedure to open it. The external female genitalia are shown in Figure 14–3. A pair of mucus-secreting glands, Bartholin's glands, are situated at the vaginal entrance. These glands produce a lubricating secretion during sexual intercourse.

The breasts, accessory organs of reproduction, consist of milk glands supported by connective tissue covered with fatty tissue and skin. Ducts of the milk glands converge at the nipple, which is surrounded by a darkly pigmented area, the **areola.** The breasts overlie the pectoral muscles of the chest.

PHYSIOLOGY OF THE FEMALE REPRODUCTIVE SYSTEM

The cyclic hormonal changes in the life of a woman prepare the uterus monthly for a possible pregnancy. The secretion of female hormones, estrogen and progesterone, is governed by the gonadotropic hormones of the anterior pituitary gland, which is controlled by the hypothalamus of the brain. Failure of the ovary to secrete sex hormones or to ovulate may result from pituitary disease or disturbances in the central nervous system.

A woman's reproductive life begins with the onset of menstruation, the **menarche,** occurring generally between ages 11 and 15. The reproductive years terminate with the cessation of menstrual periods, **menopause,** which

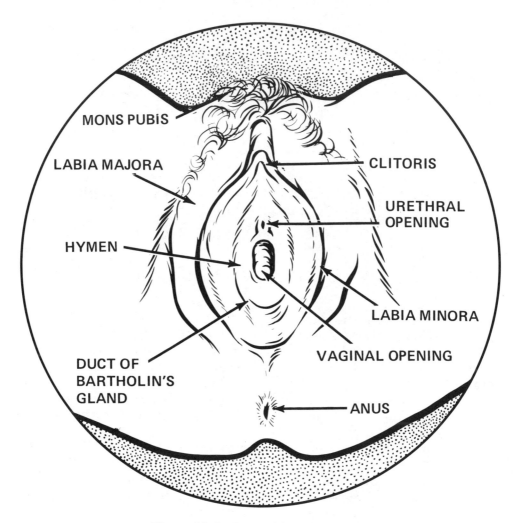

MONS PUBIS

LABIA MAJORA

HYMEN

DUCT OF
BARTHOLIN'S
GLAND

CLITORIS

URETHRAL
OPENING

LABIA MINORA

VAGINAL OPENING

ANUS

Figure 14-3. External female genitalia.

usually begins in the late 40s or early 50s. At the beginning of each monthly cycle a pituitary gonadotropic hormone stimulates ovarian follicles to develop. The particular follicles that are stimulated begin to grow and develop a fluid within. They are then called **Graafian follicles.** One of these matures first and at the midpoint of the cycle is released, which is the process of ovulation. Ovulation is also controlled by a gonadotropic hormone.

As the follicles are growing, during the first half of the cycle, the ovary secretes estrogen, which is carried by the blood to the uterus. Estrogen, stimulates the endometrium of the uterus to thicken and become more vascular. This is the first preparation for pregnancy and is called the proliferative stage.

Once the ovum has been released from the ovary, the empty follicle is converted into the **corpus luteum,** which begins to secrete progesterone. Progesterone continues the stimulation of endometrial growth and promotes the storage of nutrients for nourishing a fertilized ovum. This is the secretory phase of the uterus. Figure 14–4 shows the effect of gonadotropic hormones on the ovary, and the response of the endometrium to the female hormones.

If no fertilization occurs, the corpus luteum ceases to secrete hormones about 8 to 12 days after ovulation. At the end of the monthly cycle the level of estrogen and progesterone drops, and menstruation, the sloughing of the endometrial lining, occurs. If pregnancy occurs, the corpus luteum greatly enlarges and continues to secrete high levels of progesterone. The **placenta**

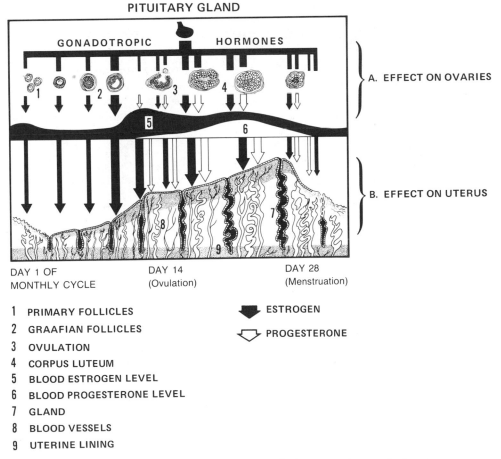

1   PRIMARY FOLLICLES
2   GRAAFIAN FOLLICLES
3   OVULATION
4   CORPUS LUTEUM
5   BLOOD ESTROGEN LEVEL
6   BLOOD PROGESTERONE LEVEL
7   GLAND
8   BLOOD VESSELS
9   UTERINE LINING

Figure 14–4. Relationship between pituitary, ovaries, and uterus.

gradually assumes the role of the corpus luteum in secreting these hormones.

The placenta is formed from both maternal and embryonic tissue. Near the site of implantation in the uterus the endometrium greatly thickens, becomes highly vascular, and develops large blood sinuses. An embryonic membrane, the chorion, develops fingerlike projections called villi, which dip into the maternal blood sinuses. This interdigitation of embryonic and maternal tissue constitutes the placenta.

The umbilical arteries extend into the chorionic villi, where the exchange of carbon dioxide for oxygen and waste material for nutrients occurs. Maternal and fetal blood do not mix; the exchange of these substances is by diffusion across the blood vessel walls. Oxygen and nutrients return to the fetus through the umbilical vein. The fetal–maternal relationship is shown in Figure 6–3 (see Chapter 6, Diseases of the Blood).

DISEASES OF THE FEMALE REPRODUCTIVE SYSTEM

The female reproductive organs are affected by disease in numerous ways. Microorganisms can invade the structures setting up infections. Tumors, both malignant and benign, and cysts develop in the reproductive organs and in the breasts. Abnormalities of the menstrual cycle and of pregnancy also occur.

■ Pelvic Inflammatory Disease (PID)

The pelvic reproductive organs become inflamed as a result of bacterial, viral, fungal, or parasitic invasion. The subsequent infection can ascend to the cervix, the endometrium, the fallopian tubes, and even to the ovaries. **Gonococcus** transmitted by a male with gonorrhea is the most common cause of pelvic inflammatory disease. Streptococcal and staphyloccocal organisms enter the female reproductive tract after an abortion or delivery in which sterile procedures were not carefully followed. The symptoms of pelvic inflammatory disease are lower abdominal pain, fever resulting from the infection, and a vaginal discharge of pus. If the infection is not treated, abscesses form. Antibiotics are prescribed to counteract the invading organisms, and aspirin is used to reduce the fever. The patient requires bed rest and fluids.

■ Salpingitis

Salpingitis is an inflammation of the fallopian tubes; the term *salpinx* refers to a tube. Untreated gonorrhea can cause this inflammation, as can a streptococcal or staphylococcal invasion. These pyogenic organisms cause a purulent, pus-producing, infection.

The fallopian tubes become red and swollen. If the outer ends remain open, the infection spreads out into the pelvic cavity to cause pelvic peritonitis. The outer ends of the tubes usually close and the tubes fill with pus. A pus-filled tube is called a **pyosalpinx.** When the inflammation subsides after treatment with antibiotics, the tube is filled with a watery fluid and is referred to as a **hydrosalpinx.** Both tubes are usually affected as the inflammation ascends through the uterus. Sterility results from salpingitis if the ends of both tubes close. Adhesions may form that affect the tubes and cause sterility. The effect of adhesion formation on the fallopian tubes is seen in Figure 14–5. Menstrual disturbances generally accompany salpingitis, as do ectopic pregnancies.

▪ Vaginitis

Vaginitis, inflammation of the vagina, is a common disease caused by several organisms. A parasite, **trichomonas,** that can be transmitted by sexual intercourse is one causative agent. Trichomonas is sometimes admitted from fecal material. *Candida albicans,* a fungus, is another cause of vaginitis. An overgrowth of fungus can develop from antibiotic treatment that destroys the normal flora. The normal flora consists of nonpathogenic microorganisms that are generally present and help keep down the number of harmful microbes. If the normal flora is wiped out by antibiotics, fungi, and viruses, antibiotic-resistant organisms thrive. A foul-smelling vaginal discharge is the principal symptom of vaginitis. The discharge causes itch-

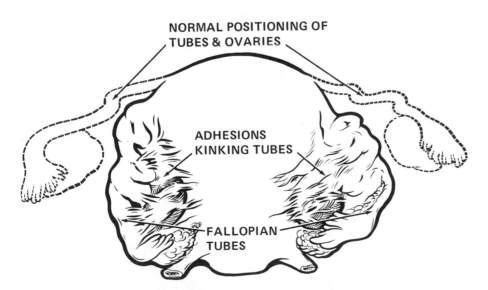

Figure 14-5. The effect of adhesions on the fallopian tubes.

ing, burning, and soreness of the surrounding tissues. Any vaginal discharge other than blood is referred to as **leukorrhea.** Atrophic vaginitis is a postmenopausal condition. The vaginal lining changes with the loss of estrogen secretion when the ovaries atrophy, and the mucosa becomes more susceptible to infection. Hormonal therapy, antibiotic salves, or steroid creams may be prescribed.

■ Inflammation of Bartholin's Glands

Bartholin's glands (see Figure 14–3) are susceptible to infections caused by gonococcal, streptococcal, and staphylococcal organisms. If the duct of the gland becomes occluded from the inflammation, pus collects in the gland and abscesses form. Such abscesses require surgical lancing to allow drainage of the pus.

■ Puerperal Sepsis

Puerperal sepsis is an infection of the endometrium after childbirth or an abortion. Danger of an infection is greater after an abortion. The puerperium is the period after childbirth, when the endometrium is open and particularly susceptible to infection. The trauma and blood loss encountered during delivery provide a portal of entry for invading microorganisms through the birth canal. The lesions of the endometrium favor bacterial growth. Streptococci are the principal causative organisms, but staphylococci and *E. coli* enter the uterus through a lack of **aseptic** technique. Necrosis of the endometrium develops from the infection.

Infected blood clots can break loose and travel as septic emboli. A systemic infection of the blood, **septicemia,** is often the result. The deep veins of the leg are frequently affected, resulting in thrombophlebitis, a condition previously described in Chapter 8. The symptoms of puerperal sepsis are fever, chills, and profuse bleeding. A foul-smelling vaginal discharge indicates infection. Pain is experienced in the lower abdomen and pelvis. Puerperal sepsis responds well to antibiotic treatment.

Neoplasms of the Female Organs

Early detection, diagnosis, and treatment of any abnormal mass or lump is extremely important in preventing the growth and spread of cancer. Many tumors and cysts are harmless, but tests are required to differentiate between malignant and benign growths.

■ *Carcinoma of the Cervix.* Carcinoma of the cervix is one of the cancers most easily diagnosed in the early stages. Incidence of this malignancy has decreased significantly since the development of the Pap smear. The Pap smear, explained in Chapter 3, enables physicians to obtain scrapings from the cervix. These scrapings are examined microscopically; cell abnormalities indicate precursors of cancer and various stages in its development. Biopsies of suspected lesions are also taken. **Carcinoma in situ** is the earliest stage of cancer. It is a premalignant lesion; the underlying tissue has not yet been invaded. Development of a carcinoma in situ to an invasive malignancy may be slow. Ulceration then occurs, causing vaginal discharge and bleeding. The cancer spreads to surrounding organs: the vagina, bladder, rectum, and pelvic wall. Widespread cancer becomes inoperable, and radiation therapy is the usual treatment. Carcinoma of the cervix appears to follow chronic irritation, infection, and poor hygiene. Promiscuity, beginning at an early age and involving many partners, is somehow related to this cancer.

■ *Carcinoma of the Endometrium.* Carcinoma of the endometrium occurs most often in postmenopausal women who have had no children. The malignant tumor may grow into the cavity of the uterus or invade the wall itself. Ulcerations develop, and erosion of blood vessels causes vaginal bleeding. Surgery and radiation are the usual treatments.

■ *Fibroid Tumors.* Benign tumors of the smooth muscle of the uterus, **leiomyomas** or fibroid tumors, are very common. Frequently these tumors cause no symptoms. Fibroids are often multiple and vary greatly in size. Fibroid tumors, some of which are stalked or pedunculated, are shown in Figure 14–6. Fibroid tumor growth is stimulated by estrogen because the tumors develop only during the reproductive years. Large tumors putting pressure on surrounding organs and nerve endings cause pelvic pain. Fibroid tumors can also interfere during delivery. Abnormal bleeding between periods or excessively heavy menstrual flow is a common symptom of fibroid tumors. A hysterectomy is generally required if bleeding continues.

■ *Ovarian Neoplasms.* The most common ovarian neoplasm is the cyst, a fluid-filled sac. Many cysts have no symptoms but are discovered during a pelvic examination. Large cysts that can interfere with blood flow are removed surgically.

Primary malignant tumors of the ovary are rare. Cancer of the ovary is usually the result of metastases from other organs. A malignant ovarian tumor can be removed surgically before metastases or treated with chemotherapy once it has spread.

A peculiar benign tumor of the ovary is the **dermoid cyst,** or **teratoma,** described in Chapter 3. The dermoid cyst contains all kinds of tissues: skin with its oil glands and hair follicles, teeth, and bone. The cyst is filled with oily material from the glands, and hair grows into the cavity. The tumor is harmless unless its size or other symptoms necessitate surgery. A teratoma is seen in Figure 14–7.

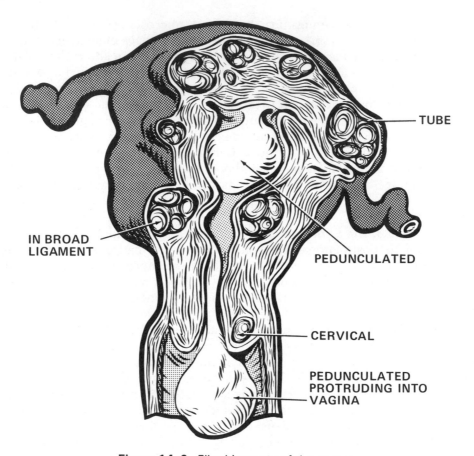

Figure 14-6. Fibroid tumors of the uterus.

■ *Hydatidiform Mole.* The **hydatidiform mole** is a benign tumor of the placenta. It can develop after a pregnancy or in association with an abnormal one. The tumor consists of multiple cysts and resembles a bunch of grapes. The tumor secretes **chorionic gonadotropic hormone (CGT),** the hormone which indicates a positive pregnancy test. The uterus enlarges greatly, although no fetus develops. Bleeding usually occurs, and the mole is expelled. Scraping of the uterus, the procedure of dilation of the cervix and curettage **(D&C),** removes any fragments of the tumor or placenta.

■ *Choriocarcinoma.* **Choriocarcinoma** is a highly malignant tumor of the placenta. A part of the placenta is formed by the embryonic membrane called the chorion. This tumor may develop after a hydatidiform mole, a normal delivery, or an abortion. A choriocarcinoma, like the hydatidiform mole, secretes large amounts of CGT. Presence of this hormone in the urine in the absence of pregnancy is significant diagnostically. The tumor is highly invasive and metastasizes rapidly. Chemotherapy rather than surgery is the usual treatment.

■ *Adenocarcinoma of the Vagina.* Adenocarcinoma of the vagina has been linked to the synthetic hormone **diethylstilbestrol (DES)** used to prevent spontaneous abortion. This rather rare cancer has developed in some young girls whose mothers were given DES during pregnancy.

Daughters of women who received DES therapy should be checked for possible cancer development, but the incidence is low. DES appears to have only slight effects in sons born to these women. Testes have been found to be smaller than normal in some cases, and some cyst formation has been found in the **epididymis.**

■ *Neoplasms of the Breast.* Adenocarcinoma, cancer of the breast ducts, is the most common breast malignancy. It occurs more often in single women, in women who have had no children, and in women with a family history of breast cancer. Adenocarcinoma of the breast usually develops around the time of the menopause. Development of this cancer seems to be

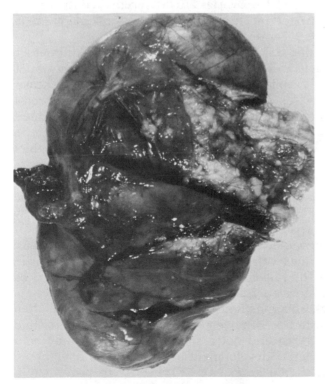

Figure 14-7. Dermoid cyst of ovary.

related to estrogen activity. Women are strongly urged to examine their breasts monthly for a possible lump. The American Cancer Society and the National Cancer Institute have done a great deal to encourage this practice, and they provide valuable information on the procedure.

The signs that indicate a malignant tumor are presented by an advanced cancer. A hard, fixed lump in the upper, outer quadrant is one such sign. Benign tumors, because they are encapsulated (Chapter 3), are not fixed to underlying structures. The nipple often retracts and the skin dimples due to contraction of dense fibrous connective tissue that extends to the chest muscles and skin.

The lymph nodes of the axillary region may be swollen. Carcinoma spreads principally through the lymph system. Metastases are frequent to the lungs, liver, brain, and bone. **Mammography** can detect small, early cancers. A biopsy of the suspected malignancy confirms the diagnosis or shows the tumor to be benign.

Treatment of breast cancer varies. In a simple mastectomy, only the breast is removed. The breast, chest muscles, and axillary lymph nodes are removed in a **radical mastectomy.** Some studies indicate that prognosis after a radical mastectomy is not necessarily better than that after a less multilating procedure. Less multilating procedures involve removal of the tumor only and radiation therapy. The ovaries are often removed to prevent the stimulating effect of estrogen on tumor growth when disease is metastatic.

Paget's disease of the nipple is a rare cancer involving inflammatory changes that affects the nipple and the areola. The nipple becomes granular and crusted with lesions resembling eczema. In advanced Paget's disease, ulceration develops and there is a discharge from the nipple. The breast becomes edematous and is characterized as having a "pigskin" appearance. Treatment depends on the extent of the disease. A significant feature in Paget's disease is that it is accompanied by an underlying infiltrating duct cancer.

■ *Benign Tumors of the Breast.* The most common benign tumor of the breast is a fibroadenoma (Figure 14–8). It is a firm, movable mass easily removed by surgery. The fibroadenoma does not become malignant.

Cystic hyperplasia or fibrocystic disease is very common and not serious. Development occurs at any age with the formation of numerous lumps in the breast. The lumps are fluid-filled cysts, not tumors. They tend to be painful at the time of the menstrual period as the breasts themselves respond to hormonal changes, enlarging and regressing. These cysts are often **aspirated:** A needle is inserted to remove fluid. The withdrawal of fluid confirms that the lump is a cyst and not a solid tumor. There may be a higher incidence of breast cancer development in women who have cystic hyperplasia. These women should be examined regularly to prevent mistaking a tumor for a cyst.

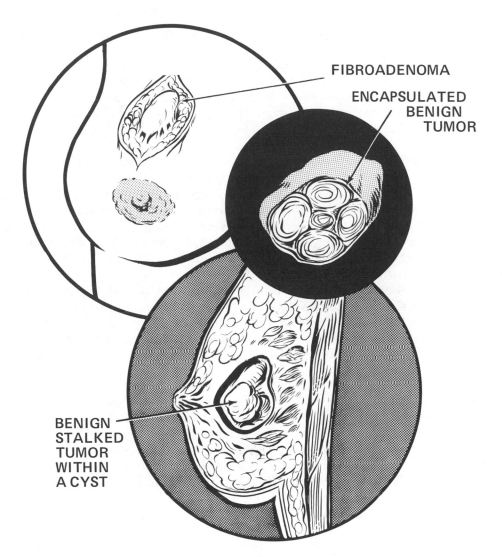

Figure 14-8. Common benign breast tumors.

■ Menstrual Abnormalities

Amenorrhea is the absence of menstrual periods. The amenorrhea is known as primary if menstruation fails to begin. Lack of gonadotropic hormones from the pituitary gland or a diseased ovary can cause the abnormality. Administration of hormones may be effective treatment. The cessation of menstrual periods for more than a year is termed secondary amenorrhea. This can result from an ovarian or uterine disease, as well as hormonal imbalance. Pituitary failure and thyroid disease can cause amenorrhea. The absence of menstruation is a symptom of a disease that must be diagnosed and treated.

Certain mental disturbances—extreme depression, worry, and continuous stress—can cause cessation of menstruation. The hypothalamus of the brain governs the release of pituitary hormones, including the gonadotropins. The condition of amenorrhea will right itself if the stressful conditions can be eliminated, or if the patient receives counseling on adjustment to the problem.

Menorrhagia is excessive or prolonged bleeding during menstruation. It can result from tumors of the uterus, pelvic inflammatory disease, or endocrine imbalance. Failure to ovulate can also cause menorrhagia. If a corpus luteum is not formed, progesterone is not secreted and estrogen continues to stimulate endometrial thickening. Treatment varies according to the cause of the disease. Tumors should be removed surgically, pelvic inflammatory disease treated with antibiotics, and hormonal therapy administered for endocrine insufficiency.

Metrorrhagia is bleeding between menstrual periods or extreme irregularity of the cycle. It results from an abnormal buildup and sloughing of endometrial tissue. Hormonal imbalance may be the cause of metrorrhagia, or the endometrial response to the hormones may be incorrect. Dilation and curettage, a D&C, is often performed, and the endometrium returns to normal.

■ *Toxic Shock Syndrome.* **Toxic shock syndrome (TSS)** is not merely a disease of menstruating women who use tampons but an infection of *Staphylococcus aureus.* The signs include high fever, rash, skin peeling, and decreased blood pressure. Other systemic involvements may include gastrointestinal complaints, elevated liver enzymes, and neuromuscular disturbances. Treatment includes fluid replacement to counteract shock and administration of selected antibiotics.

The relationship between particular tampons and development of TSS is thought to be an increase in staphylococcal toxin production in the environment of certain synthetic fibers. These fibers were found to be the ones used in "super" tampons to increase absorbancy. The fibers apparently remove magnesium from the vagina, and this produces an ideal environment for bacteria to make the toxins. These fibers are no longer used. It was found that some surgical dressings also contained the same fibers, a finding that may explain some cases of TSS in nontampon users.

Recommendations for women who use tampons include avoidance of the superabsorptive type, daytime use only, and frequent changes of tampons.

■ *Endometriosis.* **Endometriosis** is a disease condition in which endometrial tissue from the uterus becomes embedded elsewhere. The tissue may have been pushed backward through the fallopian tubes during menstruation or carried by blood or lymph. It then takes hold on some structure in the peritoneal cavity such as the ovary. The endometrial tissue by nature responds to hormonal changes even when outside the uterus. This tissue goes through a proliferative and secretory phase, along with the sloughing-off phase with subsequent bleeding. Endometriosis causes pelvic pain, abnormal bleeding, and painful menstruation **(dysmenorrhea).** Sterility and pain during sexual intercourse **(dyspareunia)** can result. Treatment of endometriosis varies according to the extent of the abnormal growth and the age of the patient. Hormonal therapy is generally used for the young patient. Pregnancy, with the absence of menstruation, tends to hold the condition in check. Extensive proliferation of endometrial tissue requires surgery. Cysts filled with blood are usually found at this time.

ABNORMALITIES OF PREGNANCY

A most important factor during pregnancy is good prenatal care. The pregnant woman should be checked regularly for weight gain, blood pressure, and urine abnormalities. She should be instructed on the importance of proper diet and exercise. Most pregnancies progress normally, but occasionally some problems do arise.

■ Ectopic Pregnancy

An **ectopic pregnancy** is a pregnancy in which the fertilized ovum implants in a tissue other than the uterus. The most common site of an ectopic pregnancy is in the fallopian tubes. The fertilized ovum becomes trapped because of a stricture or obstruction such as a tumor. Salpingitis is a predisposing condition for a tubal pregnancy due to the inflammatory effect on the mucosal lining. Embryonic development proceeds for about 2 months, at which time the pregnancy terminates. The tube often ruptures, as seen in Figure 14–9, causing severe internal hemorrhage into the abdominal cavity. Intense pain and bleeding from the uterus result, and the embryo is usually destroyed by the trauma. Once the diagnosis has been made, the ruptured tube and embryo have to be removed surgically.

■ Spontaneous Abortion

A spontaneous abortion, commonly called a miscarriage, usually results from a genetic abnormality. The fetus is expelled before it is able to live outside of the uterus. This usually occurs in the second or third month of pregnancy. The first sign is vaginal bleeding with cramping. The woman who has aborted should receive medical attention at once to reduce the hazards of hemorrhage and infection. Dilation and curretage, a D&C, is usually performed to remove any tissue that remains in the uterus.

A woman who has repeated spontaneous abortions should be examined

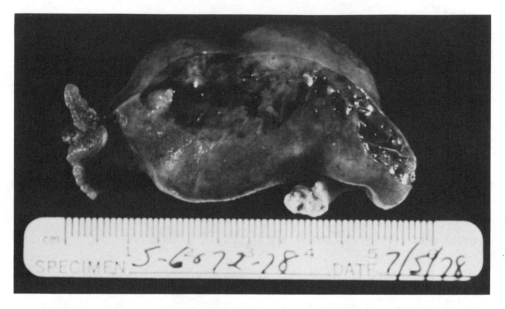

Figure 14–9. Fallopian tube ruptured from an ectopic pregnancy. *(Courtesy of Dr. David R. Duffell.)*

comprehensively to determine the cause. Hormonal imbalances are sometimes responsible and can be corrected by replacement hormones. Emotional and psychological factors may be involved, and professional counseling is advised.

■ Toxemia of Pregnancy

Toxemia of pregnancy sometimes develops during the last trimester. The condition is poorly named because no toxin appears to cause the disease. The cause of this condition is not known. The principal signs are hypertension, albuminuria, edema (particularly in the face and arms), and a significant weight gain. These signs are presented in Figure 14–10. In the first phase of toxemia, pregnancy-induced hypertension (PIH), the patient experiences headache, visual disturbances, abdominal pain, and vomiting. A spasm of blood vessels apparently causes the headache and visual disturbances. If this condition is not treated, **eclampsia** develops and the patient goes into convulsions and coma.

Preventive treatment for toxemia consists of early prenatal care, in which blood pressure is regularly checked, urine is analyzed for albumin, and weight gain is controlled. **Preeclampsia,** diagnosed early and treated, responds well. Restriction of salt (which tends to increase blood pressure), a nutritious low-calorie diet, and diuretics may be prescribed. This must be

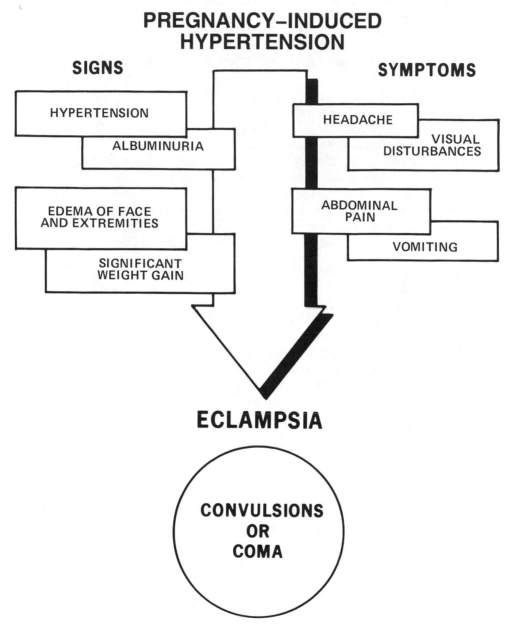

Figure 14-10. Toxemia of pregnancy.

done with great care to prevent injury to the fetus. If the patient does not respond and eclampsia with convulsions develops, anticonvulsant medications are prescribed with caution.

ANATOMY OF THE MALE REPRODUCTIVE SYSTEM

The male reproductive system consists of a pair of testes in which the sperm develop and hormones are produced, a system of tubules that convey sperm to the outside, and the penis, which transmits the sperm into the female tract. Accessory glands contribute to the formation of semen.

The testes are suspended in the scrotum, a saclike structure outside the body wall. The testes contain highly coiled tubules called the seminiferous tubules, which are the site of sperm development (Figure 14–11). When the sperm reach a certain maturity they enter the epididymis, a coiled tube that lies along the outer wall of the testis. The epididymis leads into another duct, the vas deferens, that passes through the inguinal canal into the abdominal cavity.

Near the base of the urinary bladder the vas deferens joins a duct of the seminal vesicle, an accessory gland, to form the ejaculatory duct. The ejaculatory ducts from each side penetrate the prostate gland to enter the urethra. Ducts of the prostate open into the first part of the male urethra. Another pair of glands, the bulbourethral glands, secrete into the urethra as it enters the penis. The male reproductive system is shown in Figure 14–12.

The penis consists of three cylindrical bodies of cavernous tissue also known as erectile tissue. This tissue is filled with spaces, or sinuses, that become engorged with blood. The urethra passes through one of these cylindrical bodies as it extends to the outside. Connective tissue supports the erectile structures. The distal, expanded end of the penis is the glans penis. A flap of loosely attached skin covering the glans, the prepuce or foreskin, is often removed shortly after birth, which is the procedure called circumcision.

PHYSIOLOGY OF THE MALE REPRODUCTIVE SYSTEM

Spermatogenesis, the formation of sperm, begins in the male at about age 13 and continues through life. The development of sperm and the secretion of the male hormone testosterone are processes stimulated by gonadotropic hormones of the anterior pituitary gland. Full maturation of the sperm occurs in the epididymis, where they become motile and capable of fertilizing an ovum. Sperm are stored in both the epididymis and vas deferens and can live for several weeks in the male genital ducts. Once they are ejaculated, they live for only 24 to 72 hours.

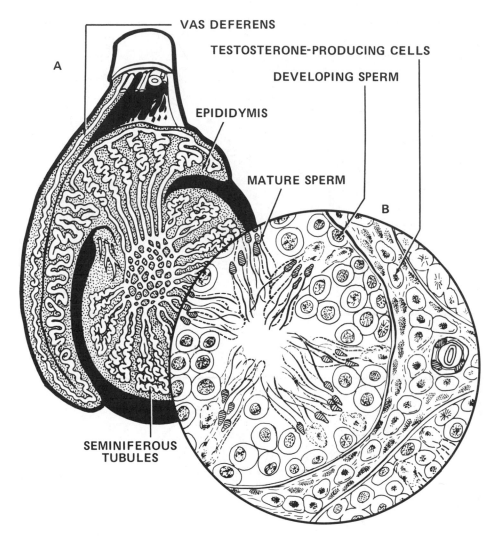

Figure 14-11. Testis. **A.** Sagittal section of testis. **B.** Cross-section of seminiferous tubule.

The accessory glands contribute to the nourishment and protection of the sperm. Mucoid secretions from these glands form the semen. The seminal vesicles provide fructose, other nutrients, and prostaglandin, which increases uterine contractions. This helps to propel the sperm toward the fallopian tubes. The seminal vesicles release their secretions into the ejaculatory ducts at the same time the vas deferens empty the sperm. The muscular prostate gland, which surrounds the first part of the urethra, contracts during ejaculation, releasing its secretions. The secretion is alkaline,

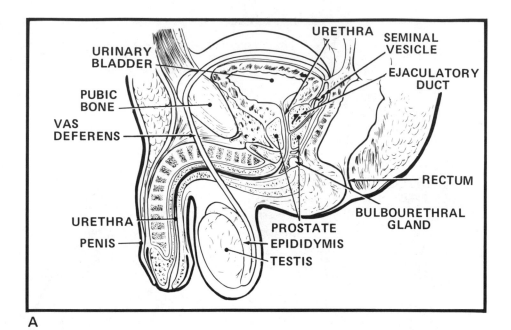

Figure 14-12. Sagittal section **(A)** and posterior view **(B)** of male reproductive system.

which is important to the motility of the sperm, since the highly acidic vaginal secretions would inhibit sperm motility.

Sexual stimulation of the male transmits impulses into the central nervous system, which initiates the male response. Erection of the penis is the first effect. Nerve impulses cause the dilation of penile arteries, allowing blood to flow under high pressure into the erectile tissue. The high pressure temporarily impedes the emptying of the penile veins, and causes the penis to become hard, elongated, and erect.

Intense sexual stimulation causes peristaltic contractions in the walls of the epididymis and vas deferens, propelling sperm into the internal urethra. The seminal vesicles and prostate gland simultaneously release their secretions, which mix with the mucous secretion of the bulbourethral glands. Semen is formed as a result. This is the process of emission. Ejaculation of the semen—the culmination of the sexual act—occurs when contraction of this musculature increases pressure on the erectile tissue, and the semen is expressed through the urethral opening.

DISEASES OF THE MALE REPRODUCTIVE SYSTEM

The most common diseases of the male reproductive system are those affecting the prostate gland. This gland can become inflamed or enlarged as a result of bacterial invasion and cause urinary problems. Cancer sometimes develops in the prostate as well as in the testes.

■ Diseases of the Prostate Gland

Inflammation of the prostate can result from urinary tract infections or sexually transmitted diseases. Conversely, an enlarged prostate can cause urinary tract infections by obstructing the outflow of urine from the bladder.

■ *Prostatitis.* The cause of **prostatitis,** inflammation of the prostate, is not always known. Infection frequently develops from gonococci in a male with gonorrhea or from *E. coli* that has caused a urinary tract infection. The patient experiences pain and a burning sensation during urination. The prostate may be tender, and pus from the tip of the penis is sometimes noted. Penicillin is the usual treatment unless hypersensitivity to the drug necessitates the use of other antibiotics.

■ *Benign Prostatic Hyperplasia.* Enlargement of the prostate gland, benign **prostatic hyperplasia,** is a common occurrence in men over 50. The incidence increases with age, and the enlargement can be felt through rectal examination.

The symptoms resemble urinary tract disturbances (see Chapter 9) as the enlarged prostate partially blocks the flow of urine from the bladder. If the bladder cannot be fully emptied, residual urine provides a medium for bacterial infection and cystitis develops. Figure 14–13 shows an obstruction of the urethra caused by prostatic enlargement.

The blockage of urine outflow places back pressure on the ureters. This causes them to become congested with urine, a condition called hydroureters. This back pressure can extend to the kidneys; they swell with fluid, and hydronephrosis results. An imbalance of sex hormones frequently causes prostatic enlargement. The level of testosterone generally decreases with age, but estrogen from the adrenal cortex continues to be secreted, changing the ratio of the two. Treatment for benign prostatic hyperplasia, which is highly symptomatic, is surgical removal.

■ *Carcinoma of the Prostate Gland.* Carcinoma of the prostate is common in old age, but the tumor may be small and asymptomatic. Rectal examination may reveal an enlarged prostate that is very hard. It will be harder than a benign enlargement. Symptoms of prostatic cancer are urinary tract

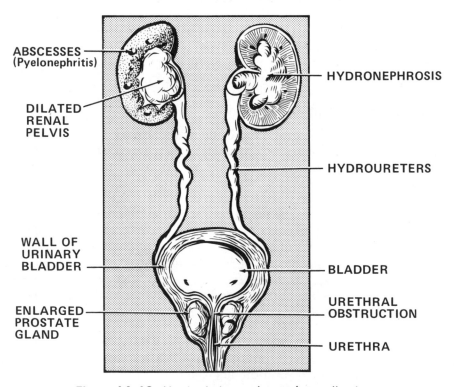

Figure 14-13. Urethral obstruction and complications.

obstruction, urinary infections, the need to urinate during the night, or nocturia, and at times urinary incontinence.

Prognosis for this carcinoma is poor, as the malignancy spreads rapidly to nearby organs like the bladder and rectum. The cancer invades the lymph and blood vessels and metastasizes to the bone and other organs. Figure 14–14 shows common sites of metastases from cancer of the prostate.

Treatment depends on the extent of the cancer, which may be inoperable. Hormonal therapy is generally prescribed. Since testosterone stimulates growth of the tumor, removal of the testes—the source of the hormone—may reduce its size. Estrogen, which has an inhibitory effect on the tumor's growth, is administered.

Diseases of the Testes and Epididymis

The testes and epididymis can become inflamed from injury, infection, or some rare tumors that develop in the testes.

■ *Epididymitis.* Inflammation of the epididymis (**epididymitis**) is frequently caused by gonococcus. A urinary tract infection or prostatitis can also be the source of epididymitis. Abscesses sometimes form, and scar tissue develops that can cause sterility if both sides are affected. Symptoms include severe pain in the testes, swelling, and tenderness in the scrotum. Antibiotic treatment is effective when combined with rest and the avoidance of irritants such as alcohol and spicy food.

■ *Orchitis.* **Orchitis,** inflammation of the testes, can follow an injury or viral infection such as mumps, with the development of inflammatory edema and pain. The most common cause of orchitis is mumps in an adult man. Swelling of the testes and severe pain usually develop about a week after mumps, an inflammation of the paraotid salivary gland. In severe cases, atrophy of the testes can occur, and if both sides are affected, sterility results.

■ *Testicular Tumors.* Tumors of the testes are rare, but when they occur it is usually in young men. These tumors are highly malignant. One such tumor is the **seminoma,** a cancer of the seminiferous tubules. The seminoma is quite radiosensitive, so the prescribed treatment is irradiation.

Another tumor of the testes is the **teratoma,** similar in form to the dermoid cyst of the ovary described previously. The teratoma evidently arises from a primitive germ cell, and the tumor contains a variety of tissues. Whereas the dermoid cyst in the ovary is benign, the teratoma of the testes is highly malignant and spreads through the lymphatics and blood vessels. Chemotherapy and radiotherapy are the usual means of treatment.

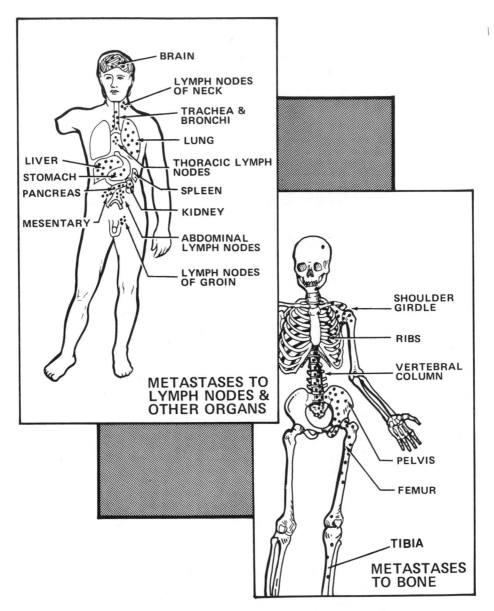

Figure 14-14. Common sites of metastases from prostatic cancer.

■ *Cryptorchidism.* **Cryptorchidism** is not a disease but a failure of the testes to descend from the abdominal cavity, where they develop during fetal life, to the scrotum. Undescended testes are shown in Figure 14–15. This condition should be corrected through surgery or hormonal therapy. Sterility results if this condition is not rectified. Maturation of the sperm cannot occur in the abdominal cavity, where the temperature is slightly higher than that of the scrotum. If the testes are not brought down into the scrotum, they should be removed. Undescended testes atrophy and may become the potential site of cancer.

■ *Hypogonadism in the Male.* Several factors can cause **hypogonadism,** that is, the decreased functional activity of the gonads. A person may be born without functional testes, the testes may fail to descend and thus atrophy, or the testes may be lost through castration. Testes fail to develop because of a lack of gonadotropic hormones.

Loss of the male gonads before puberty causes the condition of eunuchism, in which sexual characteristics do not develop. Development of male traits depends on testosterone secretion by the testes. Castration after puberty causes some regression of secondary sexual characteristics, but masculinity is retained. Hormonal therapy, the administration of testosterone, can be effective.

SEXUALLY TRANSMITTED DISEASES

The incidence of diseases transmitted by sexual intercourse has greatly increased in recent years, especially among young people. If untreated, serious conditions may develop that can gravely affect a person's life.

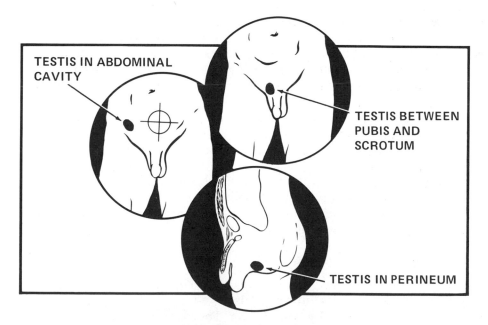

Figure 14-15. Undescended testes.

■ Gonorrhea

Gonorrhea is one of the most common and widespread of venereal diseases. It is caused by the organism gonococcus and is transmitted through sexual intercourse. Gonococci do not live outside the body. The disease is acquired by direct sexual contact with an infected person.

The initial site of infection is the genitals or urethra. Symptoms usually occur within 2 to 8 days of infection. The vaginal glands in the female are frequently affected and fill with pus; the organisms may spread to the cervix. Acute urethritis develops in the male, causing difficulty and pain during urination. A copious discharge of pus ensues. Prostatitis frequently develops with abscess formation.

Symptoms of urethritis or cervicitis may be ignored in the female or she may be asymptomatic. The female can be a reservoir for organisms and not be aware that she is infected.

Gonorrhea usually responds rapidly to penicillin but early detection and treatment are extremely important. Diagnosis of gonorrhea is made by examining pus from the urethra or vaginal discharge for the presence of gonococci.

If untreated, a chronic condition develops, and the infection spreads upward. The inflammation causes fibrosis, which can produce a stricture in the male urethra or in the vas deferens. If both vas deferens become stenotic, sterility results.

The fallopian tubes in the female are frequently affected by untreated gonorrhea, and salpingitis results. The pus-filed tubes can empty into the peritoneal cavity, causing peritonitis.

The most common cause of pelvic inflammatory disease (PID) is untreated gonorrhea. Chills, fever, and weakness develop with intestinal upset. Chronic pelvic inflammatory disease causes abscesses to develop in the fallopian tubes, with fibrous scarring and sterility resulting. Ectopic pregnancies may also result.

The baby of an infected mother can be born with acute purulent conjunctivitis, inflammation of the conjunctiva. The gonococcal organisms enter the eye during delivery, and if the cornea becomes ulcerated, blindness results. To prevent this infection from developing, a drop of silver nitrate is routinely placed in the eyes of newborn babies.

A new danger exists in treating gonorrhea with penicillin. A superinfection can develop in which the causative organisms become resistant to penicillin and actually use it as a nutrient.

■ Syphilis

Syphilis is a most serious venereal disease. The causative organism is a spirochete, ***Treponema pallidum,*** transmitted by sexual intercourse or intimate contact with an infectious lesion. The baby of an infected mother may be born syphilitic.

A **chancre,** or ulceration, develops on the genitals in the primary stage of infection. This lesion, which may vary from a small erosion to a deep ulcer, appears within a few days to a few weeks after sexual contact. The chancre usually develops on the vulva of the female and on the penis of the male as shown in Figure 14–16. The chancre may develop elsewhere: on the lips, the tongue, or anus. Anal chancres are common in male homosexuals.

The lesion, which sometimes goes unnoticed, heals after a few weeks. If untreated with penicillin, the secondary phase of the disease occurs in a matter of weeks. The principal sign of the secondary phase is a nonitching rash that affects any part of the body: the trunk, soles of the feet, palms, mouth, vulva, or rectum. The patient is still infectious at this stage, but he or she can be treated with penicillin.

An untreated case of syphilis may be dormant for many years, but the organisms are in the blood stream and a systemic spread occurs. The appearance of symptoms, years after the primary infection, marks the tertiary and most serious phase of syphilis.

The cardiovascular system is severely damaged at this stage of infection. The inflammatory response to the spirochetes in the blood causes fibrosis, scarring, and obstruction of blood vessels, particularly of the aorta. Lesions develop on the cerebral cortex, causing mental disorders, deafness,

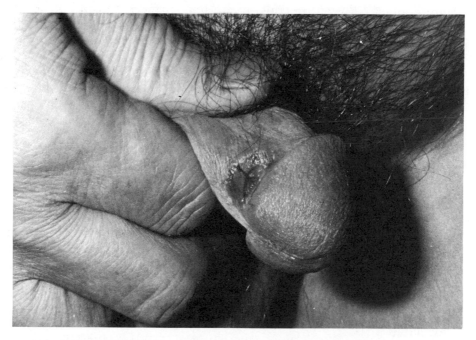

Figure 14-16. A chancre of primary syphilis seen on the penis. (*From Feinstein. Dermatology, 1975. Courtesy of Robert J. Brady Co.*)

and blindness. Loss of sensation in the legs and feet due to spinal cord damage cause a characteristic gait to develop. **Paresis,** a general paralysis associated with organic loss of intellectual function, results in death if untreated. The tertiary lesions of the syphilitic infection are irreversible.

Congenital defects are numerous in an infant born to an infectious mother. Mental retardation, physical deformities, deafness, and blindness are common. The syphilitic infection can cause death of the fetus and spontaneous abortion.

The severe consequences of syphilis point out the urgent need for early detection and treatment. Diagnostic procedures include screening tests—the **VDRL test** perfected by the Venereal Disease Research Laboratory of the United State Public Health Service, and the **Rapid Plasma Reagin (RPR) test.** The most sensitive and specific test for syphilis is the *treponema pallidum* **immobilization test (TPI),** which detects specific antibodies against the spirochete. Treatment with penicillin is successful except in reversing tertiary lesions. Development of a superinfection, described under gonorrhea, is a serious threat.

■ Genital Herpes

Genital herpes is an extremely painful, viral disease that tends to recur periodically and for which there is no cure. Herpesvirus is transmitted by intimate contact between mucous membrane surfaces, the site of herpesvirus affinity. There are two types of **herpes simplex** virus, type I causing "fever blisters" or "cold sores" and type II involving the mucous membranes of the genital tracts.

Symptoms generally appear within 3 weeks after exposure to the virus. The symptoms intensify from a burning, itching sensation to severe pain. Multiple blisters appear on the genitalia and at times on the buttocks or thigh. As the blisters rupture, they become seondarily infected and ulcerate. Painful urination and vaginal discharge are common.

The active phase subsides as the lesions heal, but the virus remains dormant until reactivated, perhaps at a time of stress or low resistance.

The disease is transmitted by contact with an active sore that is releasing (shedding) the infectious virus. The virus can be spread from a cold sore on the lips to the genitals; the reverse is also true. Great caution should be used to avoid self-infection of the mucous membrane of the eye.

Use of condoms or diaphragms provides partial protection from transmitting the virus during intercourse, but abstention from sexual contact during the active phase is essential.

Diagnosis is most accurate based on a positive viral culture on living tissue. The Tzanck smear test, which involves examination of lesion fluid, is also available.

There is no cure for a herpes infection, but secondary infections can be prevented and healing promoted. The lesions must be kept clean and dry, and ice-cold compresses may be used to relieve the pain.

Active herpes genitalis has very serious consequences during pregnancy, not only causing spontaneous abortion or premature delivery, but also increasing the risk of transmitting the infection to the newborn.

■ Chlamydial Infections

Chlamydial infections are among the most prevalent venereal diseases in the United States. Several strains of the chlamydia organism are responsible for sexually transmitted genitourinary infections in both men and women, as well as in newborns of infected mothers. The disease is a leading cause of pelvic inflammatory disease (PID) in women, with resultant infertility, and severe urethritis in both sexes. Women are often asymptomatic carriers of the infection and continue to infect partners and offspring. Improved tests for the diagnosis of chlamydia infection have recently been developed. The disease responds to certain antibiotics but not to penicillin. The infection often coexists with gonorrhea.

■ Acquired Immune Deficiency Syndrome (AIDS)

One of the most deadly diseases to affect today's population is **acquired immune deficiency syndrome, AIDS.** It attacks primarily promiscuous homosexual and bisexual men, drug users who share hypodermic needles, and, in some cases, recipients of blood transfusions. Children born to infected mothers have also contracted AIDS. There is now a significant incidence of the disease among prostitutes.

The causative agent of AIDS is a virus, HTLV-III, named for its similarity to a particular leukemia-producing virus (human T-cell leukemia virus.) The virus infects certain white blood cells of the body's immune system, namely, the T-4 lymphocytes, and destroys their ability to fight infection. The affected person becomes especially susceptible to a rare type of pneumonia, caused by *Pneumocystis carnii*, and a rare slow-growing cancer, Kaposi's sarcoma. Symptoms include unexplained weight loss, severe infections, and generalized lymphadenopathy (diseased lymph nodes).

The HTLV-III has been isolated from the blood and semen of AIDS patients and is transmitted principally by direct intimate contact involving mucous membrane surfaces. The infection may also be spread by shared contaminated hypodermic needles and blood transfusions. The virus cannot penetrate skin but enters through natural body openings and open wounds.

A long latent period increases the risk of spreading the infection. Once infected, the person is infected for life, and the mortality rate is extremely high. There have been no reported recoveries to date.

Development of a vaccine to prevent the spread of AIDS has not yet been possible. This may be due to variations of the virus or patients' inability to respond appropriately to it.

Isolation of the AIDS virus has made possible the development of a blood test to detect the presence of antibodies indicating exposure to the disease. The test can be applied to stored blood, which reduces the risk of transmission by blood transfusions.

Health care professionals must exercise great precautions when handling blood or bodily secretions of AIDS patients. It has been reported that a few have developed antibodies after an accidental cut with a contaminated needle or sharp instrument, but they have not generally developed the disease. Recommendations for protection against any blood-borne disease such as hepatitis B should be observed.

Closely related to AIDS is AIDS-related complex (ARC), in which the symptoms are similar but less severe. Many patients once diagnosed as having ARC have later developed AIDS.

Much research effort is taking place to stem the spread of this fatal disease and to treat its growing number of victims.

SUMMARY

Disease can affect the reproductive system in many ways. In the female, tumors and cysts develop in the ovary, uterus, and breast. Infections invade the vagina and vaginal glands, the fallopian tubes, and the endometrium. Menstrual abnormalities result from a diseased organ or from a hormonal imbalance. A pregnancy can develop in the fallopian tubes, a fetus can be spontaneously aborted, and toxemia can occur in a pregnancy.

Diseases of the male affect the prostate gland by infection, enlargement, or tumor formation, causing urinary complications. Infections of the testes and epididymis can result in sterility. Inadequate testosterone secretion affects the male secondary sexual characteristics.

Sexually transmitted diseases, gonorrhea, chlamydial infections, and syphilis, have far-reaching consequences if untreated. Early detection and administration of penicillin prevent numerous complications, providing that a superinfection does not develop.

STUDY QUESTIONS

1. Name three possible causes of salpingitis.
2. How can sterility result from salpingitis?

3. Explain how (a) trichomonas and (b) *Candida albicans* can cause vaginitis.
4. How does puerperal sepsis develop?
5. What are possible complications of puerperal sepsis?
6. Why is a Pap smear of great diagnostic importance?
7. What is a hydatidiform mole?
8. What are the symptoms of advanced breast cancer?
9. Name several possible causes of secondary amenorrhea.
10. What signs and symptoms accompany toxic shock syndrome?
11. What are some complications of endometriosis?
12. What causes an ectopic pregnancy?
13. How can toxemia of pregnancy usually be prevented?
14. What are some causes of prostatitis?
15. Explain the complications of benign prostatic hypertrophy.
16. Name the symptoms of carcinoma of the prostate.
17. What is the danger of mumps in an adult male?
18. Why is cryptorchidism a serious condition?
19. What are the symptoms of gonorrhea?
20. How is gonorrhea diagnosed?
21. What are the complications of untreated gonorrhea?
22. Describe the signs for each of the three stages of syphilis.
23. What are the final results of untreated syphilis?
24. Describe the complications associated with chlamydial infections.
25. Why is AIDS a fatal disease?

CHAPTER 15

Diseases of the Nervous System

The body is constantly subjected to changes in its internal and external environment. The body's response is to react appropriately to these changing conditions. How is this accomplished, often with no deliberate thought?

The body is equipped to receive all kinds of sensory information: visual, auditory, olfactory, tactile, temperature, pressure, and pain. This input is processed with lightning speed and an action results. It may be an action such as squinting in overly-bright light, a turn of the head to detect a faint sound, withdrawal from pain, or shivering to keep warm.

This response to various stimuli is accomplished through the complex nervous system. Certain nerves are specialized to receive sensory information and to convey it to the central nervous system, the brain and spinal cord. Other nerves carry messages from the central nervous system to all parts of the body and initiate action by stimulating a muscle to contract or a gland to secrete. The nervous system is basically a highly organized communication system serving the body.

Disorders of the nervous system may be manifested by such conditions as lack of sensation, paralysis, mental confusion, **seizures,** or the inability to speak. To understand the basis of the various neural disorders, understanding the structure and function of the nervous system is required.

STRUCTURE OF THE NERVOUS SYSTEM

The basic unit of the nervous system is the neuron, or nerve cell. The neuron consists of a cell body and long extensions or fibers—a single axon

295

leading from the cell body and various numbers of dendrites leading toward it. A neuron is shown in Figure 15–1. Some **neurons** are **sensory,** capable of detecting an environmental change and transmitting the message to the brain or spinal cord. Other neurons, the **motor neurons,** convey messages from the central nervous system to a muscle, causing it to contract, or to a gland, triggering its secretion. The response to a stimulus is known as a reflex arc. The fibers of sensory and motor neurons are insulated by a fatty covering called the **myelin** sheath, which increases the rate of transmission of an impulse. Deterioration of this sheath accompanies multiple sclerosis, a disease to be described. The reflex arc pattern is shown in Figure 15–2.

A nerve such as the optic or sciatic nerve consists of a bundle of neuronal fibers. Twelve pairs of nerves—the cranial nerves—enter or exit from the brain. Thirty-one pairs of nerves—the spinal nerves—enter and exit the spinal cord and innervate all parts of the body. The nervous system is illustrated in Figure 15–3.

The Spinal Cord

The spinal cord is housed within the vertebral column and is continuous with the brain stem. Numerous tracts of nerve fibers within the cord ascend to the brain, whereas others descend, carrying messages destined for muscles and glands. Three coverings, the **meninges,** protect the delicate nerve tissue. The innermost covering is the pia mater, the next is the arachnoid, and the toughest, outermost covering is the dura mater. Meningitis is an inflammation of these coverings that also surround the brain.

The Brain

The largest portion of the brain is the cerebrum, or cerebral hemispheres. The surface is highly convoluted and has many elevations and depressions. The outer surface of the brain, the cortex, consists of gray matter, where the nerve cell bodies are concentrated. The inner area consists of white matter, the nerve fiber tracts. Deep within the white matter are concentrations of nerve cell bodies known as **basal ganglia,** which help control position and automatic movements. It is the basal ganglia (also gray matter) that are disturbed in Parkinson's disease.

Within the brain are four spaces called **ventricles** that are continuous with the central canal of the spinal cord. **Cerebrospinal fluid** formation takes place in these ventricles. This fluid, derived from plasma, flows out of the ventricles through small openings and is channeled to circulate over the brain and spinal cord. It flows under the arachnoid covering, acting as a watery, protective cushion. Cerebrospinal fluid is reabsorbed into the venous sinuses of the dura mater, and new fluid is formed. Obstruction of cerebrospinal fluid circulation results in hydrocephalus, which will be described.

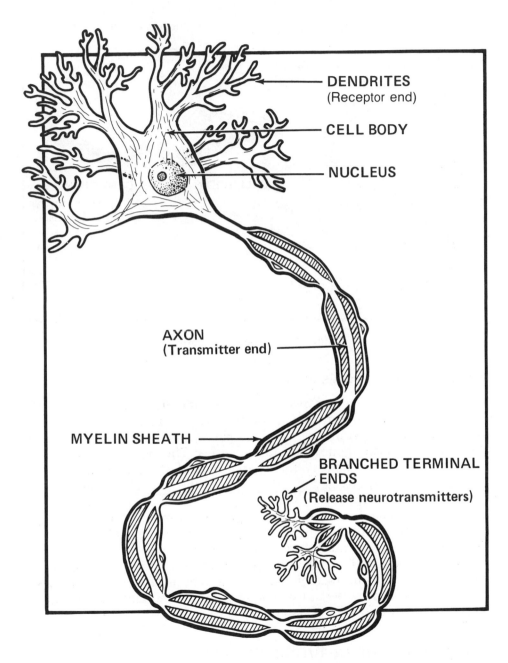

Figure 15-1. Typical neuron.

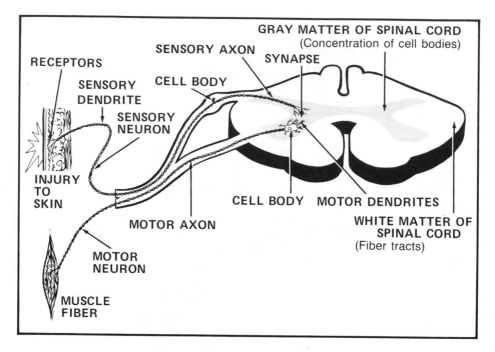

Figure 15-2. Reflex arc pattern.

The Autonomic Nervous System

Another part of the nervous system is the **autonomic nervous system.** This part controls internal functioning of the body. The autonomic nervous system contains the sympathetic and the parasympathetic nervous systems, which often work antagonistically to each other. The hypothalamus, located in the brain, controls activity for a large part of the autonomic nervous system, but it is also affected by other parts of the central nervous system.

The autonomic nervous system controls arterial blood pressure, heart rate, gastrointestinal functions, sweating, temperature regulation, and many other involuntary actions. Whereas the peripheral nerves affect skeletal or voluntary muscle, the autonomic nervous system acts on smooth or involuntary muscle and cardiac muscle. Diseases of the digestive system affected by nerves—ulcers, regional enteritis, and ulcerative colitis (Chapter 10)—are influenced by the autonomic nervous system and the response of the adrenal cortex to stress (Chapter 18).

FUNCTION OF THE NERVOUS SYSTEM

The transmission of impulses along nerve fibers is an electrical occurrence. For a detailed explanation of the transmission of nerve impulses, you might

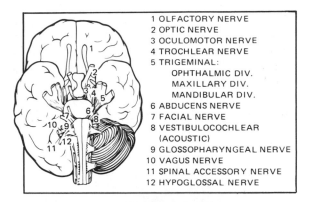

1 OLFACTORY NERVE
2 OPTIC NERVE
3 OCULOMOTOR NERVE
4 TROCHLEAR NERVE
5 TRIGEMINAL:
  OPHTHALMIC DIV.
  MAXILLARY DIV.
  MANDIBULAR DIV.
6 ABDUCENS NERVE
7 FACIAL NERVE
8 VESTIBULOCOCHLEAR
  (ACOUSTIC)
9 GLOSSOPHARYNGEAL NERVE
10 VAGUS NERVE
11 SPINAL ACCESSORY NERVE
12 HYPOGLOSSAL NERVE

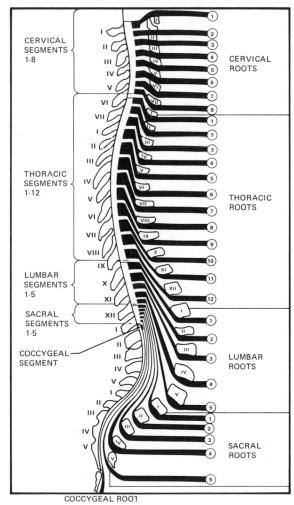

Figure 15-3. The central nervous system. **Top.** Cranial nerves. **Bottom.** Spinal nerves.

consult a physiology textbook. Impulses are passed from one neuron to another at a junction called the synapse. Transmission at the synapse is a chemical reaction in which the terminal ends of the axon release a transmitter substance that affects the dendrites of the next neuron. One-way transmission of the impulse is assured because only the axons release these chemicals. A similar phenomenon occurs when a motor neuron stimulates a muscle fiber to contract by releasing a transmitter substance, which affects the muscle fiber membrane. This junction is referred to as the neuromuscular or myoneural junction.

The Sensory Nervous System

Sensations detected by sensory neurons in the skin, the muscles, tendons, or internal organs are sent into the spinal cord, where they may trigger a simple cord response. A synapse is made with a motor neuron that will bring about an action. More complex actions require that the impulse be sent to various parts of the brain. Impulses reaching the brain stem and cerebellum bring about many automatic actions that are unconscious, but sensory information involving thought processes must reach the highest area of the brain, the cerebral cortex.

The cerebral cortex has specialized areas to receive sensory information from all parts of the body such as the foot, the hand, the abdomen. These areas are just posterior to the central sulcus. Visual impulses are transmitted to the posterior part of the brain, whereas olfactory and auditory impulses are received in the lateral parts. Association areas of the brain interpret deeper meaning of the sensations, and all the sensory messages are integrated in the "knowing area" where they may be stored as memory. Creative thought becomes possible through use of all sensory input.

The Motor Nervous System

Just as the cerebral cortex has areas specialized for the reception of sensory information, there are areas that govern motor activity. The primary motor cortex is just anterior to the central sulcus and controls discrete movements of skeletal muscles. Stimulation on one side of the cerebral cortex affects particular muscles on the opposite side of the body because the nerve fibers cross over in the medulla and spinal cord.

Anterior to the primary motor cortex is the premotor cortex, which controls coordinate movements of muscles. This is accomplished by stimulating groups of muscles that work together. The speech area is located here and is usually on the left side in right-handed people. Specialized areas of the brain are shown in Figure 15–4.

Damage to any part of the brain from trauma, hemorrhage, blood clot formation with subsequent ischemia, or infection will have varying effects depending on the degree of injury and the location of the lesion.

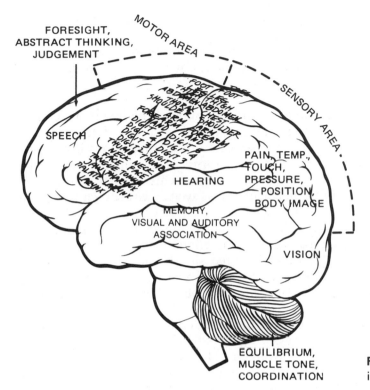

Figure 15-4. Specialized areas of the brain.

DISEASES OF THE NERVOUS SYSTEM

The nervous system is affected by disease in numerous ways. Bacteria and viruses can invade the system and cause infection. Degeneration of nerve tissue is another type of disease. Seizures result from abnormal transmission of neuronal impulses in the brain. Errors in fetal development are responsible for other neural disorders. The brain may be damaged by trauma, cerebral hemorrhages, blood clot formation, and tumors. Many diseases of the nervous system manifest themselves in abnormal muscular activity.

Only neural diseases that have a structural or physiologic basis will be treated in this book. Functional diseases such as schizophrenia, in which there is no apparent brain lesion, are better covered in a psychology text.

Infectious Diseases of the Nervous System

Many diseases are **neurotropic** in that the causative agent, a virus or bacterium, has an affinity for the nervous system. Most viruses in this class affect the nerve tissue directly, although the toxin produced by bacteria is the offending agent in another neural disease.

Infectious neural diseases have numerous causes, such as an infection elsewhere in the body, a contaminated puncture wound, a dog or insect bite, and exposure to chicken pox.

■ *Meningitis.* **Meningitis** is an acute inflammation of the first two meninges of the brain and spinal cord, the pia mater and the arachnoid. It is a disease usually affecting children and may have serious complications if not diagnosed and treated early. There are many forms of meningitis, some being more contagious than others. The most common causative organism is the *Neisseria meningitidis,* but other bacteria, as well as viruses, cause meningitis.

The infecting organisms can reach the meninges from a middle ear, upper respiratory tract, or frontal sinus infection; or they can be carried in the blood from the lungs or other infected site. Healthy children may be carriers of the bacteria and spread the organisms by sneezing or coughing. Viral meningitis may be caused by mumps, polio viruses, and occasionally by herpes simplex.

The symptoms of meningitis are high fever, chills, and a severe headache due to increased intracranial pressure. The patient has a very stiff neck and holds the head rigidly. Any movement of neck muscles stretches the meninges and increases the pain. Nausea, vomiting, and a rash may also be symptomatic. The high fever often causes delirium and convulsions in children, and they may lapse into a coma.

Diagnosis of meningitis is made through a **lumbar puncture,** or spinal tap, in which a hollow needle is inserted into the spinal canal between vertebrae in the lumbar region. This procedure is possible because the spinal cord terminates at the first lumbar vertebra but the sac containing cerebrospinal fluid extends down to the sacrum. Increased pressure of the cerebrospinal fluid with an elevated protein level, numerous polymorphs, and infecting organisms confirms the diagnosis of meningitis. The level of glucose in the cerebrospinal fluid is below normal because the bacteria use the sugar for their own growth.

Treatment with antibiotics is very effective if the meningitis is bacterial. If not treated, permanent brain damage usually results, manifesting itself by sight or hearing loss, paralysis, or mental retardation. The opening in the roof of the fourth ventricle may become blocked by the pyogenic infection. This results in the accumulation of cerebrospinal fluid in the brain, causing a form of **hydrocephalus.**

■ *Encephalitis.* **Encephalitis,** an inflammation of the brain and meninges, is caused by a viral infection. The virus may be harbored by wild birds and transmitted to man by mosquitoes. There are many forms of the disease, and they occur in epidemics. Lethargic encephalitis, or "sleeping sickness," is one type of encephalitis in which persistent drowsiness, delirium, and sometimes coma are present. Symptoms of encephalitis range from mild to severe and may include headache, fever, cerebral dysfunction, disordered thought patterns, and, often, seizures. Secondary encephalitis may develop from viral childhood diseases such as chicken pox, measles, and mumps.

Diagnosis of encephalitis is made by lumbar puncture. Treatment is essentially aimed at the symptoms, control of the high fever, maintenance of fluid and electrolyte balance, and careful monitoring of respiratory and kidney function.

In serious cases involving extensive brain damage, convalescence is slow and requires prolonged physical rehabilitation. Nerve damage may cause paralysis. Personality changes occur, as well as emotional disturbances requiring therapy.

■ *Poliomyelitis.* **Poliomyelitis,** once a crippling and killing disease that struck primarily children, has nearly been eradicated through the development of the Salk and Sabin vaccines and immunization programs to assure that all children are protected.

Polio is an infectious disease of the brain and spinal cord caused by a virus. Motor neurons of the medulla oblongata and of the spinal cord are primarily affected. Without motor nerve stimulations, muscles become paralyzed. If the respiratory muscles are affected, artificial means of respiration are required.

Symptoms of poliomyelitis are stiff neck, fever, headache, sore throat, and gastrointestinal disturbances. When diagnosed and treated early, severe damage to the nervous system is prevented.

The tremendous value of Dr. Jonas Salk's vaccine to prevent poliomyelitis cannot be measured. Salk used inactivated polio virus, injected intramuscularly, that stimulated production of antibodies against polio. The decrease in the number of polio cases with the institution of immunization programs was immediate. Dr. Albert Sabin discovered an oral vaccine against polio that is more convenient to administer, particularly to large groups, and is extremely effective. The Sabin vaccine, because it is taken orally, stimulates the production of antibodies within the digestive system, where the viruses first reside. Destruction of the viruses in the digestive system prevents their transmission and eliminates carriers, which the Salk vaccine does not do.

■ *Tetanus.* Most people are familiar with the need for a tetanus shot after a puncture wound or an animal bite. Why are these wounds particularly dangerous?

Tetanus, commonly called "lockjaw," is an infection of nerve tissue caused by the tetanus bacillus that lives in the intestines of animals and human beings. The organisms are excreted in fecal material and persist as spores indefinitely in the soil. The bacilli are prevalent in rural areas and in garden soil fertilized with manure.

The organism that enters the wound with dirt remains in the wound. This organism flourishes in the necrotic tissue of a pus infection and in the absence of oxygen. Deep wounds with ragged, lacerated tissue contaminated with fecal material are the most dangerous type. The bacillus produces a powerful toxin that circulates to the nerves. The toxin becomes anchored to motor nerve cells and stimulates them. The nerves then stimulate muscles.

Muscles become rigid, and painful spasms and convulsions develop. The jaw muscles are often the first to be affected. These muscles cannot relax, and the mouth is tightly closed. The neck is stiff, and swallowing becomes difficult. If the muscles of respiration are affected, asphyxiation occurs. Death can result from even a minor wound if the condition is not treated.

Tetanus has an incubation period ranging from 1 to a few weeks. The toxin travels slowly, so the distance from the wound to the spinal cord is significant. Treatment includes a thorough cleansing of the wound, removal of dead tissue and any foreign substance, and immediate immunization to inactivate the toxin before it reaches the spinal cord.

The type of immunization administered depends on the patient's history. If the patient has had no previous immunization, **tetanus antitoxin** is given. If 5 years have elapsed since the previous tetanus injection, the patient receives a booster injection of **tetanus toxoid** to increase the antitoxin level.

Additional treatment includes the administration of antibiotics to prevent secondary infections and the use of sedatives to decrease the frequency of convulsions. Oxygen under high pressure is also used as the bacillus is anaerobic, that is, it thrives in the absence of oxygen.

Tetanus may be prevented by adequate immunization. Tetanus toxoid, which stimulates antibody formation, should be given to infants and small children at prescribed times. This should be done in combination with diphtheria toxoid and pertussis vaccine, which prevents whooping cough.

■ *Rabies.* **Rabies** is primarily a disease of warm-blooded animals such as dogs, cats, skunks, wolves, foxes, and bats; but it can be transmitted to humans through bites or scratches from a rabid animal. Rabies is an infectious disease of the brain and spinal cord caused by a virus that is transmitted by the saliva of an infected animal.

The virus passes from the wound along nerves to the spinal cord and brain where it causes acute encephalomyelitis. The incubation period is long, 40 to 60 days or more, depending on the severity of the wound and the distance of the wound from the brain. Bites on the face, neck, and hands are the most serious. The mode of tetanus and rabies transmission to the central nervous system is illustrated in Figure 15–5.

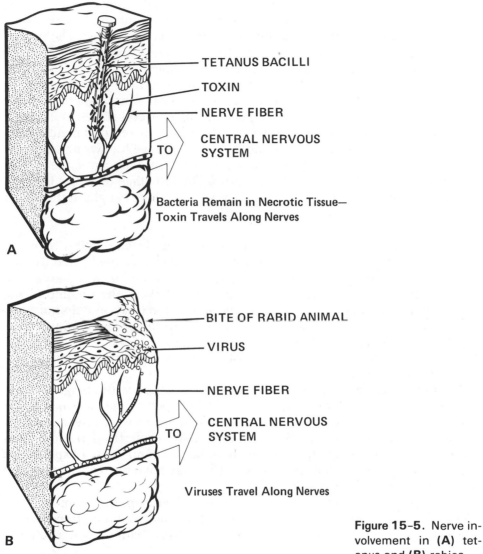

TETANUS BACILLI

TOXIN

NERVE FIBER

CENTRAL NERVOUS SYSTEM

TO

Bacteria Remain in Necrotic Tissue—
Toxin Travels Along Nerves

A

BITE OF RABID ANIMAL

VIRUS

NERVE FIBER

CENTRAL NERVOUS SYSTEM

TO

Viruses Travel Along Nerves

B

Figure 15-5. Nerve involvement in **(A)** tetanus and **(B)** rabies.

The symptoms include fever, pain, mental derangement, rage, convulsions, and paralysis. The muscles of the throat go into spasm at the sight of water, and the patient is unable to drink. Hydrophobia is an aversion to water related to rabies. A profuse, sticky saliva is secreted because of the inability to swallow.

The disease is fatal in humans once it reaches the central nervous system and the symptoms described have developed. A series of antirabies injections must be administered before the virus reaches the brain.

In the case of an animal bite, it is extremely important to know if the animal is rabid. Investigation of the animal must be made whenever possible. If rabies is suspected, immunization injections are started. The patient receives repeated injections of an altered virus to stimulate antibody production and immune serum to provide passive immunity.

The severity of rabies explains the critical need for the vaccination of dogs. In dogs the disease is fatal within a few days. Certain signs indicate that an animal is rabid. The animal goes through several stages, the first of which is an anxiety stage manifested by a change of temperament. As an example, wild animals may act friendly. A furious stage follows in which the animal bites at everything. When paralysis of the throat occurs, the animal cannot swallow and it foams at the mouth. The last stage of rabies is called the dumb stage. The animal appears to have something caught in the throat but makes no attempt to remove it. Death follows.

■ *Shingles (Herpes Zoster).* **Shingles** is an acute inflammation of nerve cells caused by the chicken pox virus, herpes zoster. It is manifested by pain and a rash consisting of small water blisters surrounded by a red area. The lesions follow a sensory nerve, forming a zone toward the midline of the body trunk, are generally confined to one side of the body, and do not cross the midline. The optic nerve can be affected, causing severe conjunctivitis. If not treated properly, ulcerations form on the cornea and scarring results. The lesions dry up and become encrusted. They cause severe itching, pain, and heal with scarring.

Shingles can develop from exposure to a patient with shingles in the infectious stage or from exposure to chicken pox within an incubation period of about 2 weeks. It sometimes accompanies another disease such as pneumonia or tuberculosis. Shingles may also result from trauma or a reaction to certain drug injections. If there has been no known exposure to the virus, it is thought that chicken pox virus may have been dormant in the body for a time and been activated.

Treatment of shingles is directed toward alleviating the symptoms, and relieving the pain and itchiness. Lotions such as calamine are often applied. Glucocorticoids may be prescribed to suppress the inflammatory reaction.

■ *Abscess of the Brain.* Pyogenic organisms such as streptococci, staphylococci, and *E. coli* can travel to the brain from other infected areas and cause a brain abscess. Infections of the middle ear, skull bones or sinuses; pneumonia; and endocarditis are potential sources of a brain abscess. Figure 15–6 shows abscesses of the brain.

The symptoms of brain abscess may be misleading. The patient has a fever and headache due to increased intracranial pressure, which can suggest a tumor. Analysis of the cerebrospinal fluid shows increased pres-

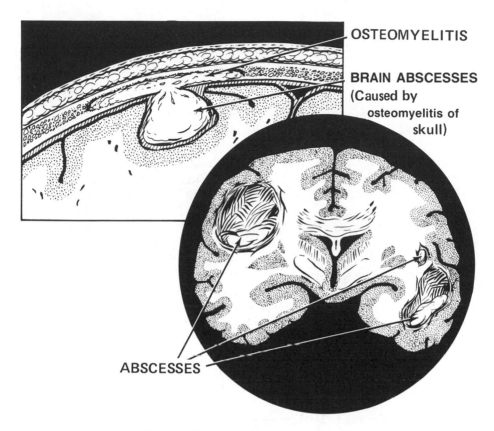

Figure 15-6. Abscesses of the brain.

sure and the presence of neutrophils and lymphocytes, indicating infection.

Once the diagnosis of a brain abscess has been made, the abscess must be opened surgically and drained and the patient treated with antibiotics. Brain abscesses are not as common today because the spread of most infections is checked by antibiotics.

Degenerative Neural Diseases

Some diseases of the nervous system involve the degeneration of nerves and brain tissue. Abnormalities in muscle function result from neural degeneration.

■ *Multiple Sclerosis.* **Multiple sclerosis (MS)** is a major disorder of the central nervous system. It is a chronic, progressive disease of unknown origin. Possible causes that have been researched are viruses, bacteria, trauma, autoimmunity, and heredity, but the findings have remained inconclusive.

The disease manifests itself at first by muscle impairment. The patient experiences a loss of balance and poor coordination. Tingling and numbing sensations progress to a shaking tremor and muscular weakness. The MS patient has difficulty in speaking clearly and bladder dysfunction frequently develops.

Vision may suddenly be impaired, and double vision frequently occurs. Lesions on the optic nerve can lead to blindness. The patient may have nystagmus, an involuntary, rapid movement of the eyeball in all directions. Emotional changes also accompany the disease.

Multiple sclerosis usually affects young adults between the ages of 20 and 40. The disease is difficult to diagnose in the early stages, as many disorders of the nervous system have similar symptoms. It is characterized by periods of remissions and exacerbations and progresses at very different rates.

The degeneration of nerve tissue in MS involves a breaking up of the neuronal myelin sheath, the white matter of the central nervous system. Patchy areas of demyelination appear and become sclerotic. The degeneration of myelin impairs nerve conduction.

There is no effective treatment for MS. Physical therapy enables the patient to use the muscles that are operable. Muscle relaxants help to reduce spasticity, and steroids are often helpful. Psychological counseling is advantageous in dealing with the emotional changes brought about by the disease.

■ *Parkinson's Disease.* **Parkinson's disease,** also known as shaking palsy, is a disease of brain degeneration that appears gradually and progresses slowly. It is a chronic disease that develops late in life and can be very disabling. Early symptoms include mild tremors of the hands and a nodding movement of the head. The patient is likely to fall frequently, as postural reflexes are lost.

As the disease progresses, muscular movements become slower and more difficult. The stiffness of the muscles affects the facial expressions, making them rigid and masklike. A characteristic tremor develops in the fingers, referred to as a pill-rolling tremor, that disappears with voluntary movement of the hands.

The posture is stooped. The forward-learning position causes a peculiar gait of short, running steps to maintain balance.

The degeneration of nerve cells occurs in the basal ganglia, the nerve centers responsible for regulation of certain body movements. It has been discovered that a neuronal transmitter substance, **dopamine,** is inadequately produced. Treatment includes the administration of L-dopa, a substance that is converted to dopamine in the brain. Although the drug therapy does not stop the neuronal degeneration, the symptoms are relieved. The drug is not recommended for patients with previous mental disorders or cardiovascular disease. Alcohol consumption should be limited because alcohol acts antagonistically to L-dopa.

Physical therapy, including heat and massage, helps to reduce muscle cramps and relieve tension headaches caused by the rigidity of neck muscles. The patient is aided by psychological support while learning to cope with the disability.

The cause of Parkinson's disease is unknown. A hereditary factor may be involved.

■ *Huntington's Disease (Huntington's Chorea).* Huntington's disease is an inherited disease, but symptoms may not appear until middle age. If either parent has the disease, all their children will have a 50 percent chance of inheriting it. (See Chapter 4 for the manner of transmission.) **Huntington's chorea** is a progressive degenerative disease of the brain that results in the loss of muscle control. The word element *chorea* means ceaseless, rapid, jerky movements, which are involuntary—an appropriate description of Huntington's symptoms. Some abnormality of the neurotransmitters causes bizarre transmission of nerve impulses.

The disease affects both the mind and body. Personality changes include carelessness, poor judgment, and impaired memory, with conditions deteriorating to total mental incompetence, dementia. The physical disabilities include speech loss and a difficulty in swallowing coupled with involuntary jerking, twisting, and muscle spasms. There is no cure for Huntington's chorea. In families afflicted with this disease, the risk for the offspring should be clearly understood.

CONVULSIONS

A **convulsion** is an involuntary contraction, or series of contractions, by voluntary muscles. Numerous factors, often involving a chemical imbalance within the body, can cause convulsions. The accumulation of waste products in the blood resulting from uremia, the toxemia of pregnancy, drug poisoning, and withdrawal from alcohol or drugs are all capable of causing convulsions.

Any irritation of the nerve cells can lead to convulsions. Infectious diseases of the brain such as meningitis and encephalitis are frequently accompanied by convulsions. They sometimes occur in infants and young children with high fevers.

The bases of convulsions are abnormal electrical discharges that spread over the brain. The excited nerves abnormally stimulate voluntary muscle to contract. Prevention of injury to the patient during a convulsion is the principal treatment.

■ Epilepsy

The seizures associated with **epilepsy** are a form of convulsion. Brain impulses are temporarily disturbed, with resultant involuntary convulsive movements. Epilepsy can be acquired as a result of injury to the brain, birth trauma, a penetrating wound, or depressed skull fracture. A tumor can irritate the brain, causing abnormal electrical discharges to be released. Most cases of epilepsy are idiopathic. A predisposition to epilepsy may be inherited.

Epilepsy may manifest itself mildly, particularly in children. Loss of consciousness may last only a few seconds, during which time the child appears absent-minded. Some muscular twitching may be noticed around the eyes and mouth and the child's head may sway rhythmically. The child does not fall to the floor. This form of epilepsy is known as **petit mal** and usually disappears by the late teens or early 20s.

Major seizures of epilepsy involve a loss of consciousness during which the person falls to the floor. Generalized convulsions are mild to severe, with violent shaking and thrashing movements. Hypersalivation causes a foaming at the mouth. The patient loses control of urine and sometimes feces. These features are characteristic of **grand mal epilepsy.**

Epileptics sometimes have a warning of an approaching seizure that gives them time to lie down or reach for support. This warning, known as an **aura,** may come as a ringing sound in the ears, a tingling sensation in the fingers, or spots before the eyes. The symptoms described are characteristic of grand mal epilepsy. After a seizure the patient is groggy and unaware of what happened. Seizures last for varying lengths of time and appear with varying frequencies.

Epileptic seizures may take different forms. The classification system adopted by the World Health Organization is called the International Classification of Epileptic Seizures. It classifies seizures into four categories.

1. Partial seizures begin locally and may or may not involve a larger area of brain tissue.
2. Generalized seizures are bilaterally symmetrical and without local onset.
3. Unilateral seizures generally involve only one side of the brain.
4. Unclassified epileptic seizures.

Diagnosis of epilepsy is made on the basis of the **electroencephalogram (EEG),** a recording of the brain waves. X-ray films are also used to identify any brain lesions. Family histories of epilepsy are very important in diagnosing the condition.

Medication is very effective in controlling epilepsy, particularly the anticonvulsant drugs. Treatment during a seizure is directed toward preventing physical injury to the patient.

DEVELOPMENTAL ERRORS

Fetal development is so complex that the relatively small number of errors is miraculous. Some errors are minor and cause no problems, but others that affect a system, such as the nervous system, can cause severe problems.

■ Spina Bifida

Spina bifida is a condition in which one or more vertebrae fail to fuse, leaving an opening in the vertebral canal. The word *bifid* means a cleft or split into two parts, which is the condition of the vertebra in spina bifida. The consequences of spina bifida depend on the extent of the opening and the involvement of the spinal cord.

One form of spina bifida, spina bifida occulta (hidden), may not be apparent at birth. Other malformations that tend to accompany this developmental error may point to the disorder. Such malformations are hydrocephalus, cleft palate, cleft lip, club foot, and strabismus (crossed eyes). The spinal cord is affected, and muscular abnormalities appearing later—such as incorrect posture, inability to walk, lack of bladder or bowel control—may signal spina bifida occulta. A slight dimpling of the skin and tuft of hair over the vertebral defect indicate the site of the lesion, usually located in the lower part of the vertebral column. The opening can be seen on x-ray films.

One form of spina bifida noticeable at birth is **meningocele.** In this condition, meninges protrude through the opening in the vertebra as a sac filled with cerebrospinal fluid. The spinal cord is not involved in this defect.

Meningomyelocele is a serious anomaly in which the nerve elements protrude into the sac and are trapped and prevented from reaching their destination. The child with this defect may be mentally retarded, fail to develop, lack sensation, or be paralyzed. The consequences of the defect depend on the part of the spinal cord affected. Surgical correction of various forms of spina bifida have been very effective.

The most severe form of spina bifida is **myelocele,** in which the neural tube itself fails to close and the nerve tissue is totally disorganized. This condition is usually fatal. The various forms of spina bifida are shown in Figure 15–7.

■ Hydrocephalus

The name **hydrocephalus** means water or fluid on the brain or head. The formation, circulation, and absorption of cerebrospinal fluid was described in the section earlier. In hydrocephalus this fluid accumulates abnormally, causing the ventricles to enlarge and push the brain against the skull.

An obstruction in the normal flow of cerebrospinal fluid is the usual cause of hydrocephalus. A congenital defect or an acquired lesion can block

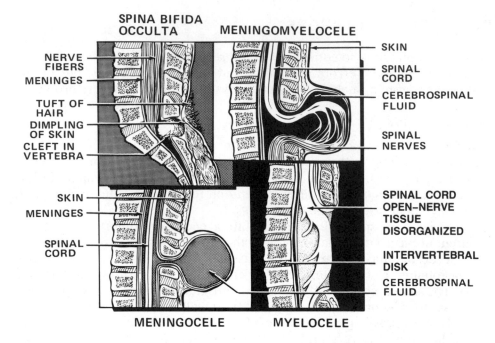

Figure 15-7. Forms of spina bifida.

the cerebrospinal fluid flow. Meningitis or a tumor may result in acquired hydrocephalus. Trauma at birth is another possible cause. Congenital stenosis of an opening from the ventricles blocks cerebrospinal fluid flow. The error may also be a failure to absorb the fluid into the circulatory system.

There are two types of hydrocephalus, called communicating and non-communicating. In the communicating type, the increased cerebrospinal fluid enters the subarachnoid space. In noncommunicating hydrocephalus, the increased pressure of the cerebrospinal fluid is confined within the ventricles and is not evident in a lumbar puncture.

The head of a child born with hydrocephalus may appear normal at birth, but it will enlarge rapidly in the early months of life as the fluid accumulates. The brain is compressed, the cranial bones are thin, and the sutures of the skull separate under the pressure. The appearance of a hydrocephalic infant is typical: The forehead is prominent and the eyes bulge, giving a frightened expression. The scalp is stretched and the veins of the head are prominent. A hydrocephalic infant is shown in Figure 15-8. The weight of the excessive fluid in the head makes it impossible for the baby to lift its head. The infant fails to grow normally and is mentally retarded.

There have been cases of self-arrested hydrocephalus in which expansion of the head stops. A balance is reached between production and absorption of the fluid. The cranial sutures fill in and the skull bones thicken. The extent of brain damage before the arrest determines the degree of retardation.

Success in relieving the excessive cerebrospinal fluid has been achieved by placing a shunt between the blockage and the heart. This allows the fluid to enter the general circulation.

BRAIN DAMAGE

The impact of damage to the brain depends on the location and extent of the injury. Manifestations of brain damage are mental retardation or muscular disorders, such as the lack of coordination and partial paralysis.

■ Cerebral Palsy

Cerebral palsy is a disease of nonprogressive brain damage that becomes apparent before age 3. The brain damage may be due to injury at or near the time of birth, an infection in the mother such as rubella (German measles), or infection of the brain even after birth. Lack of oxygen causes brain damage, as can incompatible blood. An Rh⁻ mother produces antibodies against the blood of an Rh⁺ fetus, as previously described. The

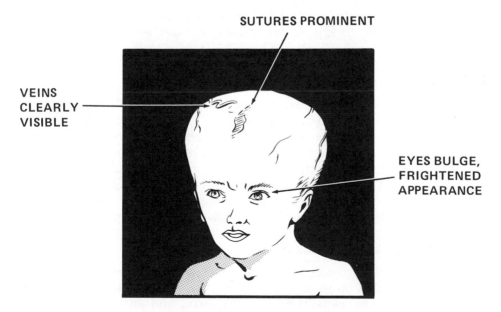

Figure 15-8. Hydrocephalus.

excessive destruction of fetal blood cells that result causes hyperbilirubine-mia, a level of bilirubin that is toxic to the brain. Often no cause is found for the brain damage in a case of cerebral palsy.

There are three forms of cerebral palsy: spastic, athetoid, and atactic. The largest number of cerebral palsy victims have the spastic type of condition. Muscles are tense, and the reflexes are exaggerated. In the athetoid form, there are constant, purposeless movements that are uncontrollable. A tremor or shaking of the hands and feet is continuous. Cerebral palsy patients with the atactic form have poor balance and are prone to fall, muscular coordination is poor, and a staggering gait is the characteristic.

Depending on the area of the brain affected, there may be seizures or visual or auditory impairment. If the muscles controlling the tongue are affected, speech defects result. Intelligence may be normal, but there is often mental retardation. Treatment depends on the nature of the brain damage. Muscle relaxants can relieve spasms; anticonvulsant drugs reduce seizures; casts or braces may aid walking; and traction or surgery is helpful in some cases. Muscle training is the most important therapy, and the earlier it is started, the more effective it is.

CEREBROVASCULAR ACCIDENTS

Vascular disturbances are the most frequent causes of brain lesions. The term stroke is used broadly to include cerebral hemorrhages and blood clot formation within cerebral blood vessels. Nerves damaged by the lack of blood flow or hemorrhage do not regenerate and are replaced by scar tissue.

■ Cerebral Hemorrhage

The main cause of cerebral hemorrhage is hypertension. Prolonged hypertension leads to arteriosclerosis explained in Chapter 8. The combination of high blood pressure and hard, brittle blood vessels is a predisposing condition for cerebral hemorrhage. Aneurysms, weakened areas in vascular walls, are also susceptible to rupture. Various aneurysms are shown in Figure 15–9. Subsequent hemorrhage into the brain tissue damages the neurons. When this occurs there is usually a sudden loss of consciousness. Death can follow, or, if the bleeding stops, varying degrees of brain damage can result.

■ Thrombosis and Embolism

Blood clots that block the cerebral arteries cause infarction of brain tissue. Thromboses develop on walls of atherosclerotic vessels, particularly in the carotid arteries. The clots take time to form, and some warning may precede the occlusion of the vessel. The patient may experience blindness in

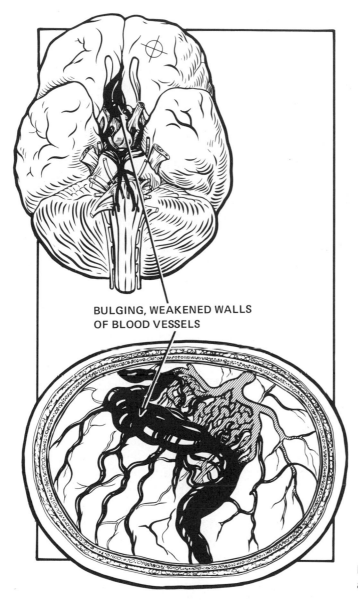

BULGING, WEAKENED WALLS
OF BLOOD VESSELS

Figure 15-9. Cerebral aneurysms.

one eye, difficulty in speaking, or a generalized state of confusion. When the cerebral blood vessel is completely blocked, the patient may lose consciousness.

Because it is a traveling clot, an embolism usually occludes a blood vessel suddenly. The embolism is most frequently a clot from the heart, but it can travel from another part of the body. Consciousness is generally lost suddenly.

The site and extent of the brain damage, regardless of its cause, determines the outcome for the patient. Consciousness is usually regained, but speech is often impaired immediately after the stroke. Loss of speech (**aphasia**) requires therapy, but the ability to speak is often restored.

Damage to the motor nerves where they are about to pass down the spinal cord causes paralysis on the side of the body opposite the brain lesion. This is because of the crossover of nerve fibers in the brain stem. Paralysis on one side of the body is referred to as **hemiplegia.**

Various techniques make it possible to determine the site of blockage in a cerebral blood vessel. Angiography, a process in which radiopaque material is injected into cerebral arteries, allows x-rays to locate the lesion.

A blockage in a carotid artery can be treated surgically. **Endarterectomy,** the more common procedure, removes the thickened area of the inner coat. Carotid bypass surgery removes the blocked segment, and a graft is inserted to allow blood flow to the brain.

TRAUMATIC DISORDERS

Physical injury to the head can damage the brain by causing a cerebral hemorrhage, by the increased pressure of resulting edema, or by creating a route for bacterial invasion.

■ Concussion of the Brain

A **concussion** is a transient disorder of the nervous system resulting from a violent blow on the head, as may occur in an automobile accident. The patient loses consciousness and cannot remember the events of the accident. The brain is not actually damaged, but the whole body is affected; the pulse rate is weak, and when consciousness is regained the patient may be nauseous and dizzy. A severe headache follows, and the patient should be watched closely as a coma may ensue.

A person suffering from a concussion should be kept quiet, and drugs that stimulate or depress the nervous system, such as pain killers, should not be administered. The condition will correct itself with rest.

■ Contusion

In a **contusion** there is an injury to brain tissue without a breaking of the skin at the site of the trauma. The brain injury may be on the side of the impact or on the opposite side, where the brain is forced against the skull. Blood from broken blood vessels accumulates in the brain, causing swelling and pain. Blood clots and necrotic tissue form, and the flow of cerebrospinal fluid can be blocked, causing a form of hydrocephalus.

The body attempts to clear the debris through phagocytosis by white blood cells and macrophages. Treatment includes the application of cold compresses to reduce the bleeding, which in turn reduces the swelling. Later, the application of heat facilitates the absorption of blood.

■ Skull Fractures

The most serious danger in a skull fracture is damage to the brain. A fracture at the base of the skull is likely to affect vital centers in the brain stem. The pressure that increases due to accumulation of cerebrospinal fluid must be reduced by medications. Another danger of a skull fracture is that bacteria may be able to reach the brain.

■ Hemorrhages

Hemorrhages can occur in the meninges, causing blood to accumulate between the brain and the skull. A severe injury to the temple can cause an artery just inside the skull to rupture. The blood then flows between the dura mater and the skull: This is called an extradural hemorrhage. The increased pressure of the blood causes the patient to lose consciousness, and surgery is required immediately to tie off the bleeding vessel and remove the blood. No blood is found in a lumbar puncture because the blood accumulation is outside the dura mater.

A hemorrhage under the dura mater, a subdural hemorrhage, is from the large venous sinuses of the brain rather than an artery. This may occur from a severe blow to the front or back of the brain. The blood clots, and cerebrospinal fluid accumulates in the cystlike clot. Pressure builds up, but the cerebral symptoms may not develop for a time. Subdural hemorrhages are sometimes chronic in alcoholics and abused children.

The surface of the brain may be torn by a skull fracture, causing a subarachnoid hemorrhage. Blood flows into the subarachnoid space in which cerebrospinal fluid circulates, and blood is found with a lumbar puncture. Rupture of an aneurysm can also cause a subarachnoid hemorrhage.

■ BRAIN TUMORS

Tumors of the brain may be malignant or benign. Even the benign tumors are serious, however, since they grow and strangle vital nerve centers. As explained in the chapter on neoplasia (Chapter 3), benign tumors are usually encapsulated and they can be completely removed surgically. Malignant tumors have extensive roots and are extremely difficult or impossible to remove in their entirety. Most malignant tumors of the brain are metastatic from other organs. Primary malignant tumors of the brain are called **gliomas,** tumors of the glial cells that support nerve tissue rather than of the neurons themselves. Figure 15–10 shows a glioma in the corpus callosum of the brain.

Brain tumors manifest themselves in different ways depending on the site and growth rate of the tumor. Brain function is affected by the increased intracranial pressure. Blood supply to an area of the brain may be reduced by an infiltrating tumor or edema causing the tissue to become necrotic.

Symptoms of brain tumors may include a severe headache due to the increased pressure of the tumor. Personality changes, loss of memory, or poor judgment in a person of normally good judgment can signal a brain tumor. Visual disturbances, double vision, or partial blindness often occur and the ability to speak may be impaired. The patient may be unsteady while standing and have seizures. A drowsy condition can progress to a coma.

Diagnostic procedures include **computed axial tomography (CAT) scans,** EEGs, and the examination of cerebrospinal fluid. Cerebrospinal fluid is drawn out by means of lumbar puncture and replaced by air in this

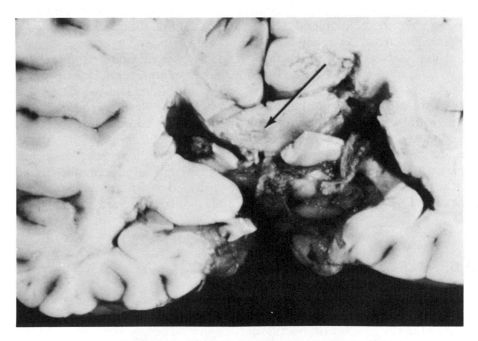

Figure 15-10. A glioma in the corpus callosum of the brain (arrow). (*Courtesy of Dr. David R. Duffell.*)

procedure. Angiography allows visualization of the cerebral circulation through the injection of radiopaque material. Scanning techniques, including the CAT scan, offer accurate information in locating the site of the tumor. The CAT scanner is a noninvasive x-ray technique used in conjunction with a computer to view cross-sectional areas of the body.

SUMMARY

The nervous system enables the human body to respond to changes in the external and internal environment. This system is affected by diseases in numerous ways. Microorganisms that enter the nervous system by various routes cause infectious diseases such as meningitis, encephalitis, polio, tetanus, rabies, and shingles.

A degeneration of nerves and brain tissue results in multiple sclerosis, Parkinson's disease, and Huntington's chorea. A manifestation of these progressively degenerative diseases is abnormal functioning of the muscles.

Convulsions often result from some chemical imbalance that causes irritation to nerve cells. The seizures of epilepsy are a form of convulsions after abnormal electrical discharges in the brain.

Hydrocephalus and the various forms of spina bifida are caused by developmental errors, obstruction to the flow of cerebrospinal fluid, and failure of the vertebral column to close. Damage to the brain during fetal life or at birth can result in cerebral palsy, which is manifested by various forms of muscular abnormalities. Cerebrovascular accidents, cerebral hemorrhages, and blood clots damage brain tissue. The result of the injury depends on the site and extent of the brain lesion.

A severe head injury that causes hemorrhaging within the brain or in the meninges has serious effects on the nerve tissue and may even be fatal. Tumors of the brain, both malignant and benign, strangle nerve fibers and obstruct blood flow. No other tissue of the body depends on a good supply of oxygenated blood as does the brain.

STUDY QUESTIONS

1. Name five infectious diseases of the central nervous system and possible routes of entry for each causative organism.
2. Explain the difference between the spread of tetanus and rabies through the body.
3. What is the relationship between shingles and chicken pox?

4. Name the principal symptoms of multiple sclerosis.
5. What are the characteristics of a patient with Parkinson's disease?
6. Contrast the seizures in petit mal and grand mal epilepsy.
7. What malformations frequently accompany spina bifida?
8. Why is meningomyelocele far more serious than meningocele?
9. Describe the head and face of a hydrocephalic infant.
10. Describe the three forms of cerebral palsy.
11. What can be accomplished through a lumbar puncture?
12. Name several symptoms that could indicate a brain tumor.
13. What determines the effect of a stroke?

CHAPTER 16

Diseases of the Bones, Joints, and Muscles

All bodily movements are the result of muscular contractions. These movements range from the wink of an eye to the acrobatic performance of a gymnast. All facial expressions—happiness, sorrow, anger, or surprise—are the result of muscle action.

The attachment of muscles to bones allows contraction, or shortening, of a muscle to move a bone. Muscles that span a joint bring about an action at that joint, and they work antagonistically to muscles on the opposite side of the joint.

Bones cannot move without muscle contractions and muscles cannot contract without nerve stimulation. Diseases of the nervous system, described in the previous chapter, are generally manifested by their effect on the musculature. In this chapter the principal diseases of bone, joints, and muscle will be explained.

THE STRUCTURE AND FUNCTION OF
BONE, JOINTS, AND MUSCLE

Bone may appear inert but it is a truly dynamic tissue, with changes constantly occurring within it. The outer surface of bone is hard and smooth due to the arrangement of its constituent protein and minerals. Bone cells, osteoblasts and osteoclasts, are situated within this bony framework and nourished by a highly organized system of blood vessels. These cells constantly remodel bone.

Bones are long, flat, or irregularly shaped, but they are all covered with a layer of compact bone. Spongy bone consisting of a different arrangement of the same material is found inside the bones. This material contains many spaces that are filled with bone marrow. The red bone marrow within flat bones and at the end of long bones is the production site for many blood cells.

The long bones found in the arms and legs contain a hollow cavity, the **medullary cavity,** that is filled with yellow bone marrow primarily consisting of fat. The growth of long bones occurs at the growth plate, an area of cartilage near each expanded end of the bone (Fig. 16–1). At this site new

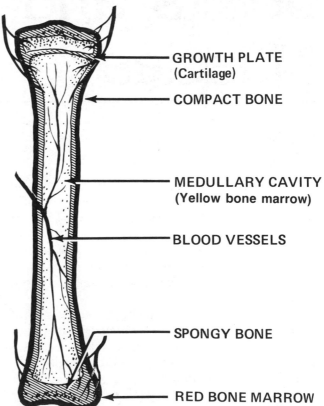

GROWTH PLATE
(Cartilage)

COMPACT BONE

MEDULLARY CAVITY
(Yellow bone marrow)

BLOOD VESSELS

SPONGY BONE

RED BONE MARROW

Figure 16-1. Cut view of long bone.

bone is formed, pushing the ends apart from each other until full growth is achieved, at which time the cartilage ossifies. Damage to the growth plate before maturity prevents the bone from reaching its proper length.

The **periosteum** is a highly vascular layer of fibrous connective tissue that covers the surface of the bones. It contains cells that are capable of forming new bone tissue and serves as a site of attachment for tendons or muscles.

Joints are the articulating sites between bones. Various degrees of movement are possible in different kinds of joints. This is referred to as range of motion. The shoulder is the most freely movable joint, but it is also the one most easily dislocated.

Articulating bones are held together by **ligaments.** A joint capsule consisting of ligaments and connective tissue surrounds the bone ends. The inner surface of the capsule is lined with a synovial membrane that secretes a lubricating fluid. Sacs of this fluid, the **bursae,** are situated near the joint to reduce friction on movement. The articulating surfaces of the bone ends are covered with a layer of smooth cartilage, which also prevents friction. A typical joint is illustrated in Figure 16–2.

Skeletal or voluntary muscles are firmly attached to bones by **tendons.** Some muscles, the muscles of facial expression, for example, are attached to soft tissue. Muscles consist of bundles of muscle fibers held together by connective tissue. When stimulated by nerves at the myoneural junction, muscle fibers contract, and the shortening of the muscles moves the bones.

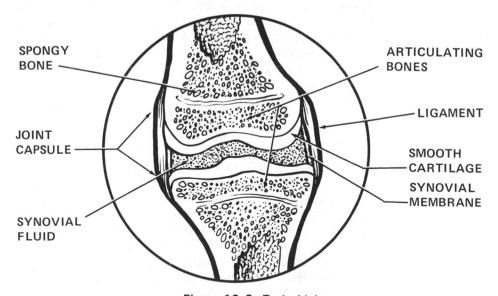

Figure 16-2. Typical joint.

The diseases of muscle described in this chapter are diseases of voluntary muscle. Smooth muscle is a different type of muscle found in the walls of the internal organs and the walls of blood vessels. Cardiac muscle is present only in the heart.

DISEASES OF BONE

Bone, which is comprised of cells, of organic material that gives some flexibility, and of inorganic salts that provide hardness, can be affected by disease in various ways. Infectious agents can enter bone through a compound fracture, transmission in the blood, or extension from an adjacent infection. Mineral and vitamin deficiencies prevent proper formation or maintenance of bone structure. Bones atrophy with disuse and fracture spontaneously in certain diseases. Tumors can also develop in bone.

Infectious Diseases of Bone

Bone infections were far more difficult to treat before the availability of antibiotics. These infections still occur and should be properly diagnosed and treated as soon as possible.

■ *Osteomyelitis.* **Osteomyelitis** is an inflammation of the bone, particularly of the bone marrow in the medullary cavity and in the spaces of spongy bone. Osteomyelitis affects principally children and adolescents whose bones are still growing. The long bones—the femur, the tibia, and the humerus—are most frequently affected in the area of the growth plate. Pyogenic organisms, such as staphylococci, carried in the bloodstream enter the bone from an infection somewhere in the body or from one adjacent to the bone. Infectious microorganisms can also enter a bone through the open wound of a compound fracture. An injury to the bone can cause small blood vessels to rupture. A clot then forms to stop the bleeding, and microorganisms invade the clot.

An abscess forms within the bone, and pus extends throughout the medullary cavity. A typical inflammatory reaction results in swelling, heat, and pain. Small blood vessels are compressed by the swelling, reducing the blood flow and causing necrosis. The infection spreads to the outer surface of the bone and extends along the bone under the periosteum. Blood supply to the bone is further reduced as the vascular periosteum is lifted from the bone. An area of bone that dies through lack of circulation and becomes separated from sound bone through necrosis is called a **sequestrum.** The periosteum attempts to make new bone around the sequestrum. Blood clots from the necrotic tissue infected with bacteria travel to other sites, initiating new abscesses.

Osteomyelitis is both a local and systemic infection. Not only is there pain at the site of the lesion, but the patient experiences chills, fever, and **leukocytosis.** The infection responds well to antibiotic therapy, particularly if it is started early, and the incidence of osteomyelitis has therefore decreased significantly. Surgery is sometimes required to clean out the dead bone tissue.

■ *Tuberculosis of the Bone.* Tuberculosis is primarily a disease of the lungs, but the infection can spread to bone. The ends of long bones, those of the arms and legs, are most frequently affected. The knee is a common site of tuberculosis infection. Similar to tuberculosis of the lung (see Chapter 12), cavity formation leads to destruction of the tissue.

When a joint such as the knee is involved, movement becomes limited. The articular cartilage is destroyed, causing pain due to friction between the articulating bones. In children, the growth plate is destroyed, resulting in the affected limb being shorter than the other.

Pott's disease is a special form of tuberculosis that affects the vertebral column of children. Vertebrae are destroyed and collapse, producing a malformation of the spine such as a humpback. The collapsed vertebrae put pressure on the spinal cord, and this can result in paralysis.

Tuberculosis of the bone responds well to antibiotic treatment. If the condition is advanced and irreversible damage to the vertebral column has already occurred, surgery may be required to correct the deformity.

Bone Diseases of Vitamin and Mineral Deficiencies

Inadequate levels of calcium and phosphorus in the blood prevent proper bone formation and maintenance. These mineral deficiencies cause the bones to become soft and deformed. The absorption of calcium from the digestive tract requires vitamin D.

■ *Rickets.* **Rickets** is a disease of infancy and early childhood in which the bones do not properly ossify, or harden. The disease is generally caused by a vitamin D deficiency. Vitamin D is necessary for proper absorption of calcium and phosphorus from the gastrointestinal tract. It is calcium and phosphorus that give hardness to bone. Calcium may be adequate in the diet, but in the absence of vitamin D it can not be used.

The bones of a child with rickets are soft and tend to bend. The weight-bearing bones of the body become deformed. The legs appear bowed or knock-kneed and the spine is curved. The sternum projects forward and nodules, referred to as "the rickety rosary," form on the rib ends. Nodular swellings also form at the joints—the wrists, ankles, and knees—and the head is often large and square. The pelvic opening in a girl may narrow, causing problems during childbirth later in life.

Other symptoms may also indicate rickets. The child's muscles are flabby because calcium, the deficient mineral, is essential for proper muscle contraction. Teething may be delayed, and the child has a characteristic pot belly.

Rickets can be prevented with vitamin D-fortified milk and sunlight. Sunlight converts a substance in the skin to vitamin D in the body. This need for sunlight explains the higher incidence of rickets in large, smoky cities where buildings are close together and shut out the sun. Children with rickets respond well to sunlight exposure and treatment with vitamin D concentrate or cod liver oil, which is high in vitamin D.

■ *Osteomalacia.* **Osteomalacia** is similar to rickets, but it is a softening or decalcification of bone in adults. It is characterized by muscular weakness, weight loss, and pain in the bones. The bones particularly affected are the spine, pelvis, and legs. They are bent, deformed, and tend to fracture with only mild stress.

A vitamin D deficiency and inadequate calcium or phosphorus in the diet causes osteomalacia. As in the case of rickets, a vitamin D deficiency prevents absorption of calcium from the digestive tract. The vitamin D deficiency may result from lack of sunshine, insufficient vitamin D in the diet, or the inability to absorb the vitamin, which is fat-soluble and is not absorbed in a disease such as the malabsorption syndrome (Chapter 10). Treatment consists of vitamin D supplements and adequate calcium and phosphorous in the diet.

Secondary Bone Diseases

Bone diseases can result from a hormonal imbalance, as in hyperparathyroidism. In the aged, particularly in patients confined to bed, bone disease develops from disuse. Immobilization of a bone in a cast for a long time can have the same effect.

■ *Osteitis Fibrosa Cystica.* The name **osteitis fibrosa cystica** may seem threatening, but each word has meaning. The word element *oste(o)* refers to bone, so *osteitis* is an inflammation of the bone. In this disease, fibrous nodules and cysts form in the bones, which become very porous and decalcified. The loss of calcium causes the bones, particularly the long bones and those of the spine and trachea to become deformed and subject to spontaneous fracture.

Osteitis fibrosa cystica generally results from hyperparathyroidism (Chapter 13). The excessive production of parathyroid hormone causes calcium removal from the bone. The blood level of calcium rises, and calcium is deposited in the form of insoluble salts. Kidney stone formation with possible renal obstruction is a complication of the condition.

Treatment involves reducing the parathyroid hormone level. A tumor of the parathyroid can be the cause of the excessive secretion and it should be removed. Orthopedic surgery may be required to correct severe bone deformities.

■ *Osteoporosis.* The word **osteoporosis** means increased porosity of the bone, which makes the bone abnormally fragile. The loss or thinning of bone tissue, due to increased calcium resorption from the bone is a predisposition to fractures, particularly of the weight-bearing bones of the vertebral column and pelvis. Compression fractures of the vertebra cause a decrease in height and bending or curvature of the spine. The compressed vertebrae cause severe pain by pressing on spinal nerves. Hip and wrist fractures also occur frequently.

Osteoporosis may develop as part of the aging process, or the condition may be related to the estrogen level reduction that occurs after menopause. Certain people seem more susceptible to osteoporosis than others. Osteoporosis is most common in patients who are bedridden. Bones that are immobilized, such as an arm or a leg in a cast, show this deterioration. This phenomenon is referred to as **disuse atrophy.** Women with small bone mass develop the condition more frequently than taller, larger women. Dietary inadequacies of calcium and protein, as well as lack of exercise, may contribute to development of osteoporosis. The manner of interaction between estrogen and the loss of bone tissue is unknown. Controversy exists between the value and the risk of estrogen therapy. Improved diet with adequate calcium and exercise are perhaps the most significant measures in preventing osteoporosis.

■ *Paget's Disease.* **Paget's disease,** or osteitis deformans, results in overproduction of bone, particularly in the skull, vertebrae, and pelvis. The disease begins with bone softening and is followed by bone overgrowth. The new bone tissue is abnormal and tends to fracture easily. The excessive bony growth causes the skull to enlarge, which often affects the cranial nerves; neurologic complications then follow. Curvatures develop in the spine from the new bone growth and the legs are deformed. The cause of Paget's disease is unknown, but it may have a hereditary basis. A complication of this disease is the development of **osteogenic sarcoma.**

Bone Fractures

Excessive stress on a bone will cause it to fracture. There are many types of fractures. A break in the bone that does not penetrate the skin is a simple fracture. A break in which the skin is pierced by the bone, resulting in an open wound, is a **compound fracture.** If the bone is splintered or crushed, it is a **comminuted fracture. A greenstick fracture** is one in which the bone is cracked, broken on one side, and bent on the other. These fractures are illustrated in Figure 16–3.

Fractures often occur spontaneously when bones are diseased, and these are called pathologic fractures. They may signal a malignancy that has metastasized from another site in the body or osteoporosis.

Some fractures are particularly dangerous because their location causes them to damage adjacent structures. A skull fracture can cause hemorrhages in the meninges and possible brain damage. A depressed skull fracture, one in which the bone has a caved-in appearance, puts pressure on the brain. The patient may become disoriented or lose consciousness. Shock often develops as a result of the injury.

A fracture of the spine can crush or sever the spinal cord, causing paralysis or death. A patient who has suffered this injury must be moved extremely carefully to prevent damage to the spinal cord by the broken bone ends.

Pelvic bone fractures suffered in the crushing injury of an automobile accident or from the pressure of a heavy weight can cause internal injury to the bladder or rectum. Internal bleeding into surrounding soft tissue results.

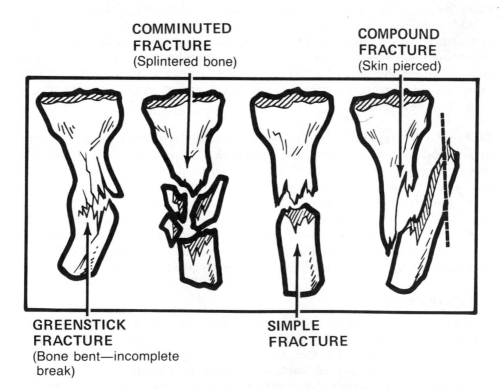

COMMINUTED FRACTURE
(Splintered bone)

COMPOUND FRACTURE
(Skin pierced)

GREENSTICK FRACTURE
(Bone bent—incomplete break)

SIMPLE FRACTURE

Figure 16-3. Common bone fractures.

Treatment of a fracture involves immediate **reduction,** which means that the broken ends of the bone are brought into proper alignment. Closed reduction is the manipulation of bone from the outside, without surgery. A compound fracture often requires open reduction, opening by exposing the wound to allow cleansing of the damaged tissue or removal of soft tissue lodged between the broken bone ends. The insertion of pins or plates to assure stability of the broken bone requires open reduction. After reduction, the bone is immobilized by a cast, splint, or traction to assure healing.

As the bone heals, new tissue is formed by osteoblasts at the fracture site. Hard material called a **bone callus** develops and unites the bone ends. New blood vessels grow into the tissue, and the fractured ends of the bone die and are resorbed. The length of time required for healing increases with the age of the patient. Bones may fail to heal due to infection or poor blood supply. Excessive motion prevents development of the bony tissue growth necessary for healing.

■ Dislocations and Sprains

A dislocated bone is forcibly displaced from its joint. Dislocations are most common in the shoulder and finger joints, but they can occur anywhere. The patient experiences pain and lack of mobility at the involved joint. The bone must be resituated and immobilized to allow healing of torn ligaments and tendons. Congenital dislocations of the hip result from an improperly formed joint, and they are treated in infancy with a cast or surgery.

Sprains result from the wrenching or twisting of a joint that injures the ligaments. Blood vessels and surrounding tissues—muscles, tendons, and nerves—may also be damaged. Swelling and discoloration due to hemorrhaging from the ruptured blood vessels occur. A sprain is very painful, and the joint should not be used while it is severely inflamed. Cold compresses reduce the swelling immediately after the injury, whereas later heat applications reduce the discoloration.

Neoplasia of Bone

Tumors of bone generally cause pain as they progress and make the bone susceptible to fractures. These tumors can be either malignant or benign.

■ *Benign Bone Tumors.* The most common benign tumor of the bone is an **osteoma.** This tumor may give no symptoms, or it may appear as a swelling. If a joint is affected, decreased motility is experienced. The tumor consists of hard, bony material, and it usually develops at the end of a long bone. Surgical removal of the osteoma is sometimes required if it causes pain or a pathologic fracture problem.

Giant cell tumors range from benign to malignant. On an x-ray film the tumor appears to consist of large bubbles. Microscopically, numerous multinucleated giant cells are seen. These tumors are usually removed through orthopedic surgery.

■ *Malignant Bone Tumors.* A primary malignancy of the bone is an **osteogenic sarcoma** (see Chapter 3). It generally affects the ends of long bones and is more common in young people. The knee is a frequent site, and expansion of the bone end is observed. The newest procedure is to pretreat with chemotherapy over weeks until the tumor stops shrinking. The extent of the surgery that follows is thus minimized, and the amputations previously performed are avoided.

Secondary tumors affecting the bone are carcinomas that have metastasized. They cause bone destruction and are very painful. The bone fractures easily, which is often the signal that carcinoma is present elsewhere. The flat bones that are highly vascular—the ribs, sternum, and skull—are the bones most affected by carcinoma.

DISEASES OF THE JOINTS

Joints are the movable parts of the body subjected to wear and tear. The joints that bear the weight of the body—the lower spine, the hip, and the knee—receive the most stress. Diseases of the joints cause pain and limit movement. Muscles, nerves, and bones can all be affected by joint disease.

■ Arthritis

The word element *arthr(o)* refers to a joint. Although arthritis means inflammation of a joint, the disease may be more or less inflammatory depending on the type. The warning signs of arthritis are persistent pain and stiffness, particularly in the morning. One or more joints may be swollen, and pain is often experienced in the neck, lower back, and hip, as well as in the joints of the arms, hands, legs, and feet.

■ *Rheumatoid Arthritis.* Rheumatoid arthritis is the most serious and crippling form of arthritis. It is a systemic disease in which more and more joints become affected and the patient feels sick all over. Rheumatoid arthritis is a chronic, inflammatory disease for which there is no cure, but early diagnosis and treatment can prevent severe crippling. Rheumatoid arthritis generally affects young adults, women more often than men. There is also a juvenile form, which can be very serious. The disease may have a sudden onset or begin slowly. Periods of exacerbation and remission are common, so that a patient may experience symptoms that disappear only to recur.

The symptoms of rheumatoid arthritis are pain and stiffness in the joints, particularly on waking. The joints are swollen, red, and warm—the typical signs of inflammation. The same joints are often affected on both sides of the body. As the disease is systemic, the patient experiences fatigue, weakness, and weight loss.

Rheumatoid arthritis begins with an inflammation of the **synovial membrane** that lines the joints, particularly the small joints of the hands and feet. The membrane thickens and extends into the joint cavity, sometimes filling the space. The inflammation affects the articular cartilage of the bone ends by eroding them. Scar tissue that can turn to bone develops between the bone ends, causing the ends to fuse. The fusion makes the joint immovable and a characteristic crippling of the hands often develops. Figure 16-4 shows the crippling effect of this disease. Rheumatoid nodules form under the skin, usually near the joints, but they sometimes develop on the white of the eye, too.

The cause of rheumatoid arthritis is not known, but a tissue hypersensitivity may be involved, such as some type of antigen–antibody reaction. The condition is aggravated by stress.

Early diagnosis and a good treatment program can reduce pain and the amount of damage done to the joints. A balance between exercise and rest should be achieved. In an acute phase the joint should be rested to prevent

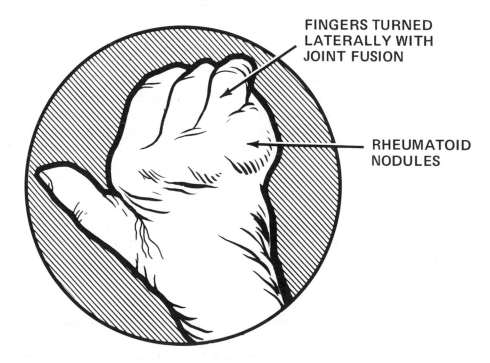

FINGERS TURNED LATERALLY WITH JOINT FUSION

RHEUMATOID NODULES

Figure 16-4. Crippling effect of rheumatoid arthritis.

further inflammation. The prescribed exercises help to maintain joint function. Exercises for good posture are directed toward removing stress on weight-bearing joints. Anti-inflammatory medications are effective when prescribed by a physician, with aspirin and similar drugs being the most commonly used. Steroids are administered with caution, as they mask the symptoms but do not stop the disease process.

■ *Osteoarthritis.* **Osteoarthritis** is the most common form of arthritis and is generally a chronic disease that accompanies aging. It results from wear and tear of the joints, chronic irritation, or a joint injury. Unlike rheumatoid arthritis, in which there is a progressive involvement of joints, osteoarthritis may affect only one joint.

The patient experiences aches, pain, and stiffness in the joint. It is pressure on the nerve endings, tense muscles, and muscle fatigue that cause the pain. Arthritis in the lower spine can exert pressure on the spinal cord or pinch a spinal nerve. Pain then radiates down the sciatic nerve of the leg. Range of motion is limited at the affected joint and the nearby muscles become weak from lack of use.

The degenerative process in osteoarthritis begins in the articular cartilage on the bone ends. As it is eroded, the underlying bone is exposed, and it degenerates. New bone forms in and around the joint, causing the bone ends to thicken and limit movement. The spicules of new bone are referred to as bony **spurs.** Small joints such as the knuckles enlarge and appear knobby.

Diagnosis of osteoarthritis is made principally by x-ray films that show the joint damage; a history of the symptoms also aids in the diagnosis.

There is no cure for osteoarthritis, but treatment can greatly relieve the pain. A combination of rest and special exercises, medication, and heat applications is generally prescribed. Steroids such as cortisone are not given orally but are sometimes injected into the joint capsule to relieve pain. Surgical replacement of a damaged joint like the hip has been very effective.

Perfectly functioning joints are least likely to become arthritic, but joints that have been injured or overworked in athletics are most susceptible. Knee and hip joints are frequently affected in a person who is overweight. Heredity may play a part in the development of osteoarthritis.

■ Gout

Gout, often called "gouty arthritis," affects the joints of the feet, particularly those of the big toe. This is a very painful condition caused by deposits of uric acid crystals in the joints. An excessively high uric acid level in the blood results in the precipitation of the crystals. Uric acid crystals are also deposited in the kidneys, stimulating kidney stone formation and irritating the kidney.

The cause of gout is unknown, but a hereditary tendency to the disease is common. It most frequently affects middle-age men. Improper metabolism of purines, a component of nucleic acids, causes the uric acid excess.

The onset of an acute attack of gout is generally sudden. It sometimes follows a minor injury or excessive eating or drinking, but there may be no accounting for the attack. The joint has the typical signs of inflammation: pain, heat, swelling, and redness. Walking is very difficult.

Various medications may be administered to reduce the uric acid level in the blood. The patient should stay off his or her feet until the inflammation subsides to prevent further irritation. Recurrent attacks are common, but if diagnosed early and treated properly, the development of chronic gout can be prevented. Chronic gout damages the affected joints, causing deformities. A complication of chronic gout is kidney damage from the uric acid deposits.

■ Herniation of Intervertebral Disks (Slipped Disk)

Cartilaginous pads or disks alternate with the vertebrae to form the spine. The disks act as shock absorbers between the vertebrae and accommodate the movement of the spine. Figure 16–5 illustrates the vertebral column. The inner core of each disk is rubbery and is surrounded by fibrous cartilage.

The intervertebral disks are subjected to constant strain. They may be injured or degenerate and lose their cushioning ability. The fibrous walls of the disk can weaken, and the inner core will bulge outward. This **herniation,** or rupture, **of an intervertebral disk** is commonly called a slipped disk.

The rupture of a disk most commonly occurs in the lower lumbar region and sometimes in the neck. The complication of a slipped disk is the pressure exerted on the spinal cord or a spinal nerve, as shown in Figure 16–6. Muscle spasms result often from the nerve stimulation.

A slipped disk in the lumbar region causes severe pain in the lower back. The pain radiates down the sciatic nerve to the back of the thigh and lower leg, making walking very difficult.

Diagnosis of a slipped disk is made principally by x-ray examination and the myelogram. The treatment depends on the nerve involvement and the age of the patient. In mild cases, bed rest on a firm mattress with an underlying board for support may be adequate. Muscle relaxants are administered to reduce muscle spasms. Careful application of heat is advantageous, and the patient is sometimes fitted with a surgical support. Some cases of slipped disk require traction. Exercises that improve posture and develop the proper use of muscles help to reduce stress on the vertebral column. Surgery is sometimes required to correct this condition.

A slipped disk in the cervical region causes severe pain in the neck,

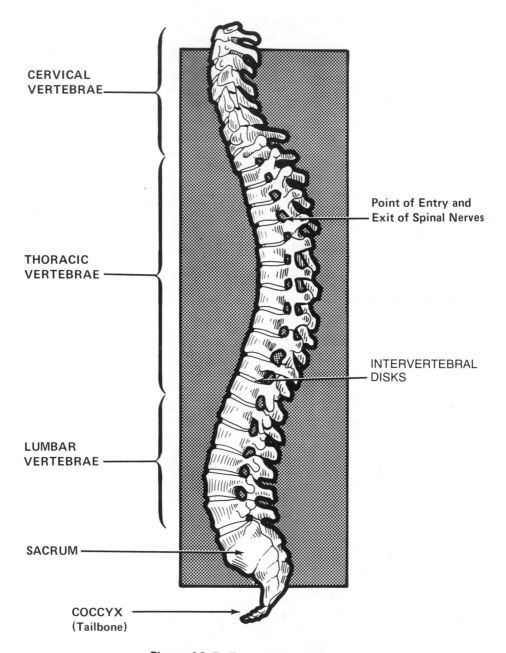

CERVICAL
VERTEBRAE

THORACIC
VERTEBRAE

LUMBAR
VERTEBRAE

SACRUM

COCCYX
(Tailbone)

Point of Entry and
Exit of Spinal Nerves

INTERVERTEBRAL
DISKS

Figure 16-5. The vertebral column.

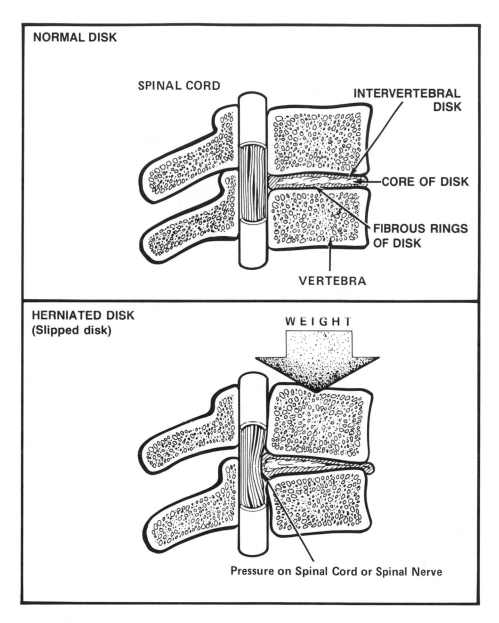

NORMAL DISK

SPINAL CORD

INTERVERTEBRAL DISK

CORE OF DISK

FIBROUS RINGS OF DISK

VERTEBRA

HERNIATED DISK (Slipped disk)

W E I G H T

Pressure on Spinal Cord or Spinal Nerve

Figure 16-6. Normal and herniated (slipped) disk.

which radiates down the arm; neck movements are restricted by the pain. Treatment is similar to that for the lower back. A collar that supports the neck often gives relief from the pain.

■ Bursitis

Bursae are small fluid-filled sacs located near the joints that reduce friction on movement. **Bursitis** is an inflammation of these bursae, and it is a very painful condition. The bursae of the shoulder joint are the most frequently affected, although bursitis can develop at any joint. Repeated irritation of a bursa or an injury to it can cause bursitis. Limitation of movement results from the pain of the inflammation. Treatment includes resting the joint and applying moist heat. Steroids are sometimes injected into the joint to reduce the inflammatory response.

DISEASES OF MUSCLES

Skeletal muscles cannot function unless they are stimulated by nerves. In the previous chapter, diseases in which the nerves fail to innervate muscles were discussed. Muscles themselves can also be diseased and lose their ability to contract. Another cause of muscle failure is the improper transmission of the impulse for contraction at the myoneural junction.

■ Muscular Dystrophy

The term **muscular dystrophy** includes several forms of the disease, all of which are hereditary. The various forms are transmitted differently and affect different muscles, but the result is the same for all forms, muscle degeneration.

Muscle fibers become necrotic, and the dead muscle fibers are replaced by fat and connective tissue. Neither of these tissues has the property of muscle cells, which is the ability to contract. Skeletal muscles are weakened by the degeneration.

The muscles of a muscular dystrophy patient lose power as they contract, but their use is regained with rest. This is different from paralysis, which results from damage to the nervous system. The disorder at the myoneural junction is in the neuronal transmitter described in Chapter 15. **Acetylcholine,** the transmitter substance, is either destroyed before it can stimulate the muscle to contract, or the transmitter is inadequately produced.

Muscular dystrophy can appear at any age, but generally it begins in childhood. A severe form can progress rapidly and affect the muscle of the heart, causing death; other forms progress slowly.

In the most severe form of muscular dystrophy, the calf muscles enlarge as a result of fat deposition. The shoulder muscles are weak, which causes the arms to hang limply. A child with this form of muscular dystrophy is very weak and thin and does not usually live to adulthood.

The genetic defect, in some way not yet known, interferes with protein metabolism. Creatine, formed from amino acids, is normally stored in muscle as **creatine phosphate.** Creatine phosphate assists in providing the necessary energy for muscle contraction. The muscular dystrophy patient is unable to store and use creatine; as a result, it is lost in the urine.

■ Myasthenia Gravis

Myasthenia gravis is a neuromuscular disorder in which neither the nerves nor the muscles are diseased. The failure is in the transmission of the impulse from the nerves to the muscles at the myoneural junction. Myasthenia gravis affects women more often than men. The cause is unknown.

The principal symptom of this disease is fatigue and the inability to use the muscles. All the voluntary muscles of the body are affected, including the muscles of facial expression. The lack of contraction in the facial muscles makes the patient's face expressionless. Simple actions such as chewing and talking become difficult.

Myasthenia gravis may be classified as an **autoimmune disease,** in which antibodies are produced against the body's own tissue. Such antibodies have been found in the serum of these patients. The thymus gland, which is involved in antibody production, at least in children, is often enlarged in myasthenia gravis patients. Removal of this gland sometimes brings about a remission but not a cure. The greatest danger in this disease is respiratory failure, because the muscles of respiration are unable to contract.

■ Tumors of Muscle

Muscle tumors are rare, but when they occur they are usually highly malignant. A malignant tumor of skeletal muscle is a **rhabdomyosarcoma.** The tumor requires surgical removal, and the prognosis is poor. The rhabdomyosarcoma metastasizes early and is usually an advanced malignancy when it is diagnosed.

SUMMARY

Bodily movements result from the interaction of muscles, bones, and joints. Diseases of these components of the musculoskeletal system cause pain and limit movement, and they can lead to structural deformities.

Pyogenic microorganisms cause bone infections and abscess formation. Tuberculosis can spread from the lungs to bone and destroy it. Other bone diseases result from mineral and vitamin deficiencies manifesting themselves by soft and deformed bones. Bone is also decalcified in hyperparathyroidism. Fractures occur under excessive stress, but when bones break spontaneously, a bone disease is indicated. A metastasized carcinoma, for example, causes pathologic fractures.

The most common joint disease is arthritis, which has several forms. Rheumatoid arthritis is the most progressive, severe, and crippling form. Osteoarthritis affects most people to some extent with age.

Muscular dystrophy is a degenerative disease in which muscles lose the ability to contract. They are unable to store creatine phosphate, an energy source for contraction. Another disease in which the muscles lose the ability to contract is myasthenia gravis, but, in this case, the failure is in the neuronal transmitter rather than in the muscles themselves. Tumors are rare in muscles, but when they occur they are usually highly malignant.

STUDY QUESTIONS

1. Name three ways in which pyogenic organisms can invade bone to cause osteomyelitis.
2. What is the result of tuberculosis in the bone of a child?
3. Why is a vitamin D deficiency the cause of rickets?
4. Describe the stature of a child with rickets.
5. What are possible causes of vitamin D deficiency in an osteomalacia patient?
6. Explain the relationship between hyperparathyroidism (Chapter 13) and osteitis fibrosa cystica.
7. What are the complications in osteoporosis?
8. Describe the various kinds of bone fractures.
9. What specific fractures are the most damaging to surrounding tissues?
10. Why is a sprain painful?
11. Which bones are most susceptible to metastases of carcinoma? Why?
12. Differentiate between rheumatoid arthritis and osteoarthritis by (a) age group affected, (b) number of joints involved, and (c) symptoms.
13. What is the difference in the use of steroids, such as cortisone, in the treatment of rheumatoid arthritis and osteoarthritis?
14. What causes the pain of gout?
15. Explain what is meant by a herniated disk.
16. Why is it so painful?
17. What are some possible treatments for a herniated disk?
18. Explain the genetic defect in muscular dystrophy.
19. What is the disorder in myasthenia gravis?
20. Why is the prognosis poor in rhabdomyosarcoma?

CHAPTER 17

Diseases of
the Skin

The skin, or integument, has many characteristics that make it an extremely effective body covering. Unbroken skin acts as a barrier to prevent microorganisms from entering the body, and the pigment of the skin, **melanin,** protects the body from harmful rays of the sun. The skin acts as a waterproof coat, preventing excessive water loss by evaporation, whereas the sweat glands and blood vessels of the skin regulate body temperature. Nerve endings in the skin sense temperature changes, pressure, touch, and pain, triggering the appropriate responses through the central nervous system. The oil glands of the skin provide a lubricant to keep it soft. The skin continually regenerates itself by sloughing off dead surface cells and forming new ones to replace them. This is significant in the healing of wounds.

The skin indicates malfunctionings within the body by color changes. Cyanosis, a blue coloration seen particularly in the lips, nose, or extremities, signals a lack of oxygen—a cardiac or pulmonary inadequacy. Jaundice indicates liver disease, bile obstruction, or hemolysis of red blood cells, in which case an accumulation of bilirubin in the blood produces the yellow coloration. An abnormal redness accompanies polycythemia (Chapter 6), carbon monoxide poisoning, and fever. Pallor, a whitening of the skin, may indicate anemia.

A total absence of melanin results from the congenital condition of **albinism.** Melanin at times disappears from patches of skin once normally pigmented, signaling an **autoimmune disease** in which the **melanocytes** are being destroyed. The loss of pigmentation is called **vitiligo.**

Diseases of the skin are numerous, and the lesions of different diseases often resemble each other. Diagnosis requires the consideration of many factors: the patient's history of disease, inherited disorders, allergies, and emotional state as well as physical examination. Many skin diseases require laboratory tests or biopsies.

STRUCTURE AND FUNCTION OF THE SKIN

The outermost layer of skin is the epidermis, consisting of stratified, or layered, squamous epithelium. Cells of the bottom epithelial layer divide, forming new cells that gradually move up to the surface. Cells at the surface die and become **keratinized,** or scalelike, providing the waterproof layer of the skin. **Keratin** is a tough fibrous protein produced by cells called keratinocytes. The keratinized cells are continually being shed. Melanocyte cells that produce the protective melanin pigment that gives color to the skin are also found in the **epidermis.** There are no blood vessels in the epidermis.

The **dermis,** or "true skin," underlies the epidermis. The dermis is composed of connective tissue supporting the blood and lymph vessels, elastic fibers, and nerves. Hair follicles, sweat glands, and **sebaceous,** or oil, **glands** pass through the dermis.

The subcutaneous tissue under the dermis connects it to underlying structures. Numerous adipose, or fat cells are in the subcutaneous tissue, and they provide a food reserve and insulation. The sebaceous glands and hair follicles arise in this tissue. Figure 17–1 shows the structure of the skin.

CLASSIFICATION OF SKIN DISEASES

The skin can be affected by diseases in numerous ways. Skin infections are caused by bacteria, viruses, fungi, and parasites, and many skin diseases result from allergies, or hypersensitivities, to various proteins. Neoplasia, or uncontrolled growth of certain cells, results in the formation of skin tumors. Hyperactivity of the sebaceous glands causes other skin diseases.

The range of lesions in skin diseases is broad. They may be small, blisterlike eruptions called **vesicles** or larger fluid-containing lesions called **bullae.** Lesions containing pus are referred to as **pustules,** and nodules and tumors are lesions that are hard to the touch. An area of skin reddened by congested blood vessels resulting from injury or inflammation is said to be erythematous. **Pruritus,** or itching, accompanies many skin diseases, especially those caused by allergies or parasitic infestation.

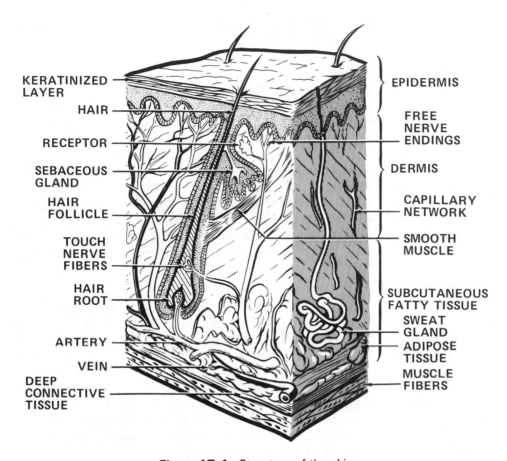

Figure 17-1. Structure of the skin.

INFECTIOUS SKIN DISEASES

Skin diseases caused by bacteria, viruses, fungi, and parasites are generally contagious. Care must be taken to prevent the spread of the infection from one part of the body to another and from one person to another.

■ Bacterial Skin Infections

■ *Impetigo.* **Impetigo** is an acute, contagious skin infection common in children. It is caused by streptococci and staphylococci organisms carried in the nose that are passed to the skin. The face and hands are most frequently affected. **Erythema,** a reddened area, develops and vesicles and pustules form. These rupture, and a yellow crust covers the lesion. Fever and enlarged lymph nodes may accompany the infection. The lesions should be washed with soap and water, kept dry, and exposed to the air. Antibiotic ointment may be used and oral antibiotics are sometimes prescribed to treat the infection systemically.

■ *Erysipelas.* **Erysipelas** is an inflammatory skin infection caused by streptococci that affects primarily the face. The strep organisms are probably transferred from respiratory discharges to the skin, entering through minute abrasions. Erysipelas can also develop if streptococci enter a surgical incision or wound.

Early symptoms of erysipelas include a sudden fever and shaking chills; reddened patches develop on the face, usually on the bridge of the nose. The redness spreads laterally, and the border is sharply defined and slightly elevated due to edema of the skin. The erythematous areas are hot to the touch and tender. If the eyelids are affected they become very swollen. Antibiotics are generally prescribed, but erysipelas is eventually self-limiting.

■ Viral Skin Infections

Cold sores or fever blisters are caused by the virus **herpes simplex.** The lesions generally form near the mouth or lips, as in Figure 17–2. The virus may be harbored in the body for a long time with no ill effect, but suddenly it becomes active and the infection develops. Cold sores frequently form when a person's resistance to infection is low or at a time of emotional stress. They often accompany a respiratory infection such as the common cold, or they develop during menstruation. A bad sunburn sometimes triggers the formation of cold sores. There is no effective medication for viral infections such as cold sores, but antibiotics are sometimes applied topically to prevent secondary bacterial invasion.

Warts, called **verucca vulgaris,** are caused by viruses affecting the keratinocytes of the skin, causing them to proliferate. A benign neoplasm develops with a rough keratinized surface. Warts are most common in children and young adults, developing particularly on the hands. They are often multiple and are contagious, being spread by scratching. Warts sometimes disappear spontaneously, but they should be removed only by a physician. If the virus remains in the body, the warts tend to recur.

Warts are not serious or painful except when they form on the soles of the feet. These warts are called plantar warts, and, in contrast to warts elsewhere on the body, which appear as an elevation from the skin, plantar warts grow inward. Pressure on the soles of the feet make them very painful, and they are often difficult to remove permanently.

■ Fungal Skin Infections

Ringworm is a highly contagious, inflammatory skin infection caused by fungi. It usually affects children and is spread by scratching. Ringworm is

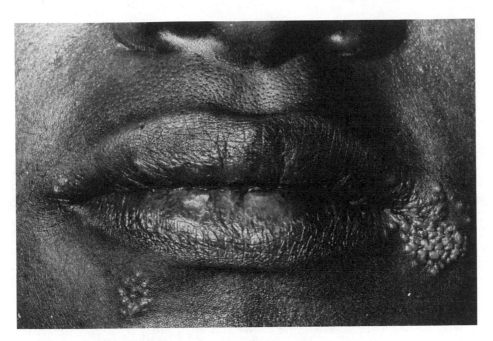

Figure 17-2. Typical cold sores or fever blisters caused by the virus herpes simplex. (*From Feinstein. Dermatology, 1975. Courtesy of Robert J. Brady Co.*)

sometimes contracted from infected pets. One form of ringworm develops on the scalp and the hairy skin of arms and legs. The lesions are red patches that are scaly or blistered. They are itchy and sore, and excessive scratching can lead to scarring and permanent hair loss.

Many different fungi cause ringworm infection on nonhairy skin. Any number of red, ring-shaped lesions can develop in an infected person. The fungi feed on perspiration and dead skin, particularly in body folds. Antifungal drugs are effective, but the disease can be prevented through cleanliness and thorough drying of the skin. Fungi thrive in a warm, damp environment.

Dermatophytosis, or athlete's foot, is also a fungal infection. In this disease the fungi attack the skin between the toes, making it red, cracked, and sore. Dermatophytosis spreads if untreated to other parts of the feet and even to distant sites on the body such as the armpits and groin. Athlete's foot is highly infectious and is often acquired from locker room floors or contaminated towels harboring the fungi.

Antifungal agents are effective in treating dermatophytosis, but it tends to recur if the fungi survive under the toenails. Drying the feet well between the toes and applying dusting powder to absorb moisture are good preventive measures against acquiring athlete's foot.

■ Parasitic Infestations

Pediculosis, or louse infestation, causes itching and irritation of the skin. The lice attach themselves to the hair of the scalp, armpit, or pubic area and live as parasites on the host's blood. The bitten area is very itchy, and the scratching that follows can open the skin to other invading organisms. Various preparations can be used to remove nits, the lice eggs, from the hair. This is followed by combing the hair with a fine-toothed comb. The infestation can be prevented by cleanliness and good hygiene.

Scabies, commonly called "the itch," is a contagious skin disease usually associated with poor living conditions. It is caused by a parasite called a mite. The female mite burrows into skin folds in the groin, under the breasts, and between fingers and toes. As she burrows she lays eggs in the tunnels, the eggs hatch, and the cycle starts again. The intense itching is caused by hypersensitivity to the mite. Blisters and pustules develop, and the tunnels in the skin appear as grayish lines. Scratching opens the lesions to secondary bacterial infection. Scabies is transmitted by close personal contact and can be linked to a venereal disease. Epidemics of scabies are common in camps and barracks.

To recover from scabies, the mites and eggs must be totally destroyed by hot baths, scrubbing, and medications to eliminate them. Underwear and bedding that harbor the eggs must be changed frequently. The itch may persist while treatment is being administered; applying calamine lotion provides relief.

HYPERSENSITIVITY DISEASES OF THE SKIN

Allergic or hypersensitivity reactions are frequently manifested by the skin. This fact serves as the basis for the scratch tests given to determine specific allergies. Some diseases of the skin develop in **atopic people,** persons with a genetic predisposition to allergies. Others occur in anyone who has been sensitized to an allergen such as poison ivy. Emotional stress frequently triggers or exacerbates an allergy-caused skin disease.

■ Urticaria (Hives)

Urticaria, or hives, results from a vascular reaction of the skin to an allergen. The lesions are **wheals,** rounded elevations with red edges and pale centers. Wheals develop most often at pressure points like those under tight clothing, but they may appear anywhere on the skin or mucous membranes. The lesions are extremely pruritic, or itchy.

The allergic response causes damage to mast cells, which then release histamine. Histamine causes blood vessels to dilate and become more permeable. Blood proteins and fluid ooze out of the capillaries into the tissues and result in edema. This irritation to the tissues causes intense itching.

Urticaria is treated with steroids, antihistamines, and lotions applied topically to reduce the itching. If the cause of the allergic reaction can be determined, that allergen should be avoided. Foods that are a common cause of hives include certain berries, chocolate, nuts, and seafood. Other allergens discussed in Chapter 2 frequently cause hives in the hypersensitive person. An attack of hives can also be brought on by emotional stress.

■ Eczema

Eczema, also called **contact dermatitis,** is a noncontagious inflammatory skin disorder. Eczema results from sensitization that develops from skin contact with various agents, plants, chemicals, and metals. Poison ivy and poison oak, dyes used for hair or clothing, and metals used for jewelry are examples of allergens that can cause eczema.

Eczema is a delayed type of allergic response in which lymphocytes are sensitized by an antigen and react with it on subsequent exposure. The typical inflammatory reaction occurs: dilated blood vessels, reddened skin, and edema. Vesicles and bullae develop from the excess tissue fluid, and the lesions are very itchy. Scratching causes the vesicles to burst and ooze, and the eczema is thus spread. Scaly crusts form on the ruptured lesions. A patient with contact dermatitis is shown in Figure 17–3.

Contact dermatitis can affect anyone and is not limited to the genetically allergic person. Skin that has been damaged is more easily sensitized by contact with allergens than healthy skin. Emotional stress can also be a factor in sensitization.

■ Lupus Erythematosus

Lupus erythematosus is a noncontagious inflammatory disease that takes one of two forms, mild or severe. The **discoid** form is only a minor disorder in which red, raised, itchy lesions develop. The lesions characteristically form the pattern of a butterfly over the nose and cheeks. Steroids are administered to relieve the inflammatory symptoms, but there is no treatment to cure the disease.

The serious form is **systemic lupus erythematosus,** which affects not only the skin but also causes the deterioration of collagenous connective tissue. Systemic lupus can affect the glomeruli of the kidney, causing abnormal excretion of albumin and blood, as well as casts (Chapter 9), in the urine. The red cell, white cell, and platelet counts are low. The lining of the heart and the heart valves may deteriorate. Hypersensitivity to an antigen is thought to be the cause of systemic lupus erythematosus. The antigen may be an allergen outside the body or the patient's own tissue to which the

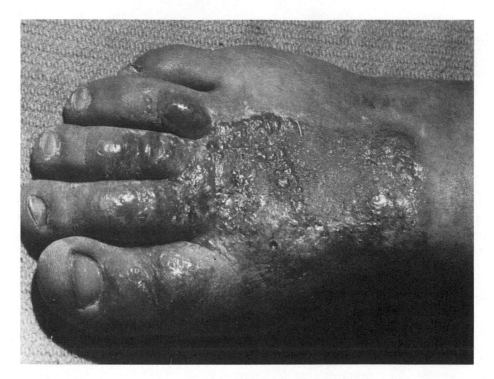

Figure 17-3. A patient with contact dermatitis from leather shoes. (*From Feinstein. Dermatology, 1975. Courtesy of Robert J. Brady Co.*)

patient has become sensitized. The latter is classed as an autoimmune disease.

Young women are most frequently affected by systemic lupus, which may begin suddenly or insidiously. The patient experiences a rash, and the skin becomes overly sensitive to sunlight. Joint and muscle pains may be accompanied by fever. The lymph nodes and spleen are frequently found to be enlarged. Periods of exacerbation and remission are characteristic of the disease.

There is no specific treatment for systemic lupus erythematosus, but, as with many inflammatory diseases, corticosteroids are administered to control the symptoms. The disease may even be fatal, death frequently being due to kidney or heart failure. The decreased number of leukocytes also reduces resistance to such diseases as pneumonia.

■ Drug Hypersensitivity

Adverse drug reactions in an atopic person are very common. The reaction may be manifested by various skin lesions, vesicles, and itchy rash, or

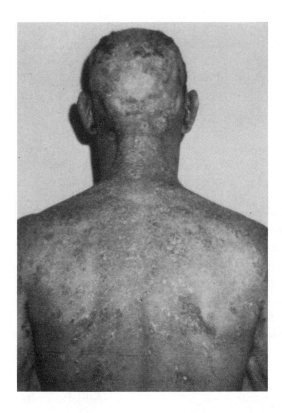

Figure 17-4. Patient experienced allergic drug eruption because of gold administered for rheumatoid arthritis. (*From Feinstein. Dermatology, 1975. Courtesy of Robert J. Brady Co.*)

erythema. The patient seen in Figure 17-4 was treated with gold for rheumatoid arthritis and developed the allergic skin reaction shown. The drug reaction may be severe enough to cause anaphylactic shock and death.

Penicillin, effective in treating bacterial infections, is an antigen to some atopic patients that triggers serious vascular reactions. Patients allergic to penicillin should never receive it and should carry identification warning of their sensitivity.

NEOPLASTIC SKIN DISEASES

Tumors of the skin range in seriousness from the benign mole to melanoma, a potentially fatal disease. The development of skin cancer is frequently linked to excessive sun exposure in the fair-skinned. Irritating chemicals and various radiations have also been associated with skin cancer.

■ Nevus (Mole)

Melanocytes in the epidermis produce the pigment melanin that gives color to the skin and protects the body against harmful rays of the sun. The neoplastic growth of melanocytes causes an excessive production of melanin, resulting in a **nevus,** or mole. A nevus is a benign skin tumor that is not present at birth but develops later. Most people have several nevi. The moles themselves are harmless but they can become malignant, as was described in Chapter 3.

■ Basal Cell Carcinoma

The most common skin cancer is **basal cell carcinoma**—a slow-growing, generally nonmetastasizing tumor. It generally develops on the face of people with light skin who do not tan in the sun but have been exposed to the sun. Figure 17–5 shows patients with basal cell carcinoma. The lesion begins as a pearly nodule with rolled edges that may bleed and form a crust. Ulceration occurs and size increases if it is neglected. This tumor is treated by surgical removal or radiation therapy.

■ Squamous Cell Carcinoma

Squamous cell carcinoma is more serious than basal cell carcinoma because it grows more rapidly, infiltrates underlying tissues, and metastasizes through lymph channels. Squamous cell carcinoma is a malignancy of the keratinocytes in the epidermis of people who have been excessively exposed to the sun. The lesion is a crusted nodule that ulcerates and bleeds. This cancer develops in any squamous epithelium of the body, including the skin or mucous membranes lining a natural body opening. It should be completely excised surgically or treated with radiation.

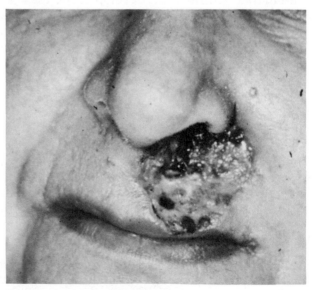

Figure 17-5. A. Basal cell carcinoma removed by Moh's microscopically controlled excision for skin cancer. Reconstruction planned because of loss of lip function. (*Courtesy of Dr. Barry A. Goldsmith.*)

A

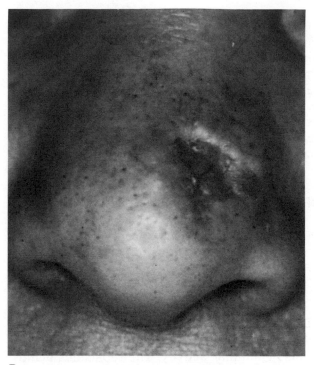

B

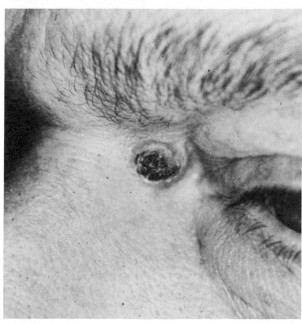

C

Figure 17-5. B. A 48-year-old woman with progressive growth of whitish plaquelike lesion with central indentation over a 5-year period. Patient underwent three stages of microscopically controlled surgical excision. Wound extended down to cartilage layer. A skin graft was applied. (*Courtesy of Dr. Barry A. Goldsmith.*) **C.** A 62-year-old man with basal cell carcinoma recurrent after prior treatment with electric needle. Gross tumor was excised. Margins clear after one layer of Moh's microscopically controlled surgical excision. Excellent healing in this area. (*Courtesy of Dr. Barry A. Goldsmith.*)

■ Malignant Melanoma

The most serious skin cancer is **malignant melanoma,** which arises from the melanocytes of the epidermis. It is highly malignant and metastasizes early. A malignant melanoma of the skin is seen in Figure 17–6. Melanoma sometimes develops from a mole that changes its size and color and becomes itchy and sore. It is usually excised with the surrounding lymph nodes to reduce metastasis. Prognosis depends on the depth of infiltration, previous spread, and how completely the tumor is excised. Figure 17–7 shows a malignant melanoma that metastasized to the brain.

METABOLIC SKIN DISORDERS

Hyperactivity of the sebaceous glands causes acne and chronic dandruff. Raised, horny lesions result from an excessive production of keratinocytes.

■ Acne (Vulgaris)

Many adolescents suffer at some time or another from acne: blackheads, pimples, and pustules. Acne is the result of hormonal changes that occur at puberty. The increased level of estrogen and testosterone stimulates not only growth at this time but also glandular activity. The sebaceous glands increase their secretions of **sebum,** the oily fluid that is released through the hair follicles. If the duct becomes clogged by dirt or make-up, the sebaceous secretion accumulates, causing a little bump or white head. Sebaceous accumulation at the surface becomes oxidized and turns black, causing the familiar blackhead. Blackheads should not be squeezed or picked because the broken skin offers an entry to bacteria that are always present on the

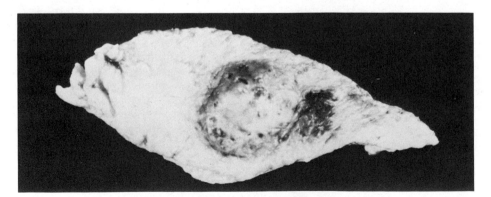

Figure 17-6. A malignant melanoma of the skin. (*Courtesy of Dr. David R. Duffell.*)

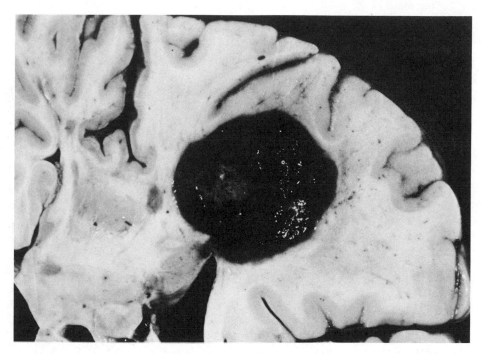

Figure 17-7. Malignant melanoma that metastasized to the brain. (*Courtesy of Dr. David R. Duffell.*)

skin surface. Once pyogenic bacteria enter the skin, pus forms and a pimple or pustule results. Squeezing the pimple spreads the infection.

There is no cure for acne, but various treatments can control the lesions. Acne generally corrects itself with maturity, but it may persist as a chronic condition that is aggravated by stress. Severe chronic acne is seen in Figure 17–8. The most important measure for controlling acne is frequent, thorough washing of the skin to remove excess oil and bacteria. Creams and heavy make-up that clog the pores should be avoided. Severe cases of acne are best treated by a dermatologist, who may prescribe topical steroids or antibiotics to prevent secondary bacterial infection.

■ Seborrheic Dermatitis (Chronic Dandruff)

The cause of dandruff is similar to that of acne: the excessive secretion of sebum from the sebaceous glands. The person with **seborrheic dermatitis** has an oily scalp, and the excessive secretion of sebum forms the familiar scales of dandruff. This condition can spread to the face and ears, and the eyebrows are often affected. Frequent shampooing, particularly with medicated shampoo, is the most effective treatment. Thorough brushing of the hair loosens the dandruff scales, and they will wash out easily.

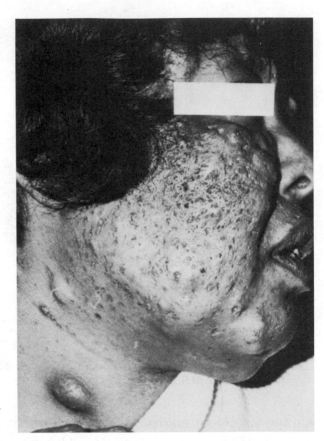

Figure 17-8. A patient with severe chronic acne. Note deep scarring and prominent cysts. (*From Feinstein. Dermatology, 1975. Courtesy of Robert J. Brady Co.*)

■ Sebaceous Cysts

Sebaceous cysts form when a sebaceous gland duct becomes blocked, and the sebum accumulates under the surface of the skin, forming a lump. Sebaceous cysts are not considered serious but they can rupture, allowing bacteria to enter the body. These cysts can be incised and drained, although they tend to recur, or they can be removed surgically.

A cyst that forms in the crease between the buttocks is the **pilonidal cyst.** This cyst begins as an ingrown hair and is very painful if it becomes infected and abscessed. A pilonidal cyst should be removed surgically.

■ Seborrheic Keratosis

The keratinocytes produce the fibrous protein keratin in the surface layers of the epidermis, making it waterproof. Proliferation of the keratinocytes, with resultant keratin excess, produces a benign, raised, horny lesion. This hyperplastic condition is called **seborrheic keratosis** and occurs with aging. The lesions, which are harmless, vary in color from yellow to brown, with edges that are sharply marked. No treatment is necessary.

■ Psoriasis

Psoriasis is a chronic skin disease with a hereditary basis, but the cause is unknown. The lesions are red patches with sharply marked edges, covered with white or silvery scales. Psoriasis lesions primarily form on the elbows and knees (the extensor surfaces of joints), but other parts of the body, such as the trunk, arms, legs, and scalp, can be affected. Typical lesions of psoriasis are seen in Figure 17–9.

There is no permanent cure for psoriasis, but the lesions can sometimes be controlled. The application of steroids and the use of antihistamines are the most effective treatments. Periods of exacerbation and remission are characteristic.

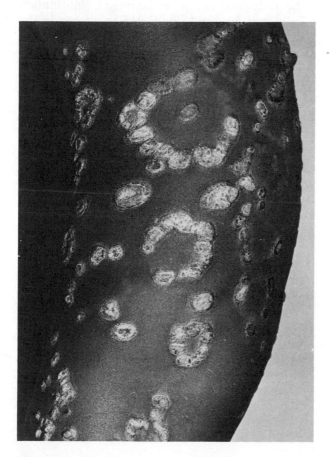

Figure 17-9. Psoriasis patient. Note the silvery scaling and the definite borders of individual lesions. (*From Feinstein. Dermatology, 1975. Courtesy of Robert J. Brady Co.*)

SUMMARY

The skin, which protects the body from various elements in the environment, can become diseased in numerous ways. Streptococci and staphylococci cause such bacterial infections as impetigo and erysipelas. Cold sores and warts result from viral infections. Ringworm and athlete's foot are caused by a fungus. Even parasites such as the louse and mite can infest the skin.

Allergies are frequently manifested by skin diseases. Hives, eczema, and lupus erythematosus are examples of skin eruptions caused by hypersensitivity to various antigens. Allergic drug reactions often result in the development of skin lesions. Abnormal growth or neoplasia of the skin cells causes malignant and benign tumors, ranging from the common mole to malignant melanoma, a potentially fatal disease. Hyperactivity of the sebaceous glands results in acne and chronic dandruff.

Skin lesions take many forms, each of which is significant in diagnosing the disease. The lesions may be reddened areas, indicating inflammation and congested blood vessels. They may be fluid-filled, due to edema in the skin, or pus-filled, a result of a pyogenic bacterial infection. The location of the lesion, whether it tends to recur, and whether it itches, are also factors in the diagnosis.

STUDY QUESTIONS

1. What do impetigo and erysipelas have in common?
2. What are the symptoms of erysipelas?
3. Name two skin diseases caused by viruses.
4. Explain how warts develop.
5. What is the principal difference between warts on the hand and plantar warts?
6. What is the causative agent of ringworm?
7. Explain how dermatophytosis develops giving the (a) causative organism, (b) initial site of attack, and (c) possible means of acquiring it.
8. Describe the parasitic infestation causing scabies, including the (a) parasite, (b) method of infestation, and (c) treatment.
9. Describe the typical lesions of urticaria.
10. What is the usual treatment for urticaria?
11. Explain the poison ivy rash in terms of physiologic response.
12. Distinguish between discoid lupus erythematosus and systemic lupus erythematosus.

13. Explain the development of a nevus.
14. Differentiate between basal cell carcinoma and squamous cell carcinoma.
15. What is the most serious form of skin cancer?
16. What do acne and seborrheic dermatitis have in common?
17. Explain the danger in squeezing or picking blackheads.
18. Describe the lesions of psoriasis.

CHAPTER 18

Stress and Aging

The body is constantly striving to maintain a constant internal environment in the midst of ever-changing conditions. For example, excess acidity or alkalinity that develops in the blood and body fluids is removed through the kidneys. Normal body temperature is maintained despite climate extremes, and the proper amount of water is conserved to prevent dehydration or hydration of tissues. This maintenance of a steady state is called **homeostasis.**

The regulation of the internal functioning of the body is controlled by the hypothalamus of the brain, which governs the autonomic nervous system and the master endocrine gland, the pituitary. Not only does the hypothalamus control homeostasis, it senses when the body or a body part is under stress and directs the proper response through nerves and glands.

How are the maintenance of homeostasis and the response to stress related to disease? The body is frequently subjected to forces requiring greatly increased internal activity. In responding or adapting to the stress, abnormal conditions can result.

Consider the phenomenon of inflammation previously described in Chapter 2. Although it produces pain that may be severe and the typical characteristics of swelling, heat, and redness, inflammation is a positive protective body response. It prevents the spread of an infection by barricading it and attempting to overcome foreign invaders such as pathogenic organisms or toxic substances.

Closely related to the mechanism of inflammation is the allergic reaction, or hypersensitivity. In this case, the inflammatory response is against a generally harmless invader such as pollen, dust, or a particular food, and the patient suffers from the disease of hay fever, asthma, or hives. The inflammation is more harmful than helpful under these conditions. Some diseases represent inappropriate responses to a stimulus.

Disease is more than being overcome by a disease-producer. It includes the body's fight against it. The symptoms of respiratory tract diseases, coughing and sneezing, are reflex actions that aid in ridding the throat and nose of irritants. Vomiting, a symptom of gastrointestinal distress, is a reflex action to relieve the distress. The seriousness of any disease largely depends on the patient's defenses against it.

EFFECTS OF STRESS ON THE BODY

Many diseases have been described throughout this book as being stress related. Diseases of the gastrointestinal system, the respiratory system, and the skin are often aggravated, if not caused, by stress. Hypertension is another disease greatly affected by stress.

A wide range of situations in a person's life may be stressful, including living conditions, occupation, injury, inadequate diet, and prolonged exposure to cold. Worry, fatigue, and alcoholism also cause stress. Signs of damage caused by stress are often the result of the body's defense against or adaptation to it.

What are some changes that occur in the body when it is subjected to stress such as an injury? The blood sugar level rises, providing an additional energy supply needed for repair of the damaged tissue. The injured site becomes inflamed due to the increased blood flow to the area. The neutrophil count increases, enabling the phagocytic cells to engulf foreign matter and cellular debris.

If the injury is severe and blood loss results, the patient may go into shock (Chapter 8). The reduced blood volume lowers the blood pressure, and venous return to the heart is poor. Cardiac output then becomes inadequate to meet the demands of the body, and the patient loses consciousness because insufficient blood reaches the brain.

The response of the body to this stress is to increase blood pressure. Specialized neural receptors sense the low pressure, and through a neural mechanism, which will be explained, the blood pressure increases. The kidneys, sensing the reduced blood pressure due to the loss of blood, release a substance called renin that aids in restoring proper pressure. The adrenal glands are stimulated to release adrenalin, which also increases blood pressure and heart activity.

FUNCTION OF THE AUTONOMIC NERVOUS SYSTEM IN RESPONSE TO STRESS

We are all familiar with our bodily response to a stressful situation, a frightening experience, or an emotional upset. Our heart beat increases to the point of pounding, blood pressure rises, respiration quickens, and perspiration increases. These changes, which occur through the action of the autonomic nervous system, provide us with additional energy to meet the stress.

Large portions of the sympathetic nervous system are stimulated simultaneously by stress. The first response is redistribution of blood to where it is most needed: the heart, the brain, and the muscles of respiration. This is accomplished by a constriction of skin and gastrointestinal blood vessels and a dilation of those to the heart, brain, and active muscles. The constriction of the blood vessels elevates blood pressure, causing greater venous return to the heart and increased cardiac output.

The liver releases stored glucose into the blood when stimulated by the sympathetic nervous system, thus providing an increased energy source for actively metabolizing cells. The rate of cellular metabolism increases as the thyroid gland is stimulated under stress to secrete additional thyroxine. The adrenal medulla releases adrenalin (epinephrine), enhancing the stimulatory effect of the sympathetic nervous system. Glucocorticoids from the adrenal cortex also increase the level of blood glucose. This overall excitation of the body in response to stress is known as the alarm reaction. Figure 18–1 illustrates the function of the autonomic nervous system in stress.

STRESS AND THE ADRENAL CORTICAL HORMONES

Signals of an alarm reaction are sent to the hypothalamus, which in turn sends releasing factors to the pituitary gland (Chapter 13). The pituitary secretes ACTH (adrenocorticotropic hormone) and thyrotropin, which stimulate the thyroid gland and the adrenal cortex to release thyroxine and the corticosteroids. This hormonal response to stress is illustrated in Figure 18–2.

Cortisol, a glucocorticoid, is anti-inflammatory and inhibits unnecessary defense reactions. In the case of hay fever or rheumatoid arthritis, inflammation is actually the disease. In diseases of this type there are no pathogens or toxins to be barricaded, and the inflammatory response is harmful rather than beneficial.

It is necessary that a proper balance of aldosterone and anti-inflammatory cortisol be maintained. An excess of **anti-inflammatory hormones** produced during stress can actually cause the spread of an infection by

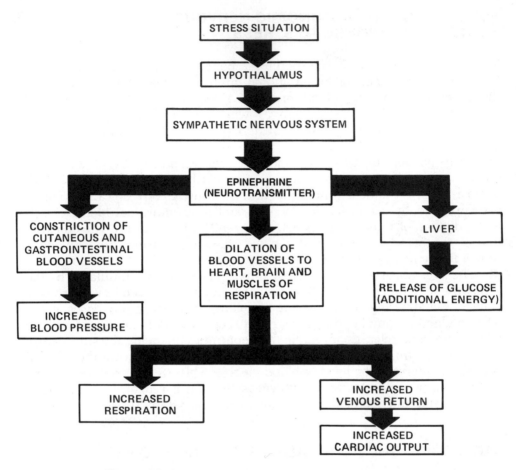

Figure 18-1. Function of the nervous system in stress.

weakening the barricade around infectious organisms. Stress can be a predisposing factor in the spread of tuberculosis for this reason. Tubercle bacilli can be held at bay until excessive cortisol is circulated. Nonpathogenic organisms that normally live in the respiratory tract, the intestines, or on the skin become dangerous when the defense mechanism against them is reduced.

The anti-inflammatory cortical hormones not only suppress the immune reaction against microorganisms, but they also suppress the tendency to reject foreign tissue in graft or transplantation procedures. These hormones are extremely important in preventing unnecessary inflammation in the typical inflammatory diseases.

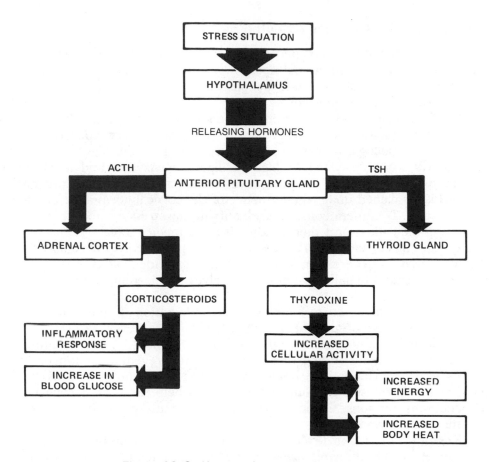

Figure 18-2. Hormonal response to stress.

TREATMENT WITH CORTICAL HORMONES

The effectiveness of corticosteroids as treatment for many inflammatory diseases has been described throughout the book. Caution is always required because of the side effects from these hormones. High dosages or prolonged use of cortisol or cortisone reduces a patient's response to infection, which can therefore go unnoticed and become very widespread in the absence of inflammatory symptoms.

STRESS-RELATED DISEASES

The symptoms, causes, and treatment of many of the diseases aggravated by stress have already been described. This section will try to explain how the stress or alarm reaction affects a particular disease.

Gastrointestinal Diseases Affected by Stress

The gastrointestinal system is particularly affected by stress, as most people have experienced. An emotional upset, worry, or fear can cause vomiting, diarrhea, or constipation. Some people under stress lose their appetite, whereas others eat compulsively.

Peptic ulcers are a prime example of a stress-related disease. The ulcer patient is frequently nervous, prone to worry, and very conscientious. Prolonged physiologic or psychological stress triggers the alarm reaction, and gastric secretion, which is high in digestive enzymes and acidity, is increased. In other people the protective barrier of the gastric or duodenal mucosa is weakened under the influence of the cortical hormones secreted during stress. Treatment consists of identifying the stress or anxiety, as well as placing the patient on a diet or administering medications.

Certain ulcers, called "stress ulcers," develop suddenly after a shock or trauma, such as severe burns or surgery. These ulcers differ from the chronic types and usually manifest themselves by bleeding rather than by pain.

Ulcerative colitis, an inflammation and ulceration of the colon, is a disease of unknown origin that is aggravated by stress. Severe diarrhea with blood and mucous accompanies the disease. Treatment for this inflammation includes a nonirritating diet, antibiotics to prevent infection of the lesions, and rest. The patient should be kept free from emotional stress, and psychological counseling should be offered to help the person cope with anxieties and tensions. Corticosteroids are frequently prescribed for their anti-inflammatory effect.

Regional enteritis or Crohn's disease is similar to ulcerative colitis. It is not caused by a pathogenic organism but is aggravated by stress, such as emotional upsets. Regional enteritis is an inflammation of the large or small intestine. The patient experiences abdominal pain, diarrhea, and weight loss. Corticosteroids are used with caution to prevent side effects from overdosage.

■ Migraine Syndrome

The migraine sufferer knows the effect of the disease on the body is more extensive than periodic headaches. A migraine headache usually begins in the temple on one side, spreads to the other side, and becomes generalized. It can last for a short time or for days, and the range of severity is very broad. Gastrointestinal disturbances frequently accompany the headache, including nausea or vomiting and diarrhea or constipation.

Certain symptoms often precede the migraine headache: visual changes such as a sensation of flickering lights, dizziness, and a flushing or paling of the skin. Changes occur in the cranial arteries before the onset of the headache with a vasoconstriction, followed by a vasodilation, which causes the throbbing, aching pain. The eyes may become red, swollen, and show excessive tearing.

Treatment is aimed at constricting the dilated arteries. Aspirin is effective in relieving the pain if the headache has a low intensity, but other medications may be required to dilate the arteries. Dosages of these vasoconstricting medications must be carefully controlled to prevent side effects.

People subject to migraine headaches are generally hard-working and like order. A threat or a conflict causes them to become tense and fatigued. Frequently, stress or emotional upset precedes the onset of the headache. Migraines often occur during a woman's menstrual period.

The stress or alarm reaction causes a generalized accumulation of body fluid. This is probably due to the increased secretion of aldosterone by the stimulated adrenal glands. Aldosterone causes the retention of sodium and water and the excessive fluid retention precipitates the vascular changes that cause the pain. There may be abnormalities in the level of certain neurotransmitter substances such as **serotonin** just before the attack.

The migraine sufferer should be aided in recognizing the source of the stress that causes the syndrome. Counseling may enable the sufferer to express inner feelings of anger, depression, or conflict and so to cope with thcm better.

Closely related to migraine headaches are cluster headaches, named for their tendency to occur in clusters, often several within a day or longer period of time. The intense, throbbing pain of these headaches is generally confined to one side and may last for a few hours. Men are more often affected by cluster headaches than are women, who are more prone to migraines. The treatment is similar to that of migraines.

The Cardiovascular System and Stress

The response of the sympathetic nervous system to stress is a constriction of peripheral blood vessels that elevates the blood pressure. The adrenal cortex, responding to stress, also causes blood pressure elevation by excessive secretion of aldosterone. Sodium and water are retained under the influence of aldosterone, and the increased fluid volume causes increased blood pressure. A person predisposed to hypertension and subjected to prolonged stress will probably develop chronic high blood pressure. This is usually accompanied by arteriosclerosis (discussed in Chapter 8), which overworks the heart. The risk of a heart attack under these circumstances increases, particularly if the person is obese, smokes, and is sedentary.

A special case of hypertension is eclampsia of pregnancy, in which there is a sudden, intense increase in blood pressure. Eclampsia usually occurs in the third trimester and is accompanied by an increase in the level of serum albumin, which appears in the urine. Convulsions develop that can lead to a coma. The cause of eclampsia is unknown, but it is thought to be aggravated by stress (see Chapter 14).

Sexual Abnormalities Related to Stress

Prolonged and intense stress causes changes in the sex organs. The ovaries and testes shrink and decrease their activity. Menstruation becomes irregular and may even stop, as often experienced by women subjected to the stress of prison. In men, sperm production is decreased, and both men and women may experience a decline of libido (sex urge). The depressed activity of the gonads may result from decreased stimulation by the gonadotropic hormones of the pituitary gland. During prolonged periods of stress, the pituitary may secrete an excessive amount of ACTH at the expense of the gonadotropins.

■ *Impotence.* **Impotence,** the inability of the male to achieve and maintain an erection sufficient for sexual intercourse, is usually caused by emotional disturbances. Stress decreases the output of gonadotropic hormones, and, consequently, testosterone production and spermatogenesis are diminished. The dilation of penile arteries that leads to engorgement of the erectile tissue of the penis and then erection is under the control of the autonomic nervous system. Anxiety, fear, and worry are emotions that affect the nervous system.

Impotence is said to be primary if the man has never been able to complete intercourse successfully. The inability to maintain an adequate erection may stem from worry about satisfactory sexual performance or from psychological concerns about events in adolescence. Impotence is secondary if intercourse has been achieved successfully at least once. The onset of impotence may be due to fatigue, a form of stress, or distraction. Premature ejaculation and alcoholism are also possible causes of impotence. This condition is not generally the result of a physical disorder, but it may be.

Treatment should be directed toward the source of the stress, which requires openness on the part of the patient with the physician or therapist. The man must be helped to overcome his personal insecurity and frustration, and his partner should also be supported and instructed about the problem. With good counseling, impotence can usually be overcome.

The Respiratory System and Stress

The respiratory system is frequently affected by disease when a person's defenses against it are lowered by stress. The cause of the stress may be emotional factors like worry, depression, and conflict or physical factors such as trauma, prolonged exposure to cold, or inadequate nutrition. Stress reduces the body's ability to fight infection as previously mentioned in the case of tuberculosis.

Development of the common cold during a time of stress is within the experience of most people. The alarm reaction, with its release of the cortical hormones, is probably related to this phenomenon. Infectious diseases of the respiratory system are not the only conditions affected by stress.

Asthma, a disease characterized by marked changes in the diameter of the bronchi and obstruction of the air passageways, usually has an allergic basis. A wide variety of allergens or irritants can precipitate an asthma attack. The antigen–reagenic antibody complex (Chapter 2) attaches to the surface of the bronchial mast cells, causing the release of histamine and other **spasmogens,** substances that cause spasmodic contractions of the bronchial musculature.

An asthma attack—with its coughing, wheezing, and shortness of breath—can be aggravated by emotional or psychological stress. The asthmatic manifests a hyperactivity of the bronchi through an exaggerated response to autonomic nervous activity.

Other factors that aggravate an asthmatic condition are overexertion and viral respiratory tract infections. A young child's asthma can appear to be worse for a combination of reasons as school begins. The new experience is emotionally stressful, the school environment increases the child's exposure to respiratory infections, and school play can involve overexertion.

The treatment of asthma begins by reducing exposure to allergens or irritants wherever possible. Allergy shots aimed at desensitization are helpful for some people. The use of a bronchodilator such as epinephrine is generally quite effective. Severe cases may require administration of corticosteroids or ACTH to reduce the inflammatory reaction, edema, and excessive mucous secretion.

Skin Diseases Affected by Stress

Diseases of the skin may be caused by infectious agents, allergies, or abnormal cellular activity, but many of them are affected by stress (Chapter 17). A cold sore or fever blister, which is a viral infection, often develops when resistance to infection is low. The virus may be present and silent for a long time, only to become actively infective at the time of an emotional or physical stress.

Hives are an allergic skin disease that can be aggravated by stress. The relationship between hypersensitivity and stress has already been discussed. Treatment for hives often includes the administration of corticosteroids to reduce the inflammatory response. Eczema is another inflammatory skin disease of an allergic nature that is affected by emotional stress.

The cause of psoriasis is unknown, but it does have a hereditary basis and can be aggravated by stress. Application of corticosteroids and other medications is quite effective in controlling the lesions.

Systemic Changes Produced by Stress

Various stress diseases or diseases of adaptation have been discussed: cardiovascular, respiratory, and gastrointestinal disorders, as well as allergies and the migraine syndrome. Experimentation has shown other marked changes resulting from prolonged stress. The adrenal cortex becomes enlarged from overwork by excessive stimulation to secrete its hormones. Lymphoid tissue, which is important in immune reactions and the removal of foreign invaders, atrophies. Ulceration of the gastric and duodenal lining frequently develops.

EFFECTS OF AGING

Aging is not a process that begins at retirement but one that occurs continuously throughout a lifetime. The body constantly replaces wornout cells but the rate of replacement gradually slows down in adulthood. Cellular activity is reduced, tissues lose moisture, and flexibility declines. Noticeable body changes occur in the eyes, the skin, and the endocrine glands as early as the 30s and 40s. Distance vision may remain good, but the ability to accommodate for close vision decreases. Connective tissues lose their elasticity, and muscles lose their speed of response and strength, making the body less agile. Hair often begins to gray as less melanin pigment is produced for the hair follicles.

Heredity and environment greatly affect the aging process. A person's ability to withstand or adapt to stress significantly influences the rate at which the aging process occurs. The diseases that a person has had, the amount of activity and exercise he or she engages in, and his or her nutritional habits all affect the physiologic changes that accompany aging.

Many diseases that make old age difficult begin in the middle years. Diagnosis and treatment of such diseases as diabetes, hypertension, and arthritis early in their course can prevent much discomfort and suffering in later life.

Common Diseases of the Elderly

The elderly patient frequently has a combination of several diseases, some of which are interrelated. Hip fractures are common, and most aged people develop some degree of arteriosclerosis, which affects circulation to the heart, brain, and legs. As coronary arteries become atherosclerotic, the risk of myocardial infarction, a heart attack, increases. Hypertension, which frequently accompanies arteriosclerosis, is a predisposing factor for stroke.

Poor blood flow through narrowed, hardened cerebral arteries causes a form of senility.

Debilitating changes occur in the musculoskeletal system. Osteoarthritis, a degenerative joint disease (Chapter 16), generally develops in the normal aging process, affecting those joints most subjected to stress during a lifetime. The pain and stiffness of the disease tend to restrict movement, and the immobility increases the risk of thrombosis and embolism. Lack of exercise causes muscles to become thin and weak, a condition known as disuse atrophy. An elderly person may become more accident prone as sight and hearing fail and the reflexes slow. Bones become more brittle and fracture easily under slight stress, and they heal slowly.

Gastrointestinal complaints stem from a number of diseases: gallbladder malfunction, diverticulitis, ulcers, and various malignancies. Decayed teeth, poorly fitting dentures, or the inability to wear dentures makes chewing difficult or impossible.

Prostatic hyperplasia (Chapter 14) in males causes urinary complaints. The inability to eliminate urine adequately results in stasis and predisposes to cystitis, inflammation of the bladder, and other urinary tract infections. Symptoms of painful urination, a change in frequency, and nocturia are common in elderly men.

The prevalence of cancer in the elderly is high. Many malignancies go undetected and are only discovered at autopsy. The exposure to carcinogenic agents through a lifetime no doubt takes its toll.

Visual acuity can diminish from a number of causes, but one eye disease that particularly affects the elderly is cataracts. Cataract formation is a clouding of the eye lens to the point of opacity. The patient experiences blurred and dimmed vision and may see double. These symptoms do not necessarily signal a cataract, but the eyes should be examined. Removal of cataracts has become a simple procedure, one that can often be performed on an outpatient basis. Intraocular lens implants have been very successful, eliminating the need for thick glasses.

In addition to the physical diseases that are common to the elderly, **senility** often causes a loss of memory, disorientation, and personality changes. Senility is defined as the loss of mental, physical, or emotional control and is manifested by delusions of persecution, apathy, slovenliness, and at times sudden emotional outbursts. The patient's recent memory may be poor but long-standing memories are very vivid. The past is confused with the present, and the patient may fail to recognize loved ones.

The cause of senility may be physical, such as brain damage resulting from inadequate blood flow through hardened cerebral arteries. Psychological factors may also foster senility. A feeling of worthlessness, loss of interests, and the stress of worrying about health and future security may be underlying causes of senility. Lack of interest and attention can account for the failure to recall recent events.

Many of the problems of aging can be prevented through preparation for retirement time. Maintaining an interest in life by engaging in hobbies, community service activities, and part-time employment are effective in preventing withdrawal from society and in fulfilling the need to be useful.

■ *Alzheimer's Disease.* **Alzheimer's disease** is the most common form of senility, affecting $1\frac{1}{2}$ to $2\frac{1}{2}$ million Americans. The cause of Alzheimer's disease is not known; however, there is some familial tendency to develop it, perhaps because of a combination of acquired genes. Women are slightly more susceptible to the disease than are men. The disease usually manifests itself in persons over age 65, but it can occur in the late 40s or 50s. Alzheimer's disease manifests itself in the early stages by forgetfulness, failing attention, and declining mathematical ability, such as the inability to balance a checkbook. Later, the patient exhibits personality changes, speech difficulties, and general confusion. There is a tendency toward depression, irritability, and severe anxiety. Symptoms may be more noticeable to the casual observer than to family members. When the disease becomes severe, the patient experiences hallucinations at night, and the resulting sleeplessness causes the person to wander aimlessly.

Extensive research on the changes that take place in the nerve cells of these patient's brains has been done on autopsy findings. Abnormalities include a loss of neurons in regions essential for memory and understanding, and accumulations of twisted filaments and nerve tangles in the cortex. Aggregates of protein interfere with cerebral circulation, and degenerating nerve endings disrupt transmission of nerve impulses. A deficiency in enzymes required to produce neurotransmitters has also been found.

There is no known prevention, treatment, or cure for Alzheimer's disease. Symptoms may be reduced, however, through physical activity—walking, dancing, rocking in a chair—which reduces the patient's restlessness. Counseling and support for family members is extremely important in dealing with this irreversible and progressive disease that leads to complete mental and physical disability of loved ones.

Diagnosis of Alzheimer's disease is based on family histories and interviews with family members. Tests are used to determine the patient's orientation and mood, recent and old memory, and the ability to solve problems and make judgments.

Care of the Elderly

Advances in medical science enabling people to live longer than in the past, and a decrease in the birth rate, have raised the median age in our society. A higher percentage of people are in an older age bracket and require proper attention and health care. **Geriatrics** is the branch of medicine that deals with the problems of aging and the diseases of the elderly.

Research in **gerontology,** the study of aging problems, has revealed the need for psychological support and counseling as well as physical care of the elderly. The aging patient must experience a sense of dignity, worth, and acceptance, whether the person is living with relatives or friends, at home, or in a health-care facility. The elderly should be supervised carefully to prevent accidents and should be kept alert and aware of their surroundings.

An important physical need of the elderly is proper nutrition: a diet that includes an adequate supply of protein, vitamins and minerals, fruits, vegetables, and milk. If a digestive problem exists, small and more frequent meals may be desirable. Food may have to be chopped or strained because of the inability to chew.

Another need of the aged is a rest and exercise program that helps maintain circulation. The elderly person should be encouraged to engage in a walking program that takes into account the person's strength limitations and does not cause exhaustion. Rest should include short naps or sitting in a chair with the feet elevated. Staying in bed for long periods is harmful, and anemia can develop in the absence of exercise since the mechanism for red blood cell production is not stimulated (Chapter 6).

A good understanding of the changes that occur in the aging process makes one better able to give proper health care to the elderly patient. The slowed rate of metabolism, with its decreased production of energy, makes the aged very sensitive to temperature changes. The elderly may require warmer clothing or extra blankets.

Resistance to infection is reduced in the elderly as the activity of lymphoid tissue decreases. Bronchopneumonia caused by staphylococci commonly develops in the aged after the flu. Early signs of infection should be noted and the proper medication prescribed. The chance of death naturally increases with age, and although many of the diseases that have been mentioned in this chapter do not cause death themselves, the slightest stress can bring it about.

SUMMARY

The body responds to stress in a variety of ways in the attempt to maintain homeostasis or adapt to the stress. The autonomic nervous system is extensively stimulated, and its response provides the body with additional energy to meet the emergency. Blood pressure is elevated, heart activity is increased, and blood rich in oxygen is provided to active muscles. The liver releases stored glucose needed by the actively metabolizing cells. Adrenalin is secreted by the adrenal medulla, enhancing the effect of the sympathetic nervous system.

The hypothalamus responds to stress by stimulating hormonal activity of the pituitary gland, which in turn stimulates the thyroid gland and the adrenal cortex. The rate of cellular metabolism and that of concurrent energy production is greatly increased by the elevated thyroxine level.

Hormones of the adrenal cortex have important functions in responding to stress. The mineralocorticoids such as aldosterone cause retention of sodium and water, increasing the volume of body fluid—an effect that elevates blood pressure. Aldosterone stimulates the inflammatory response that walls off infection and attempts to counteract it.

The glucocorticoids such as cortisol increase the level of circulating glucose and prevent an unnecessary inflammatory and immune response. This is important in allergic reactions and rheumatoid arthritis, in which no pathogen is present. Cortisol also suppresses the immune reaction that causes rejection of tissue grafts and transplants. Excessive cortisol can cause the spread of infection by reducing the protective barrier around an infectious agent and preventing the symptoms which signal an infection. Administration of cortisol, cortisone, or ACTH to reduce the inflammatory response in such diseases as regional enteritis, asthma, and rheumatoid arthritis must be done with caution to prevent side effects.

Many diseases are aggravated by stress, particularly those of the cardiovascular system, the skin, the respiratory, and digestive systems. Psychological and emotional factors, as well as physical factors, can trigger the alarm reaction, and the response to it exacerbates the disease. The treatment of these diseases includes identification of the source of stress and removing it where possible or counseling, which can enable the patient to adapt to the stress. Medication is prescribed as warranted.

Physiologic changes that are part of the aging process begin early in life. Heredity and environment significantly affect the rate at which these changes occur. A person's ability to withstand stress or adapt to it influences the manner in which aging occurs.

Elderly patients often suffer from cardiovascular problems: heart conditions, hypertension, and arteriosclerosis, which are interrelated. Wear and tear on the body cause degenerative diseases such as osteoarthritis, the pain and stiffness of which decrease mobility and predispose to circulatory problems, muscle atrophy, and anemia. The incidence of cancer is high among the elderly, although many malignancies are detected only at autopsy.

Mental changes also occur with aging. Memory may fail in the elderly patient, and the person becomes disoriented. Personality changes, inappropriate behavior, and the inability to recognize loved ones indicate the altered mental state of senility. Senility can have a physical basis of brain damage due to the lack of blood flow through cerebral arteries or Alzheimer's disease, or it can stem from psychological factors such as depression, worry, or a sense of uselessness. Thoughtful preparation for retirement age and suitable counseling can help to maintain an interest in life and provide a feeling of worth.

STUDY QUESTIONS

1. Describe the general changes that occur when the body is subjected to stress.
2. How does the body counteract the effect of shock due to blood loss?
3. What is the role of the hypothalamus in responding to stress?
4. What is the action of cortisol and related steroids?
5. How can stress predispose to tuberculosis?
6. How are peptic ulcers related to stress?
7. What are "stress ulcers?"
8. Describe the symptoms of the migraine syndrome.
9. Explain the cardiovascular problems aggravated by stress and their interrelationship.
10. What sexual abnormalities are often associated with stress?
11. Give several examples of the effect of environment on the aging process of a person.
12. What is a cataract and how is it treated?
13. What are possible causes of senility?
14. Describe the effects of Alzheimer's disease.
15. How should a person prepare for old age physically and psychologically?
16. Why is stress particularly significant in the aged?

References

American Medical Association: The Illness Called Alcoholism. Chicago, American Medical Association, 1977.

American Medical Association: Manual of Alcoholism, 3rd ed. Chicago, American Medical Association, 1977.

Beeson PB, McDermott W: Textbook of Medicine, 14th ed. Philadelphia, Saunders, 1975.

Boyd W, Sheldon H: An Introduction to the Study of Disease. Philadelphia, Lea & Febiger, 1977.

Goodhart RS, Shills ME: Modern Nutrition in Health and Disease, 6th ed. Philadelphia, Lea & Febiger, 1980.

Groer ME, Skekleton ME: Basic Pathophysiology, 2nd ed. St. Louis, C.V. Mosby, 1983.

Guyton AC: Human Physiology and Mechanisms of Disease, 3rd ed. Philadelphia, Saunders, 1982.

Guyton AC: Textbook of Medical Physiology. Philadelphia, Saunders, 1986.

Kent TH, Hart MN, Shires TK: Introduction to Human Disease. New York, Appleton-Century-Crofts, 1979.

Kosowicz J: Atlas of Endocrine Diseases. Bowie, Md., Charles Press, 1978.

Laurence J: The immune system in AIDS. Sci Am 253:84–93, December 1985.

Nester EW, Roberts CE, Lidstom ME, et al: Microbiology. Philadelphia, Saunders, 1983.

Netter FH: Ciba Collection of Medical Illustration. West Caldwell, N.J., Ciba Pharmaceutical Co, Vols 1–7, 1983.

Price SA, Wilson L: Pathophysiology: Clinical Concepts of Disease Processes. New York, McGraw-Hill, 1982.

Purtilo DT: A Survey of Human Diseases. Menlo Park, Calif., Addison-Wesley, 1978.

Sandritter W, Thomas C, Kirsten WH: Color Atlas and Textbook of Macropathology. Chicago, Year Book Med Pub, 1979.

Selye H: The Stress of Life. New York, McGraw-Hill, 1978.

Sherlock DS, Summerfield JA: Color Atlas of Liver Disease. Chicago, Year Book Med Pub, 1979.

Sloan E: Biology of Women, 2nd ed. New York, Wiley, 1985.

Tortora GJ, Anagnostakos NP: Principles of Anatomy and Physiology, 4th ed. New York, Harper & Row, 1984.

Walter JB: An Introduction to the Principles of Disease, 2nd ed. Philadelphia, Saunders, 1982.

Wurtman RJ: Alzheimer's disease. Sci Am 252:62–75, January 1985.

Young CG, Barger JD: Introduction to Medical Science. St. Louis, C.V. Mosby, 1977.

Glossary of Terms

Abscess. Collection of pus in a cavity

Acetylcholine. Neuronal transmitter substance

Achlorhydria. Absence of hydrochloric acid from gastric juice

Achondroplasia. Disorder of cartilage formation in the fetus

Achondroplastic dwarf. Undersized person with short arms and legs but normal trunk

Acidosis. Excessive acidity of the blood and body fluids (pH of blood less than 7.3)

Acromegaly. Disease caused by excessive growth hormone in an adult

ACTH. See Adrenocorticotropic hormone

Active immunity. Bodily produced antibodies

Acquired immune deficiency syndrome (AIDS). Viral infection of certain white blood cells that destroys a person's immune system

Acute. Sudden onset, short duration

Addison's disease. Disease of adrenal cortical hypoactivity

Adenocarcinoma. Cancer of a gland

Adenohypophysis. Anterior pituitary

Adenoma. Benign glandular tumor

Adenomatous or nodular goiter. Enlargement of thyroid due to tumors

ADH. See Antidiuretic hormone

Adhesions. Union of two surfaces normally separate

Adrenal diabetes. Hyperglycemia due to hyperadrenalism

Adrenocorticotropic hormone (ACTH). Hormonal stimulant of adrenal cortex

Adrenogenital syndrome. Adrenal virilism; excessive masculinization

Agglutination. Clumping of red blood cells

AIDS. See Acquired immune deficiency syndrome

Albinism. Congenital absence of melanin

Albuminuria. Plasma protein (albumin) in the urine

Aldosterone. Principal mineralocorticoid of adrenal cortex

Alkalosis. Excessive alkalinity of the blood and body fluids (pH of blood more than 7.4)

Alleles. One of two or more alternative forms of a gene at the same site on a chromosome

Allergen. Foreign protein causing an allergic reaction

Allergy. Hypersensitivity to normally harmless proteins

Alpha cells. Glucagon-producing cells of pancreas

Alveoli. Tiny, thin-walled air sacs of the lung

Alzheimer's disease. Premature senility

Amenorrhea. Absence of menstruation

Amphetamines. Drugs sometimes used as an appetite depressant

Amylase. Carbohydrate enzyme

Anaphylactic shock. Circulatory failure resulting from an allergic reaction

Anaplasia. Lacking differentiation and form

Androgens. Male hormones

Anemia. Disease of insufficient hemoglobin

Aneurysm. A dilation or saclike formation in a weakened blood vessel wall

Angina pectoris. Acute chest pain due to inadequate cardiac oxygen supply

Angiocardiography. X-ray examination of the heart using opaque dyes

Angioma. A benign tumor of blood vessels

Anomaly. Deviation from the normal

Anorexia. Loss of appetite

Anorexia nervosa. Nutritional disease of psychoneurotic origin

Antibody. Molecule produced by the body in response to the presence of an antigen

Anticoagulants. Substances that prevent blood clotting

Antidiuretic hormone (ADH). Hormone of posterior pituitary affecting kidney tubules

Antihistamine. Drug that counteracts the effect of histamine

Anti-inflammatory hormones. Hormones that inhibit the inflammatory or immune response, e.g., cortisol

Antigen. Protein not normally found in the body

Antineoplastic agents. Substances that inhibit the growth of cancer cells

Anuria. Absence of urine formation

Aphasia. Loss of speech

Aplastic. Lacking new development

Areola. Darkly pigmented area surrounding the nipple

Arrhythmia. Abnormal rhythm of the heart beat

Arteriosclerosis. Hardening of the arteries

Ascites. Abnormal accumulation of fluid in the abdominal cavity

Aseptic. Free from infectious material

Aspirate. To withdraw fluid from a body cavity

Asymptomatic. Showing no symptoms

Atelectasis. A collapsed or airless state of the lung

Atherosclerosis. Development of lipid deposits in arterial walls

Atopic person. One with a genetic predisposition to allergies

Atresia. Absence or closure of a normal body opening

Atrial fibrillation. Rapid, uncoordinated impulse over the atria

Atrophy. Decreasing in size; wasting

Aura. Warning preceding an epileptic seizure

Auscultation. Listening for sounds inside the body, usually with a stethoscope

Australia antigen. Antigen present in serum of hepatitis virus type B patient

Autoimmune disease. Disorder in which antibodies act on a person's own tissue

Autonomic nervous system. Nerve network that controls smooth muscle and internal organs

Autosomes. All chromosomes other than sex chromosomes

Azotemia. Presence of nitrogen-containing compounds in the blood

Barium. Opaque substance used in some x-ray examinations

Basal cell carcinoma. A nonmetastasizing skin tumor

Basal ganglia. Areas deep in the cerebrum that control much automatic action

Benign. Nonmalignant

Beriberi. Disease caused by a thiamine deficiency

Beta cells. Insulin-producing cells of the pancreas

Biliary calculi. Gallstones

Biliary cirrhosis. Liver degeneration due to chronic bile duct disease

Bilirubin. Orange pigment derived from hemoglobin

Biopsy. Microscopic examination of cells and tissues to detect the presence of cancer

Blood urea nitrogen (BUN). Indicator of kidney function

B-lymphocytes. Stimulate plasma cells to produce immunoglobulins

Bone callus. Network of woven bone formed between broken bone ends

Bowman's capsule. Site of initial urine formation

Bradycardia. Abnormally slow pulse rate

Bronchi. Branching air tubules from trachea to bronchioles

Bronchiectasis. Chronic dilation and distention of the bronchi with subsequent infection

Bronchioles. Smallest bronchi terminating in alveoli

Bronchogenic carcinoma. Lung cancer

Bronchoscope. Lighted tube designed to view bronchial interior

Bulimia. A gorge and purge syndrome

Bulla. A large, fluid-containing lesion

Bullae. Blisterlike structures formed by fusion of alveoli in emphysema

BUN. See Blood urea nitrogen

Bursa or bursae. Fluid-filled sacs that reduce friction near joints

Bursitis. Inflammation of a bursa

Cachexia. State of profound ill health; emaciation

Candida albicans. Fungus capable of causing vaginitis

Capillary fluid shift mechanism. Movement of fluid from the blood into tissue spaces

Carcinoma. A malignant tumor of epithelial or glandular tissue

Carcinoma in situ. Premalignant stage of cancer

Cardiac arrest. Sudden stoppage of heart action

Cardiac arrythmia. Disturbance of heart rhythm

Cardiac catheterization. Procedure for examining the chambers of the heart

Cardiac sphincter. Valve at entrance to stomach

Caseation. Destructive process forming cavities in lungs in tuberculosis

Caseous. Cheeselike mass resulting from destruction of tissue

Casts. Molds of kidney tubules consisting of protein and blood cells

Cataract. Opacity of the eye lens

CAT scan. See Computed axial tomography

Cerebral palsy. Muscular disorder caused by brain damage at or near the time of birth

Cerebral vascular accident (CVA). Stroke

Cerebrospinal fluid. Protective fluid around the brain and spinal cord

CGH. See Chorionic gonadotropic hormone

Chancre. Characteristic lesion of primary syphilis

Chemical carcinogens. Cancer-causing agents

Chemotherapy. Treatment of a disease with chemicals

Chlamydial infection. Prevalent venereal disease

Choleangiogram. X-ray films of bile duct system using radiopaque dyes

Cholecystitis. Inflammation of the gallbladder

Cholecystogram. X-ray films of gallbladder using radiopaque dyes

Cholelithiasis. Formation or presence of gallstones

Choriocarcinoma. Highly malignant tumor of the placenta

Chorionic gonadotropic hormone (CGH). Hormone secreted by the placenta

Chronic condition. Gradual development, long term

Chronic obstructive pulmonary disease (COPD). Disorder in which the exchange of respiratory gases is deranged

Chronic ulcerative colitis. Inflammation of the large intestine due to unknown cause

Chymotrypsin. A proteolytic enzyme

Cilia. Hairlike structures that sweep the respiratory mucosa

Cirrhosis. Chronic degenerative liver disease with nodular regeneration and scarring

Coarctation. Stricture or narrowing

Collateral circulation. Accessory blood vessels

Colostomy. Artificial abdominal opening to allow evacuation of colon

Comminuted fracture. Bone fracture in which the bone is shattered or crushed

Complication. A new disease that develops concurrently with an existing one

Compound fracture. Bone fracture in which the skin is pierced

Computed axial tomography (CAT scan). Noninvasive x-ray technique for obtaining a cross-sectional view of the body

Concussion. Transient disorder of the nervous system resulting from a severe blow to the head

Congenital. Present at and existing from birth

Congenital disease. Disorder present at birth

Congestive heart failure. Inadequate heart action resulting in edema

Conjunctiva. Membrane that lines the eyelids and covers the eyeballs

Conn's syndrome. Disease of adrenal cortical hyperactivity

Consolidated. Solidified

Contusion. Injury to the brain from a severe impact

Convulsion. Involuntary contraction, or a series of contractions, of voluntary muscles

COPD. See Chronic obstructive pulmonary disease

Coronary thrombosis. Blood clot in coronary artery

Cor pulmonale. Right-sided heart failure due to chronic lung disease

Corpus luteum. Yellow glandular mass in the ovary formed from ruptured Graafian follicle

Cortisol. Principal glucocorticoid of adrenal cortex

Cortisone. Glucocorticoid usually converted to cortisol in humans

Creatine phosphate. Form of energy storage in muscles

Creatinine. Waste product of protein metabolism

Cretinism. Mental and physical retardation due to congenital thyroid deficiency

Cryptorchidism. Failure of the testes to descend into the scrotum

Cubic millimeter (mm³). Unit of measure

Cushing's syndrome. Disease of adrenal cortical hyperactivity

CVA. See Cerebral vascular accident

Cyanosis. Blue coloration of tissue due to lack of oxygen

Cyst. A fluid-filled sac

Cystic fibrosis. Disease of the exocrine glands

Cystic hyperplasia. Multiple cysts in the breast

Cystitis. Inflammation of the urinary bladder

Cystoscope. Instrument used to examine the bladder interior

D&C. Dilation of the cervix and curettage, scraping of the endometrium

Debilitated. Totally weakened

Deciliter. See Grams per 100 milliliter

Defibrillator. Device to correct ventricular fibrillation

Delirium tremens (DTs). An acute mental disturbance resulting from long-standing alcohol abuse, marked by shaking, delirium, and halucinations

Dementia. Organic loss of intellectual function

Dermatophytosis. Athlete's foot

Dermis. The true skin

Dermoid cyst. Teratoma; ovarian cyst containing skin, hair, oil glands, and teeth

DES. See Diethylstilbestrol

Desensitization. Reduction of sensitivity to an allergen, as in allergy shots

Detoxify. Make poisonous substances harmless

Diabetes insipidus. Disease resulting from antidiuretic hormone deficiency

Diabetes mellitus. Disease resulting from lack of insulin

Diagnosis. Determination of the nature of the disease

Dialysis. Method of artificially clearing blood of waste products

Diastole. Relaxing, filling phase of the heart

Diastolic pressure. Lowest pressure in the arteries

Diethylstilbestrol (DES). Synthetic hormone, formerly administered to prevent spontaneous abortion

Diffuse colloidal goiter. Endemic goiter caused by insufficient iodine in diet

Dilation. Widening

Disease. The unhealthy state of a body part or physiologic system

Disuse atrophy. Shrinkage or wasting through inactivity

Diverticulitis. Inflammation of diverticula (sacs)

Diverticulosis. Formation of pouches, or sacs, by the mucosa

Dominant gene. Gene that will always be expressed

Dopamine. A neuronal transmitter substance that is deficient in Parkinson's disease

Down's syndrome. Mongolism

DTs. See Delirium tremens

Duodenal ulcer. Peptic ulcer of first segment of small intestine

Dysentery. Severe inflammation of the colon

Dysmenorrhea. Painful menstruation

Dyspareunia. Pain during sexual intercourse

Dyspepsia. Indigestion

Dysphagia. Difficulty in swallowing

Dyspnea. Shortness of breath

Dysuria. Painful urination

Ecchymosis. A bruise; superficial discoloration caused by escape of blood into the tissue

Eclampsia. Toxemia of pregnancy resulting in convulsions

Ectopic. Misplaced or malpositioned

Ectopic pregnancy. Implantation of fertilized ovum outside the uterus

Eczema or contact dermatitis. A noncontagious inflammatory skin disorder

Edema. Excess of fluid in the tissues

EEG. See Electroencephalogram

Electroencephalogram (EEG). Electrical recording of brain waves

Electrolyte balance. Balance of salts: sodium, potassium, calcium, and others

Embolism. A detached thrombus

Emphysema. Inflation of the lungs with trapped air

Empyema. Accumulation of pus in the pleural cavity

Encephalitis. Inflammation of the brain and meninges

Endarterectomy. Surgical procedure to remove blockage in carotid artery

Endocarditis. Inflammation of heart lining

Endocrine glands. Ductless glands of internal secretion

Endometriosis. Proliferation of endometrial tissue outside of the uterus

Endoscope. Lighted instrument used to view interior of digestive tract

Epidermis. Outermost layer of skin

Epidermoid carcinoma. A cancer of epithelial tissue, skin, or mucous membranes

Epididymitis. Inflammation of epididymis

Epilepsy. Disease of abnormal electrical discharges in the brain

Epinephrine (adrenalin). Bronchial dilator and hormone

Epistaxis. Bleeding from the nose

Erysipelas. An inflammatory skin infection caused by streptococci

Erythema. Skin area reddened by inflammation or infection

Erythroblastosis. Abnormal increase of erythroblasts, immature red cells

Erythrocytosis. Abnormal increase of erythrocytes (red blood cells)

Erythropoiesis. The process of red cell development

Erythropoietin. Hormone-stimulating red cell production

Esophageal varices. Varicose veins of the esophagus

Esophagitis. Inflammation of the esophagus

Esophagoscope. Endoscope used to view interior of esophagus

Estrogen. Female hormone

Etiology. Cause of disease

Exacerbation. Period in which symptoms become more severe

Exfoliative cytology. Study of cells shed or scraped from a body surface

Exocrine glands. Glands of external secretion through ducts

Exophthalmos. Protrusion of eyeballs due to postocular edema

Extrinsic factor. Vitamin B_{12}

Fetal alcohol syndrome. Disease of babies born to alcoholic mothers

Fibrin. Plasma protein essential for blood clotting

Fibroblasts. Connective tissue cells capable of producing fibers

Flatus. Gas of the intestinal tract

Foramen ovale. Fetal opening between atria

Friable. Breakable

Fulminating. Disease of sudden onset and rapid progression

Galactosemia. Disease in which galactose cannot be used

Gangrene. Death of tissue due to loss of blood supply followed by bacterial invasion

Gastric ulcer. Peptic ulcer of the stomach

Gastritis. Inflammation of the stomach

Gastroscope. Endoscope used to view stomach interior

Gastroscopy. Inspection of stomach interior using a gastroscope

Genital herpes. Viral infection spread by intimate contact

Geriatrics. Branch of medicine dealing with the aged

Gerontology. Study of the problems of aging

Glioma. Malignant brain tumor

Glomerulonephritis. Kidney disease affecting glomeruli

Glomerulus. Tuft of capillaries through which blood filtration occurs

Glycogen. Storage form of glucose

Glycosuria. Sugar present in the urine

Goiter. Enlargement of the thyroid

Gonadotropins. Hormonal stimulant of sex glands

Gonococcus. Gonorrhea-producing organism

Gout. Joint disease resulting from excessive uric acid

Graafian follicle. Saclike structure containing ova

Grams per 100 milliliter (deciliter) (g/dl). Unit of measure

Grand mal epilepsy. Severe form of epilepsy

Graves' disease. Disease of severe hyperthyroidism

Greenstick fracture. A cracked bone

Group A hemolytic streptococci. Organism causing infection that leads to rheumatic fever

Gynecomastia. Enlargement of breasts in the male

Hematemesis. Bloody vomitus

Hematocrit. The volume percentage of erythrocytes in whole blood

Hematuria. Blood in the urine

Hemiplegia. Paralysis on one side of the body

Hemoglobin. Oxygen-carrying pigment of erythrocytes

Hemolysis. Rupture of red blood cells

Hemoptysis. Coughing up of blood

Hemorrhoids. Varicose veins of the rectum

Hepatavax B. Vaccine providing immunity against virus type B hepatitis

Hepatic coma. State of unconsciousness due to liver dysfunction

Hepatitis. Inflammation of the liver

Hepatocarcinoma. Cancer of the liver

Hereditary. Genetically determined

Hermaphrodite. Person with ovarian and testicular tissue

Herniation of intervertebral disk. Slipped disk

Herpes simplex. Causative agent of cold sores

Heterozygous. Having different alleles for a given trait

Hiatal hernia. Protrusion by part of the stomach through the diaphragm near the esophagus

Hirsutism. Abnormal hairiness, especially in women

Histamine. Substance released from damaged tissue causing dilation and increased permeability of blood vessels

Hodgkin's disease. A malignant disease of the lymph nodes

Homeostasis. Maintenance of stability amidst changing conditions

Homozygous. Having identical alleles for a given trait

Hormones. Chemical messengers secreted by the endocrine glands

Huntington's chorea. Hereditary disease causing mental and physical deterioration

Hyaline membrane disease. Disorder of premature newborn infant resulting in lung collapse

Hydatidiform mole. Benign tumor of the placenta

Hydrocephalus. Excessive fluid in or around the brain

Hydrolithotripsy. Nonsurgical laser beam procedure that crushes kidney stones in patients who are immersed in a tank of water

Hydronephrosis. Dilation of renal pelvis with urine

Hydrosalpinx. Fluid-filled tube

Hydroureters. Distention of the ureters with obstructed urine

Hymen. Membranous fold that partly or completely closes the vaginal opening

Hyperactive bone marrow. Excessive production of blood cells

Hyperadrenalism. Overactivity of adrenal cortex

Hypercalcemia. Excessive calcium in the blood

Hyperemia. Increased amount of blood in an area

Hyperglycemia. Elevated blood glucose level

Hypernephroma. Carcinoma of the kidney

Hyperparathyroidism. Overactivity of parathyroids

Hyperpituitarism. Overactivity of pituitary

Hypertension. High blood pressure

Hypertensive heart. Enlarged heart due to high blood pressure

Hyperthyroidism. Overactivity of thyroid

Hypertrophy. Enlargement of a structure

Hypervitaminosis. Excessive vitamin intake, particularly of vitamins A and D

Hypoadrenalism. Underactivity of adrenal cortex

Hypoalbuminemia. Albumin deficiency in the blood causing edema

Hypocalcemia. Abnormally low calcium level in the blood

Hypochromic. Lighter than normal color

Hypoglycemia. Abnormally low blood glucose level

Hypogonadism. Decreased functional activity of the gonads

Hypoparathyroidism. Underactivity of the parathyroids

Hypophysis. Pituitary gland

Hypopituitarism. Underactivity of the pituitary

Hypoproteinemia. Deficiency of blood proteins

Hypothyroidism. Underactivity of thyroid

Hypovolemic shock. Disruption of circulation due to severe blood volume reduction

Hypoxia. Decreased availability of oxygen to the tissues

Idiopathic. Cause of a disease is unknown

Idiopathic thrombocytopenia purpura (ITP). A severe platelet deficiency

Immune. Not susceptible to a particular disease

Immunoglobulin. Antibodies carried in plasma against a particular antigen; protective immunity

Immunoglobulins, IgE. antibodies that cause allergic diseases; reagins

Impetigo. An acute contagious bacterial skin infection

Impotence. Inability to achieve and adequately maintain an erection

Inflammatory exudate. Fluid that has oozed out of blood vessels as a result of inflammation

Influenza. Inflammation of the mucosa of the upper respiratory tract

Insulin. Hormone secreted by pancreas in order to regulate carbohydrate metabolism

Insulin-dependent diabetes mellitus (IDDM). Juvenile-onset diabetes

Insulin shock. Hypoglycemic shock

Intima. Inner lining of blood vessels

Intravenous pyelogram. X-ray examination of kidney and ureters using contrast dye

Intrinsic factor. Substance in gastric juice

Intussusception. Telescoping of an intestinal segment into the part forward to it

Ischemia. Inadequate blood supply to an organ or tissue

ITP. See Idiopathic thrombocytopenia

Jaundice. Yellowish discoloration of skin and tissues due to excessive bilirubin in the blood

Juxtaglomerular apparatus. Cells that secrete renin

Karyotype. Chromosomal composition of the nucleus

Keloid. Hard, raised scar

Keratin. Tough fibrous protein produced by keratinocytes

Keratinize. To fill with keratin

Ketone bodies. Acetone and related byproducts of fat metabolism

Klinefelter's syndrome. Sexual anomaly due to an extra X chromosome

Kupffer cells. Phagocytic cells lining blood spaces in the liver

Kwashiorkor. Disease of young children caused by protein deficiency

Leiomyoma. A fibroid tumor, benign tumor of smooth muscle

Lesion. Structural abnormality

Leukocytes. White blood cells

Leukocytosis. Excessive production of white blood cells

Leukorrhea. Vaginal discharge other than blood

Ligament. Band of fibrous tissue connecting bones and strengthening joints

Lipoma. A benign fatty tumor

Lithotripsy. Nonsurgical crushing of kidney stones

Lower respiratory diseases. Diseases of the trachea, bronchi, and lungs

Lumbar puncture. Spinal tap; removal of cerebrospinal fluid for diagnostic or therapeutic purposes

Lumen. Channel through a tube or tubular organ

Lupus erythematosus (discoid). A noncontagious inflammatory skin disease

Lupus erythematosus (systemic). An autoimmune or collagen disease

Lymphatic (lymphocytic). Pertaining to the lymph nodes

Lymphocytes. White blood cells produced in lymphoid tissue

Lymphoid tissue. Lymph nodes, thymus gland, spleen

Lymphomas. Malignancies of lymphoid tissue

Lymph tissue. Specialized tissue for filtering out and removing bacteria

Malabsorption. Inability to absorb normal nutrients

Malignant. An invasive tumor capable of metastasis

Malignant melanoma. A highly malignant skin tumor

Mammography. X-ray of the breast

Mast cells. Cells that release histamine in an inflammatory response

Medullary cavity. Cavity within long bones filled with yellow bone marrow

Melanocytes. Epidermal cells that produce the pigment melanin

Melena. Stools darkened by blood pigments

Menarche. Onset of menstruation

Meninges. Protective coverings on the brain and spinal cord

Meningitis. Inflammation of the meninges

Meningocele. Saclike protrusion of meninges and cerebrospinal fluid through a vertebral opening

Meningomyelocele. Protrusion of nerve fibers into a blind sac through a vertebral opening

Menopause. Time during which menstrual cycle wanes and stops

Menorrhagia. Excessive or prolonged bleeding during menstruation

Metastasis. Spread of cancer to a distant site

Metrorrhagia. Bleeding between menstrual periods

mg. See Milligram

Milligram (mg). Unit of measure

Milliliter (ml). Unit of measure

Millimeter of mercury (mm Hg). Unit of measure

ml. See Milliliter

mm Hg. See Millimeter of mercury

Monocytes. Macrophages; large phagocytic leukocytes

Motor neurons. Neurons that carry impulses to muscles and glands

MS. See Multiple sclerosis

Mucosa. Mucous membrane lining digestive tract

Mucus. Thick fluid secreted by mucous membranes

Multiple sclerosis (MS). Demyelinating disease of the central nervous system

Muscular dystrophy. Degenerative muscle disease

Mutation. Permanent change in the DNA structure

Myasthenia gravis. Disease of the neuromuscular junction

Myelin. Lipid sheath on neuronal fibers, destroyed in multiple sclerosis

Myelocele. Open neural tube with disordered nerve fibers

Myelogenic (myelocytic). Produced in the bone marrow

Myocardial infarction. Dead portion of heart muscle tissue

Myoma. A benign tumor of muscle

Myxedema. Disease of severe hypothyroidism

Necrotic. Dead cells or tissue

Negative feedback mechanism. Control of hormonal secretion by inhibition of the stimulator

Neisseria meningitidis. Most common causative organism of meningitis

Neoplasia. New and abnormal growth

Neoplasm. A tumor

Nephron. Functional unit of the kidney where urine is formed

Nephrotripsy. Nonsurgical laser beam procedure in which kidney stones are crushed without use of a water tank

Neurogenic shock. circulatory failure due to generalized vasodilation

Neurohypophysis. Posterior pituitary

Neurotropic. Organisms having an affinity for the nervous system

Nevus. A mole, a benign, pigmented skin tumor

Nondisjunction. Failure of chromosomes to separate during cell division

Nonhemolytic Streptococci. Organisms causing infectious endocarditis

Non–insulin-dependent diabetes mellitus (NIDDM). Maturity-onset diabetes

Normoblasts. Nucleated red blood cells

Nystagmus. Involuntary, rapid movement of the eyeball

Occluded. Closed

Occult blood. Blood in stools observed by means of chemical tests

Oliguria. Diminished urine secretion

Orchitis. Inflammation of the testes

Organic obstruction. Material blockage

Osteitis fibrosa cystica. A decalcifying bone disease caused by hyperparathryoidism

Osteoarthritis. Chronic joint disease

Osteoblasts. Bone-forming cells

Osteoclasts. Bone-dissolving cells

Osteogenic sarcoma. Primary bone malignancy

Osteoma. Benign bone tumor

Osteomalacia. A decalcifying bone disease in adults due to a dietary deficiency

Osteomyelitis. Infectious bone inflammation

Osteoporosis. Deterioration of the bone

Oxytocin. Hormone of posterior pituitary

Pacemaker. Patch of tissue setting heart rate; sinoatrial node

Paget's disease. (1) Cancer of the nipple and areola; (2) disease of excessive bone formation

Palpitations. Noticeably rapid heartbeat

Pancreatitis. Inflammation of the pancreas

Panhypopituitarism. Total absence of anterior pituitary hormones

Papilloma. A polyp or a benign epithelial tumor

Paralytic obstruction. Blockage due to failure of peristalsis

Parathormone. Parathyroid hormone

Paresis. Paralysis associated with organic loss of intellectual function

Parkinson's disease. Degenerative disease of the basal ganglia

Passive immunity. Administration of preformed antibodies in immune serum

Pathogenic organisms. Disease-producing organisms

Pathologic fracture. A fracture due to a diseased bone

Pediculosis. Louse infestation of the hair

Pellagra. Disease caused by niacin deficiency

Peptic ulcer. Gastric or duodenal ulcer

Periosteum. Vascular connective tissue layer covering the surface of bone

Peripheral resistance. Resistance encountered by the blood from the walls of the vessels

Peristalsis. Rhythmical waves of smooth muscle contractions

Peritonitis. Inflammation of abdominal cavity lining

Petit mal epilepsy. Mild form of epilepsy

Phagocytic cells. Cells capable of digesting bacteria and other harmful substances

Phenylketonuria. Disease in which phenylalanine cannot be used

Phlebitis. Inflammation of a vein

Pilonidal cyst. A sebaceous cyst formed in the buttocks

Placenta. Structure joining fetus and mother in the uterus

Plaques. Fatty deposits

Platelets. Formed elements of the blood that initiate the clotting mechanism

Pleural cavity. Space between lungs and inner chest wall

Pleural membrane. Double-layered membrane forming pleural cavity

Pleurisy. Inflammation of the pleural membranes

Pleurocentesis. Surgical puncture and drainage of the pleural space

Pneumothorax. Entrance of air or gas in the pleural cavity

Poliomyelitis. Viral disease affecting motor neurons

Polycystic kidney. Congenital kidney disease associated with multiple cyst formation

Polydactyly. Extra fingers or toes

Polydipsia. Excessive thirst

Polymorphs. Polymorphonuclear leukocytes, neutrophils

Polyuria. Excessive urination

Pott's disease. A form of tuberculosis affecting the vertebral column of children

Preeclampsia. First phase of toxemia of pregnancy

Primary hypertension. Elevated blood pressure not caused by another disease

Proerythroblasts or erythroblasts. Primitive red blood cells

Progesterone. Female hormone

Prognosis. Predicted course and outcome of the disease

Prostatic hyperplasia. Benign enlargement of the prostate

Prostatitis. Inflammation of the prostate

Pruritus. Itching

Psoriasis. A chronic hereditary skin disease

Psychogenic factors. Emotional or psychological factors

Puerperal sepsis. Infection of the endometrium after childbirth or abortion

Purpura. Petechiae; flat, red spots caused by small hemorrhages

Pustule. Pus-containing lesion

Pyelitis. Inflammation of the renal pelvis

Pyelonephritis. Suppurative inflammation of the kidney and renal pelvis

Pyloric sphincter. Valve at entrance to small intestine

Pyogenic organisms. Pus-forming bacteria

Pyosalpinx. Pus-filled tube

Pyuria. Pus in the urine

Rabies. Hydrophobia, fatal viral disease transmitted by a rabid animal

Radical mastectomy. Removal of breast, chest muscles, and axillary lymph nodes

Radiopaque dyes. Dyes used to show contrast on x-ray films

Rapid plasma reagin (RPR) test. Diagnostic procedure for syphilis

Reagins. Antibodies formed by allergy sufferers

Recessive gene. Gene that is expressed in the homozygous condition

Reduction. Alignment of broken bone ends to promote healing

Reflux. Backward flow

Regional enteritis. Inflammation of the intestine due to unknown cause

Regurgitation. Abnormal back flow of fluid

Relapse. Return of a disease

Releasing factors. Stimulatory substances sent from hypothalamus to anterior pituitary

Remission. Period in which symptoms subside

Renin. Enzyme secreted in kidney to raise blood pressure

Resolution. Return to normal state, as in a lung after lobar pneumonia

Respiratory epithelium. Mucous membrane lining respiratory tract

Resuscitation. Restoration to consciousness after respirations have ceased

Reticulocytes. Red blood cells with endoplasmic reticulum

Rhabdomyosarcoma. Malignant muscle tumor

Rh factor. A protein factor; an antigen present on the red blood cells of about 85 percent of the population

Rhodopsin. Light-absorbing pigment in the rods of the retina

Rickets. Bone disease of infancy and early childhood caused by a vitamin D deficiency

Ringworm. A contagious skin infection caused by fungus

RPR. See Rapid plasma reagin

Salpingitis. Inflammation of the fallopian tubes

Sarcoma. A malignant tumor of connective tissue

Scabies. A contagious skin disease caused by a parasite

Sclerotic. Hard

Scurvy. Disease caused by a vitamin C deficiency

Sebaceous glands. Oil glands

Seborrheic dermatitis. Chronic dandruff

Seborrheic keratosis. Horny lesions of excess keratin

Sebum. Oil secretion of sebaceous glands

Secondary hypertension. Elevated pressure due to another disease

Seizures. A form of convulsions

Seminoma. Highly malignant tumor of the seminiferous tubules

Senility. Loss of mental, physical, or emotional control

Sensory neurons. Neurons that convey impulses to the central nervous system

Septic embolism. A detached clot containing pus-forming bacteria

Septicemia. Systemic infection of the blood

Sequela. One disease condition resulting from another

Sequestrum. Piece of dead bone separated from sound bone by necrosis

Serotonin. A neurotransmitter substance and vasoconstrictor

Sex-linked inheritance. Acquisition of traits on the sex chromosomes

Shingles. Herpes zoster; viral infection of sensory neurons

Shock. Failure of circulatory system to meet tissue needs

Signs. Objective evidence of disease

Simmond's syndrome. A premature senility

Somatotropin. Growth hormone of the anterior pituitary

Somnolence. Unnatural sleepiness or drowsiness

Spasmogen. Substance that causes spasmodic contraction of the bronchial musculature; histamine

Spastic colon. Irritable bowel; colitis

Specific gravity. Measure of fluid concentration

Spheroidal. Round

Spina bifida. Incomplete closure of the vertebral column

Spirometer. Instrument used to measure lungs' ability to move air in and out

Splenomegaly. Enlargement of the spleen

Sprain. A joint injury resulting from wrenching or twisting

Spur. Spicule of projecting bone formed in arthritic joints

Squamous cell carcinoma. A malignant skin tumor

Staphylococci. Microorganisms always present on the skin

Stasis. Stoppage or slowing of flow

Status asthmaticus. Severe asthma attack that does not respond to usual treatment

Stenosis. Narrowing of an opening

Streptococci. Microorganism present in the throat

Suppurative. Inflammation with pus formation

Symptoms. Subjective evidence of disease

Syncope. Failing due to cerebral anemia

Syndrome. Symptoms occurring concurrently

Synovial membrane. Lining of joint capsule

Systole. Contracting phase of the heart

Systolic pressure. Highest pressure in the arteries.

Tachycardia. Rapid heart beat

T-cells. Whole cell antibodies

Tendon. Band of strong fibrous tissue that connects muscle to bone

Teratoma. Highly malignant tumor of the testes

Tetanus. Lockjaw; disease characterized by muscle spasms and convulsions

Tetanus antitoxin. Passive immunization against tetanus

Tetanus toxoid. Active immunization against tetanus

Tetany. Sustained contraction of muscle

Thrombocytopenia. Scarcity of platelets

Thrombophlebitis. Blood clot in an inflamed vein

Thrombosis. Development of blood clots on the inner wall of a blood vessel

Thyrotropin. Anterior pituitary stimulant of thyroid gland

Thyroxine. Thyroid hormone (T_4)

Toxic shock syndrome (TSS). Infection of *Staphylococcus aureus*

Toxins. Poisonous substances produced by pathogenic organisms, certain animals, and some plants

Toxoid. Chemically altered toxin

TPI. See *Treponema pallidum* immobilization

Tracheobronchitis. Inflammation of the trachea and bronchi

Tracheotomy. Surgical opening of the trachea to free the air passageway

Trauma. Wound or injury

Treponema pallidum. Spirochete causing syphilis

Treponema pallidum **immobilization (TPI).** Test for the presence of antibodies against *Treponema pallidum*

Trichomonas. Parasite causing vaginitis

Triiodothyronine. Thyroid hormone (T_3)

Trisomy 21. Chromosome 21 in triplicate

Trypsin. Proteolytic enzyme

TSS. See Toxic shock syndrome

Tubercle. Small, rounded nodule characteristic of tuberculosis

Tubercle bacillus. Organism causing tuberculosis

Turner's syndrome. Sexual anomaly due to missing Y chromosome

Upper respiratory diseases. Diseases of the nose and throat

Urea. Waste product of protein metabolism

Ureters. Pair of urinary tubes connecting kidneys to bladder

Urethra. Single urinary tube from the bladder to body exterior

Urethritis. Inflammation of the urethra

Urinary calculi. Stones in the kidney system

Urticaria. Hives

Vaccine. Dead or deactivated pathogens that can engender immunity

Vaginitis. Inflammation of the vagina

Valvular insufficiency. Inability of valve to close

Varicose veins. Swollen, dilated veins

VDRL test. Screening procedure for syphilis

Vegetations. Small growths on diseased heart valves

Ventricles. Spaces within the brain in which cerebrospinal fluid is made

Ventricular fibrillation. Rapid, irregular, ineffective twitches of ventricles

Verucca vulgaris. Warts

Vesicle. Small, blisterlike lesion

Vitamin K. Essential to blood-clotting mechanism

Vitiligo. Loss of skin pigmentation

Volvulus. Twisting of the intestine on itself

Vulva. Female external genitalia

Wernicke's encephalopathy. Brain disease associated with chronic alcoholism

Wheal. Lesion of hives

Wheezing. Respiratory sound indicating narrowed air passageways

Wilms' tumor. Malignant tumor of the kidney occurring in young children

Index